Diagnostic Interviewing
Second Edition

D0068905

Diagnostic Interviewing
Second Edition

Edited by

MICHEL HERSEN
Nova Southeastern University
Fort Lauderdale, Florida

and

SAMUEL M. TURNER
Medical University of South Carolina
Charleston, South Carolina

PLENUM PRESS • NEW YORK AND LONDON

Library of Congress Cataloging-in-Publication Data

Diagnostic interviewing / edited by Michael Hersen and Samuel M.
  Turner. -- 2nd ed.
       p.   cm.
    Includes bibliographical references and index.
    ISBN 0-306-44755-X
    1. Interviewing in psychiatry. 2. Mental illness--Diagnosis.
  I. Hersen, Michel. II. Turner, Samuel M., 1944-   .
    [DNLM: 1. Interview, Psychological. 2. Mental Disorders-
  -diagnosis.   WM 141 D53664 1994]
  RC480.7.D5 1994
  616.89'075--dc20
  DNLM/DLC
  for Library of Congress   94-33280
                                                              CIP

---

10 9 8 7 6 5 4 3 2

ISBN 0-306-44755-X

©1994, 1985 Plenum Press, New York
A Division of Plenum Publishing Corporation
233 Spring Street, New York, N.Y. 10013

Printed in the United States of America

Contributors

HAGOP S. AKISKAL, Department of Psychiatry, University of California at San Diego, La Jolla, California 92093-0603

KAREEN AKISKAL, Department of Psychiatry, University of California at San Diego, La Jolla, California 92093-0603

JEFFREY B. ALLEN, University of Mississippi, University, Mississippi 38677

SUSAN E. BARKER, Department of Psychology, Louisiana State University, Baton Rouge, Louisiana 70803

DEBORAH C. BEIDEL, Department of Psychiatry and Behavioral Sciences, Medical University of South Carolina, Charleston, South Carolina 29407-7274

GARY R. BIRCHLER, Department of Veterans Affairs Medical Center, and University of California at San Diego School of Medicine, San Diego, California 92161

THOMAS J. BOLL, University of Alabama at Birmingham, Birmingham, Alabama 35294

JUDITH A. COHEN, Medical College of Pennsylvania, Allegheny General Hospital, Pittsburgh, Pennsylvania 15212

LARRY W. DUPREE, Florida Mental Health Institute, University of South Florida, Tampa, Florida 33612

JOHN P. FOREYT, Nutrition Research Clinic, Baylor College of Medicine, Houston, Texas 77030

G. KEN GOODRICK, Nutrition Research Clinic, Baylor College of Medicine, Houston, Texas 77030

ALAN M. GROSS, University of Mississippi, University, Mississippi 38677

MICHEL HERSEN, Center for Psychological Studies, Nova Southeastern University, Fort Lauderdale, Florida 33314

KEVIN J. LAPOUR, Department of Psychology, Louisiana State University, Baton Rouge, Louisiana 70803

ANTHONY P. MANNARINO, Medical College of Pennsylvania, Allegheny General Hospital, Pittsburgh, Pennsylvania 15212

NATHANIEL MCCONAGHY, School of Psychiatry, University of New South Wales, Kensington 2033 Australia

JESSE B. MILBY, Veterans Administration Medical Center and Behavioral Medicine Unit, Division of Preventative Medicine, University of Alabama School of Medicine, Birmingham, Alabama 35233

KIM T. MUESER, Dartmouth Medical School, Hanover, New Hampshire 03301

ROGER L. PATTERSON, Department of Veterans Affairs, William V. Chappell, Jr. Outpatient Clinic, Daytona Beach, Florida 32117-5115

STEVEN L. SAYERS, Medical College of Pennsylvania at Eastern Pennsylvania Psychiatric Institute, Philadelphia, Pennsylvania 19129

JOSEPH E. SCHUMACHER, Behavioral Medicine Unit, Division of Preventative Medicine, University of Alabama School of Medicine, Birmingham, Alabama 35233

LAUREN SCHWARTZ, Department of Rehabilitation Medicine, University of Washington, Seattle, Washington 98195

JENNIFER-ANN SHILLINGFORD, Toronto General Hospital, Toronto, Ontario, Canada M5G 2C4

LINDA C. SOBELL, Addiction Research Foundation, Toronto, Ontario, Canada M5S 2S1; Department of Psychology, University of Toronto, Toronto, Ontario, Canada M5S 1A1; and Department of Behavioural Science, University of Toronto, Toronto, Ontario, Canada M5S 1A8

MARK B. SOBELL, Addiction Research Foundation, Toronto, Ontario, Canada M5S 2S1; Department of Psychology, University of Toronto, Toronto, Ontario, Canada M5S 1A1; and Department of Behavioural Science, University of Toronto, Toronto, Ontario, Canada M5S 1A8

PAUL H. SOLOFF, Western Psychiatric Institute and Clinic, University of Pittsburgh School of Medicine, Pittsburgh, Pennsylvania 15213

TONY TONEATTO, Addiction Research Foundation, Toronto, Ontario, Canada M5S 2S1; and Department of Behavioural Science, University of Toronto, Toronto, Ontario, Canada M5S 1A8

SAMUEL M. TURNER, Department of Psychiatry and Behavioral Sciences, Medical University of South Carolina, Charleston, South Carolina 29425-0742

CHARLES VAN VALKENBURG, Mental Health Clinic, Veterans Administration Hospital, El Paso, Texas 79925

DONALD A. WILLIAMSON, Department of Psychology, Louisiana State University, Baton Rouge, Louisiana 70803

Preface

Perhaps the most difficult milestone in a young clinician's career is the completion of the first interview. For the typical trainee, the endeavor is fraught with apprehension and with some degree of dread. If the interview goes well, there is considerable rejoicing; if it goes badly, much consternation results. Irrespective of the amount of preparation that has taken place before the interview, the neophyte will justifiably remain nervous about this endeavor. Thus, the first edition of *Diagnostic Interviewing* was devoted to providing a clear outline for the student in tackling a large variety of patients in the interview setting.

In consideration of the positive response to the first edition of *Diagnostic Interviewing*, published in 1985, we and our editor at Plenum Press, Eliot Werner, decided that it was time to update the material. However, the basic premise that a book of this nature needs to encompass theoretical rationale, clinical description, and the pragmatics of "how to" once again has been followed. And, as in the case of the first edition, this second edition does not represent the cat's being skinned in yet another way. Quite to the contrary, we still believe that our students truly need to read the material covered herein with considerable care, and once again the book is dedicated to them. We are particularly concerned that in the clinical education of our graduate students, interviewing has been given short shrift. Considering that good interviewing leads to appropriate clinical and research targets, we can only underscore the importance of the area.

Almost a decade has passed since publication of the first edition, and many developments in the field have taken place, including the appearance and obsolescence of DSM-III-R. Therefore, we have asked our eminent contributors to direct their discussions on diagnosis to DSM-IV changes. The basic structure of the new edition remains identical to that of the first edition, in that Part I deals with General Issues, Part II with Psychiatric Disorders, and Part III with Special Populations. In some instances, the contributors are identical; in others, coauthors have been changed; in still others, we have entirely new contributors. However, all the material is either updated or completely new. Part III has been expanded and now contains chapters on interviewing strategies for marital dyads, children, sexually and physically abused children, organically impaired patients, and older adults.

Of the sixteen chapters in the book, three are completely new (Chapters 12, 14, and 15). Eight chapters have been totally updated (Chapters 1, 2, 4, 6, 8, 10, 13, and 16). In addition, five chapters that originally appeared in the first edition have been written by different authors in the second edition (Chapters 3, 5, 7, 9, and 11).

Many individuals have contributed to the development and production of this book. First, we thank our contributors for sharing with us their clinical and research expertise. Second, we thank Burt G. Bolton, Jane Null, Christine Apple, and Christine Ryan for their technical assistance and help with the preparation of the index. Finally, we thank Eliot Werner for his appreciation of the need for this revision.

MICHEL HERSEN
SAMUEL M. TURNER

Contents

PART III. SPECIAL POPULATIONS

I

General Issues

The Interviewing Process

SAMUEL M. TURNER AND MICHEL HERSEN

INTRODUCTION

The foundation for all clinical enterprises is the interview. It is during the interview that one learns of the difficulties experienced by a client and lays the foundation necessary for a productive relationship with the client. Also, it is during the course of the interview that one obtains critical information needed to make decisions regarding diagnosis and, in some cases, disposition. One cannot be a good diagnostician or clinician without proper interviewing skills; indeed, a clinician who, without appropriate interviewing skills, makes critical decisions about what a client needs and does not need represents a threat to the health of those being served.

It is our experience from many years of working with psychology graduate students, interns, and other mental health trainees that not enough attention is focused on the interviewing enterprise in our training programs. Indeed, some offer little or no formal or practical training. In order to become a good interviewer, one must have a broad knowledge of psychopathology and of our current diagnostic schema. But this knowledge is only one of the tools that a good interviewer must possess. In addition to formal knowledge, basic social skills and sensitivity to a host of parameters are needed in order to garner the cooperation of clients and properly evaluate information obtained during the course of the interaction.

The first diagnostic interview is perhaps the most difficult milestone in a young trainee's career, and no amount of preparation can completely abolish the apprehension associated with this task. However, having some practical guidelines to follow can alleviate some of the anxiety and further the likelihood that the initial interviewing experience will be a positive one. One of the purposes of this chapter is to elucidate some of the factors that can facilitate the interviewing process for the novice as well as the more experienced clinician.

SAMUEL M. TURNER • Department of Psychiatry and Behavioral Sciences, Medical University of South Carolina, Charleston, South Carolina 29425-0742. MICHEL HERSEN • Center for Psychological Studies, Nova Southeastern University, Fort Lauderdale, Florida 33314.

Diagnostic Interviewing (Second Edition), edited by Michel Hersen and Samuel M. Turner. Plenum Press, New York, 1994.

We will address a number of issues that confront the clinician in the interview setting. These issues include the type of setting and its influence on the interview, confidentiality, methods of gathering information, therapist behavior, problems posed by specific diagnostic groups, and issues pertaining to ethnic minority populations. It is our intent to discuss these issues in a clinical fashion, supporting our discussion with information from our own clinical experience.

CLINICAL ISSUES IN THE INTERVIEW SETTING

The setting in which an interview is conducted is perhaps the first critical factor that needs to be addressed before the actual interview commences. The setting is critical because it will dictate how a client should be approached, what types of questions need to be asked, and what degree of cooperation might be expected from him or her. For example, interviewing a client in an emergency room requires a different approach than would interviewing a regularly scheduled client in the confines of a private practice office. Similarly, interviewing a client on a medicine unit in a general hospital would dictate an approach somewhat different from that to an interview conducted on a psychiatric unit. The reason for these differences is that the circumstances of how each client comes to be interviewed are different, and each no doubt brings a different set of expectations given the context in which the interview takes place. In order to address the issue of the interview setting more fully, we will now discuss some of the characteristics of patient populations seen in various types of settings.

Emergency Diagnostic Centers and Crisis Settings

Emergency diagnosis takes place in general hospital emergency rooms, diagnostic centers within psychiatric facilities, intake centers in comprehensive mental health clinics, and crisis centers via telephone or actual contact in the community. Such settings frequently serve as the first mental health contact for persons who decide on their own to seek mental health services, those who are hospitalized for related and unrelated medical disorders, those who are brought for evaluation by law enforcement or emergency medical personnel, those who are persuaded to seek help by relatives or friends, those who are remanded by the judiciary through involuntary commitment proceedings, and those who are encountered in volatile crisis situations. In any of these settings, a wide variety of mental disorders will be confronted, including psychotic disturbances (e.g., schizophrenia, bipolar affective illness); organic brain syndromes caused by substance abuse, disease, and injury; drug and alcohol problems; other affective (e.g., major depression) and anxiety (panic disorder) disorders; and a host of personality and adjustment difficulties. Table 1 lists the types of disorders seen in a major psychiatric evaluation center located in a metropolitan area during a 1-year period.

In emergency settings, clinicians must be aware that clients are often frightened by their perceptions and feelings, as well as by the surroundings in which they find themselves. Hence, they may not be lucid enough or they may be too frightened to provide detailed histories. The goal in such situations should be to

TABLE 1.   Distribution of Diagnostic Categories for a
1-Year Period in an Emergency Diagnostic Center

Axis I: Diagnostic category	Frequency of diagnosis
Mental retardation	36
Attention deficit disorders	28
Conduct disorders	99
Anxiety disorders of childhood or adolescence	19
Eating disorders	26
Stereotyped movement disorders	2
Other disorders with physical manifestations	5
Pervasive developmental disorders	23
Other disorders of childhood and adolescence	41
Senile and presenile dementia	48
Substance-induced organic mental disorders	36
Organic brain syndrome	72
Alcohol use disorders	145
Other substance abuse disorders	88
Schizophrenic disorders	206
Paranoid disorders	16
Other psychotic disorders	118
Bipolar disorder, manic	55
Bipolar disorder, mixed	26
Bipolar disorder, depressed	30
Major depression, single episode	294
Major depression, recurrent	344
Dysthymic disorders	122
Other affective disorders	55
Phobic disorders	99
Anxiety states	76
Other anxiety disorders	18
Somatoform disorders	9
Dissociative disorders	2
Psychosexual disorders	14
Factitious disorders	1
Impulse-control disorders	13
Adjustment disorders	280
Factitious disorder with physical symptoms	11
Unspecified mental disorders	9
Condition not a mental disorder	74
Deferred	209
No diagnosis	87

gain enough information to make a reasonable diagnostic decision in order to arrange a rational and proper disposition. Thus, it would be sufficient to determine that a person is psychotic and in need of hospitalization without being certain of the exact nature or cause of the psychosis. Similarly, it would be sufficient to determine that a patient is suffering anxiety symptoms as a result of situational stress and that the individual could best be served on an outpatient basis.

It is particularly important in interviews conducted in emergency settings to make a careful examination of mental status, rather than take a detailed social history or undertake an evaluation with formal psychological tests. As noted above, the clinician needs to understand that patients in emergency settings are frequently frightened by their symptoms as well as by the situation in which they find themselves. Such pronounced apprehension is often a particularly acute problem with those who are psychotic. Inexperienced clinicians are frequently surprised to learn that even the most psychotic individuals are concerned and frightened by the unusual thoughts and perceptual experiences that they are encountering. Although actively psychotic, they are often keenly perceptive and sensitive to interpersonal interactions. A calm and understanding attitude on the clinician's part can serve to mitigate fear in such persons and increase their comfort level enough to allow the interviewer to obtain a reasonable sense of the nature of the problem.

At times, it may be necessary to supplement information from the client with comments from family members, the police, or court records. Finally, an important source of information is the observation of the client's behavior prior to and during the interview. Frequently, in fact, the client's behavior is the single most important source of information in the emergency room.

Crisis situations might altogether supersede concern about a diagnosis. Frequently, the goal is to prevent an impending tragedy, and thus the interview is devoted to that end. For example, a trainee under supervision by one of us (Turner) recently received a call from a client who had been seen only once previously. This patient expressed a desire to die and articulated a specific plan by which she might commit suicide. Because she had access to several firearms, the interviewer's immediate task was to get her to move the weapons to a place where she could not easily get at them on impulse. A second strategy was to engage the client in conversation while the police were sent to take her to an emergency room. Needless to say, another crisis situation might dictate a different course of action.

Outpatient Settings and the Private Consulting Office

Because clients seen regularly in outpatient settings and private offices are likely to be somewhat less acute, as well as less severe, than those seen in emergency and crisis settings, the nature of the interview will be considerably different. Similarly, the goal of the interview will also be different. Although the mental status remains an important issue and diagnosis is still an objective, disposition normally is not a major concern because the client is already in a setting in which ongoing treatment can be provided. Therefore, the client can be approached in a more inquiring manner and there should be sufficient time for detailed questioning. The objective is to learn as much about the client's emotional functioning as possible and to ascertain the reasons for seeking consultation.

Of course, the nature of any interview is governed by what is perceived to be tolerable for each individual. Thus, one would choose not to pressure a patient with paranoid features about his or her sexual behavior in an initial interview because paranoid patients are known to be exquisitely sensitive in this area. In general, interviews conducted in these settings should allow ample time for establishing rapport and laying the groundwork for a fruitful therapeutic relationship.

Many clients seen in these settings are more inquisitive about the causes of their disorders as well as treatments that might be available. They typically bring a medical model conception to the initial interview. When one goes to the doctor, it is expected that the doctor will tell you what is wrong and provide treatment. Although diagnosis and prescription of treatment typically cannot be accomplished on the basis of the initial psychological interview, clinicians still should provide some information to clients regarding their condition at the end of the first interview. Also, it might be appropriate to discuss the best possible treatment options, or at least what is believed to be the best course of action to follow.

Thus, the clinician will have to engage in much more of an information-exchange process than is typical in emergency or crisis situations. For example, it is not uncommon for many anxiety-disordered clients to engage the clinician in protracted discussions concerning their distress, why they rather than someone else developed the symptoms, what types of treatments can be used, what the "cure" for their condition is, how many people have problems identical to theirs, what their prognosis is, how long treatment will take, and how much it will cost. Frequently, the directness with which these questions are answered will determine whether or not a client will remain in treatment. The manner in which these questions are addressed is also important in helping the individual develop a "proper" perspective on his or her treatment, as to what can and cannot be done, and what long-term prognosis entails. Although relatively infrequent in comparison to other settings, emergency situations may arise in outpatient settings as well (e.g., suicide attempts, homicidal ideation).

Medical Settings

Interviewing clients in a general medical setting presents a unique type of challenge. In many cases, medical patients have not requested to see a mental health professional. Rather, referral is frequently the decision of the treating physician, sometimes without consulting or explaining to the client. Thus, on occasion, clients in this setting will be reluctant to communicate and may refuse to be interviewed. A critical factor in such a case is to introduce oneself and explain the nature of the consultation and who requested it and what the relationship with the patient is to be at this point. An important factor to remember in these situations is that patients see themselves as suffering from a medical disorder, and frequently they do have various medical illnesses. Because they have defined their problems as being medical, they do not understand why a mental health professional has been sent to see them. Also, depending on their medical condition, they may be in considerable discomfort, which may influence their ability to respond to questions and the type of response that they give. Thus, the clinician will need to adjust the format and length of questioning based on these factors.

In approaching patients in general medical settings, we have found it advisable to present oneself as an information gatherer, acknowledging the patient's physical condition without suggesting that there is a psychological disturbance, even if one is suspected. These clients may require a period of cultivation before they are willing to discuss their emotional state. Thus, several visits may be warranted before the interviewing task can be completed.

A potential major problem in this setting can arise if clinicians allow themselves to be manipulated into siding with the patient against the physician or other caregiver. Patients in these settings will sometimes complain about physicians and nursing personnel to mental health professionals, and in some cases may seek to prove the physician wrong by getting the interviewer to agree with them or their conceptualization of the presenting problem. It is critical that the clinician assume no specific position in such cases, but rather maintain the stance of investigator with no particular point of view. Consultants must remember that they are invited in by the treating physician to render their expert advice on a particular problem. Statements and judgments about other aspects of the patient's care can have a negative impact on the doctor–patient relationship and can well reduce the interviewer's credibility and effectiveness.

CONFIDENTIALITY

The issue of confidentiality is one of the most critical to be faced in the interview setting. Guidelines for psychologists regarding confidentiality can be found in *Ethical Principles for Psychologists* (American Psychological Association, 1992). In addition, there are numerous other publications of the American Psychological Association that offer guidance in this area. Finally, state laws regulating the practice of psychologists typically have provisions about confidentiality and guidelines pertaining to the doctor–patient relationship in the particular states. It is essential that clinicians become familiar with the laws of the states in which they practice.

The issue of confidentiality will arise in a number of ways. First, clients enter into the interview with the expectation that in divulging information, they do so in confidence. Furthermore, in many cases, whether patients reveal highly personal information will depend on whether or not they feel they can do so in confidence. To some degree, the setting will likely dictate the level of confidence expected. For example, those being interviewed in an emergency room might be seen by more than one clinician, and the interviewer might involve other sources, such as significant others or employers, in an effort to gather information necessary to render a diagnosis and make a disposition. On the other hand, in the private consulting room, in many cases, no one else will be involved in the interview. Listed below are a number of other factors that impinge on the confidentiality issue.

Age

The age of consent or individual responsibility varies among the states. Thus, a 15-year-old adolescent seeking mental health services without parental consent might be able to do so legally in one state but not in another. In a state in which it is legal to provide services to 15-year-olds, all confidentiality laws of that state would apply. On the other hand, in some states, persons this age would be considered minors, and no services could be dispensed without parental consent. In this case, the clinician should inform the client of this requirement before rendering services. The interviewing of minors normally requires parental consent, and parents have a legal right to know the results of such an interview or assessment.

Confidentiality of Records

Written records of psychological interviews are confidential documents. Such records may be released to others (including other professionals) only with the client's written consent. Confidentiality is governed by American Psychological Association guidelines as well as by state law. It is the responsibility of each professional to provide adequate safeguards for such material. Even though records are normally considered privileged information, they are subject to court subpoena in certain types of criminal cases. This liability holds even though the communication between doctor and patient may be privileged information under state law.

Despite the enormous amount of time and resources required to maintain proper records, this documentation should not be taken lightly for a number of reasons. First, records may be important to a client for future treatment or third-party reimbursement. Second, the information contained in a record might prove helpful to a clinician reviewing the history of illness and the client's treatment history. Third, the record conveys the clinician's thoughts about the illness as well as the rationale for treatments used. As such, the record could be extremely important in any disagreement or malpractice claim arising from an interview or treatment. Thus, it behooves the clinician to maintain up-to-date, detailed, and accurate records of each client contact.

The security of client records is the responsibility of everyone in the clinical setting, and in particular the clinician. Records often contain highly personal and intimate information and, as such, should be handled as confidential documents. Written information should not be left lying in open view, but rather should be filed promptly and properly. Records should be kept in locked files with limited access.

Duty to Warn and Protect

During the course of their work, mental health professionals will at times confront the issue of dangerousness. This issue concerns danger that clients represent to themselves (i.e., suicide potential), danger to the clinician, and danger to society in general or to specific persons. It is the latter that we are concerned with in this section. What are the obligations of a clinician who interviews a client and learns that the client harbors aggressive feelings toward others? Also, how does this potential danger relate to the issue of confidentiality of the doctor–patient relationship?

Although clinicians have a legal and ethical obligation to maintain confidentiality of information between themselves and their clients, the straightforward application of the legal and ethical responsibility for confidentiality has been blurred since the landmark Tarasoff vs. Regents of University of California case in 1976. Basically, the decision by the California Supreme Court requires clinicians to take steps to protect individuals who are potential victims of their clients. Thus, if an interviewee informs the interviewer of plans to harm an identifiable person, the clinician might incur the responsibility not only to warn but also to take steps to protect the intended victim. For example, it might be sufficient to inform the intended victim and hospitalize the patient. Obviously, this is a serious and complex issue with many ramifications, and our intent here is merely to alert the clinician to it. For more complete coverage of this issue, the reader is referred to Bennet, Bryant, Vandenbos, and Greenwood (1990), Stromberg et al. (1988), Stromberg, Schneider, and Joondeph (1993), and *Ethical Principles for Psychologists and Code of Conduct* (American Psychological Association, 1992).

ETHNIC AND RACIAL CONSIDERATIONS

The role of ethnic and racial variables in psychopathological states, diagnosis, and the therapeutic relationship remains poorly understood, but there has been a continuous, albeit slow, increment of data over the past three decades. Unfortunately, most of our clinical training programs do not provide any systematic education on either of these issues, and few of our textbooks address them in any depth. Since the civil rights movement of the 1960s, major societal changes have taken place. Nevertheless, not much in the way of understanding the psychology of minority groups has been taught. In other words, we still do not have a psychology that addresses the diversity of the American population. Thus, clinicians often find themselves thrust into service settings that largely serve ethnic minorities (i.e., groups they are ill prepared to serve). In these cases, the best that can be hoped is that these clinicians will learn from supervisors in the particular settings or that a course of self-education will be pursued.

How important are ethnic and racial variables in the interview process? Although it is difficult to answer this question in a general sense, there are enough data to suggest that both can be important in certain circumstances. Race consistently has been found to bias diagnosis and clearly has implications for treatment decisions (Adebimpe, 1982). Lopez and Hernandez (1986) noted that there is a consistent tendency to "overpathologize" symptoms found in African Americans and Hispanic Americans. There is a consistent pattern of overdiagnosis of schizophrenia and underdiagnosis of affective disorder in African Americans (e.g., Jones & Gray, 1986). Generalized anxiety disorder in African Americans is sometimes misdiagnosed as paranoid schizophrenia because anxiety is often masked by hostility, machismo, and false pride (Mayo, 1981). Loring and Powell (1988) reported that both race and gender significantly influenced diagnoses rendered by psychiatrists. The misdiagnosis problem for African Americans exists even when they display the same symptom pattern as whites.

In a review of the literature, Neighbors, Jackson, Campbell, and Williams (1989) concluded that the diagnoses of African Americans based on open clinical interviews were much less accurate than those made with the aid of structured interview schedules. Structured and semistructured interviews ensure that certain questions are asked and that specific criteria are met before a diagnosis is made and thus seem to control to some degree the influence of race or ethnicity. This means, of course, that when there is nothing to structure the course of the interview, race influences the interviewer as to the assignment of diagnoses.

One finding that might be related to the issue is that the perception of social behavior is influenced by race (Turner, Beidel, Hersen, & Bellack, 1984). One frequent problem encountered by the interviewer with respect to race or ethnicity is that culture- or race-specific behavior patterns will not be understood (or will be misunderstood). An example of this problem was discussed by Adebimpe (1982) when he noted that the cultural relevance of various religious patterns might be misinterpreted as psychotic behavior in the diagnostic interview.

In recent years, a number of works have appeared that address ethnic and minority issues with respect to interviewing as well as the therapeutic process itself. These works have focused on such issues as race of interviewer and interviewee, black therapists and white patients, white patients and black therapists, and the particular psychology of the various minority groups. Issues regarding race and ethnicity are highly complex and poorly understood, and here we will limit our discussion to some of the issues related to interviewing. For in-depth coverage, the interested reader is referred to a number of sources that cover this area more comprehensively (cf. Block, 1984; Boyd-Franklin, 1984; Comas-Diaz & Griffith, 1988; Jones, 1984; Jones & Block, 1984; Jones & Korchin, 1982; Stewart, 1981; Turner & Jones, 1982).

We have found that when racial and ethnic issues arise during an interview, it is best to acknowledge them without dwelling on the topic and making them the focus of the interview. If racial or ethnic issues clearly become the paramount focus of attention, it is unlikely that the interview will prove to be useful. Interviewers must be prepared to acknowledge racial or ethnic biases of their own, as well as those that might be harbored by the interviewee. In some cases, it might be advisable to bring in an interviewer of the same race or ethnic background as the interviewee either for consultation or to conduct the interview. Decisions in these matters must be made by each individual clinician.

Interview Process

A number of studies have examined racial variables as they affect the interview process. Most have been analog studies involving college-student populations. With respect to self-disclosure, a number of these studies indicated that subjects tend to prefer counselors of their own race, whereas others indicated that race was not a significant variable (e.g., Burrell & Rayder, 1971; Casciani, 1978). How much these analog studies reflect problems faced in the consulting room is unclear, although an early study involving a clinic sample tended to support the view that clients racially most similar to the counselor tended to engage in greater self-exploration (Banks, 1971; Carkhuff & Pierce, 1967). If self-exploration can be considered a positive behavior for successful outcome in therapy, then the studies would seem to suggest that same-race pairs of patients and therapists probably would be best. On the other hand, a similar study by Banks, Berenson, and Carkhuff (1967) seemed to indicate that the therapist's experience and not race was the more critical variable, although the findings were not unambiguous. This study pointed to what we believe is a crucial factor: that race is probably not a major factor with respect to self-disclosure in all cases. Yet, when it is an issue, the clinician must be able to identify the problem.

Perhaps more crucial to a successful initial interview are factors that might impede communication. A number of variables have been noted to affect communication. One is the perception that many African Americans have about psychological intervention. Psychological services are often viewed as being available only to the white privileged classes (Mitchell, 1978). Furthermore, the dominant cultural pattern among the black population is toward self-help rather than help from mental health professionals (Maultsby, 1982), although this preference likely depends a great deal on socioeconomic status. Given the existence of a cultural norm toward self-help, and a skeptical attitude toward psychological services, clinicians will confront many skeptical African Americans in the interview setting.

Mitchell (1978) noted a second variable that can have a negative influence in the interview setting. This factor is the language barrier, although this too is partly a socioeconomic issue. For example, African-American clients often use the phrase "That's alright" when asked questions about their motives for engaging in certain behaviors. This phrase is used to mean, "Although I know exactly how to answer you, I have no intention of doing so." Under such circumstances, direct questioning in an interrogative fashion may not be the best course of action. Clinicians should also be alert to a tactic used by African-American patients that involves what appears to be nonverbal ability, inability to conceptualize, mumbling, or display of other negative behaviors that have sometimes been used to describe such patients. Jones and Seagull (1977) pointed out that this might well be a 300-year-old defense mechanism used by field slaves against their masters. The behavior pattern is referred to as "shucking." Similar behavior among prisoners has been referred to as "dummying up" (Spewack & Spewack, 1953). Such behavior was also seen in concentration camp survivors (Bettelheim, 1960; Frankl, 1963). Thus, this behavior is a method of exerting control by those who feel they have no control. We believe it is particularly important to remember this point when interviewing clients from lower socioeconomic groups. Hence, it might be wise for the clinician to devote more time to cultivating trust when such cases are confronted. Also, highly personal or emotionally charged questions might have to take a back seat to more general and superficial questioning and discussion until the patient is perceived to be comfortable.

The cultural norm of self-sufficiency and denial of emotional problems mentioned previously can be a significant factor when interviewing African-American clients. This attitude can be seen in patients who verbally deny the depth of their problems and the need for help. Block (1984) noted that this tactic might be part of a coping style aimed at avoiding the appearance of being helpless and dependent. The patient's presence at a mental health facility is considered to be enough proof that he or she needs help. Therefore, the clinician should not assume that the patient is unwilling to receive or uninterested in receiving help. Moreover, the interviewer should not be dissuaded by such behavior and should proceed to complete a diagnostic assessment.

Diagnosis

Although the core symptoms of many emotional disorders have been found to be similar cross-culturally, secondary symptom patterns can vary markedly. Even within a particular culture, some diversity of symptomatic expression can be seen. For example, Canadians of British origin differ from Canadians of French ancestry with respect to patterns of symptomatology and a host of other dimensions relevant to treatment (Murphy, 1974a,b). That race particularly is an important factor in the diagnostic process was noted earlier. We will note a number of differences here, but the reader is referred elsewhere for more extended discussions (Adebimpe, 1982; Singer, 1977).

In the case of depression, it has been noted that African Americans, particularly those from the lower socioeconomic strata, often do not present with a depressed mood when they are in fact depressed. Rather, multiple somatic complaints predominate (Carter, 1974; Schwab, 1975). How much of this behavior is a function of race as opposed to social class is unclear. It is clear, however, that the clinician must be able to recognize the potential importance of somatic complaints in these patient groups. It also has been reported that African-American patients who are depressed are likely to be more active and self-destructive and to overeat as opposed to having appetite loss. They also are less likely to have crying episodes and more likely to appear agitated (Block, 1984). Among African-American patients who commit suicide, there is a strong association with concomitant alcohol use (Thomas & Lindenthal, 1975). This association is in contrast to what is seen in white populations.

Stress-related disorders occur at an alarmingly high rate among African Americans. Therefore, clinicians are likely to see many African-American patients with such disorders. African-American clients with panic disorder appear to have a greater rate of comorbidity with isolated sleep paralysis (ISP) (Bell, Dixie-Bell, & Thompson, 1986), a condition characterized by awakening in the night with an acute onset of inability to move. The condition occurs during periods of rapid eye movement (REM) and non-REM sleep and is more prevalent in African Americans than in white and Nigerian populations (see Neal & Turner, 1991). In addition to the comorbidity of ISP with panic disorder, the condition also appears to be present in African Americans with hypertension. Because hypertension and panic are known to be associated with emotional distress, it has been hypothesized that stress might be the mediator of all these conditions (e.g., Neal & Turner, 1991). The point is that African Americans suffering from panic might present with a complaint of any one of these syndromes or other stress-related conditions, and one might need to be more cognizant of the possible interrelationships of the stress-related conditions when interviewing African Americans. Although the causes of hypertension are complex, a number of variables have been found to be highly correlated with the incidence and rising mortality rates. These include poor education and low occupational status (Jenkins, 1977). A large percentage of people meeting such criteria are indeed African American and in many cases Hispanic. This issue is being raised here because when stress-related disorders are seen in African Americans, the primary source of stress is often environmental as opposed to intrapsychic. Hence, the clinician needs to be sensitive to such issues if a correct assessment is to be made.

It is not our purpose in this chapter to provide the necessary background material for one to adequately assess clients from different cultural or racial groups. Rather, it is to alert the clinician to the importance of these issues. Training programs in psychology, psychiatry, social work, and other mental health professions need to devote the necessary time to these issues in their curricula to ensure that their trainees have some minimal level of knowledge. Currently, minority clinicians are frequently as ignorant as their white colleagues in these matters because they have been trained in the same programs. Most clinical training programs give lip service to the need for training of this type, but few ever implement serious empirically based curriculum and experiential training. Training programs for all the mental health disciplines have the responsibility to ensure that their graduates have some level of knowledge and competence to serve racial and ethnic minorities. If they do not, in our view this represents programmatic and training malfeasance.

METHODS OF OBTAINING INFORMATION

In recent years, a large number of structured and semistructured schedules have been used to enhance interrater reliability in the interview. Such schedules have also improved the diagnostic process by delineating specific targets and types of information that the interviewer must uncover. These schedules have been developed for interviewing both children [e.g., Kiddie Schedule for Affective Disorders and Schizophrenia in Present Episode (Chambers et al., 1985), Child Assessment Schedule (Hodges, McKnew, Cytryn, Stern, & Klein, 1982), Interviewing Schedule for Children (Kovacs, 1983)] and adults [e.g., Schedule for Affective Disorders and Schizophrenia (Endicott & Spitzer, 1978), Rating Scale for Depression (Hamilton, 1960), Present State Examination (Wing, Birley, Cooper, Graham, & Isaacs, 1967), Child Abuse and Neglect Interview Schedule (Ammerman, Hersen, Van Hasselt, Lubetsky, & Sieck, in press), Anxiety Disorders Interview Schedule—Revised (Klosko, DiNardo, & Barlow, 1988)]. The fully structured interview schedules enable the interviewer to follow an established format and sequence. In the semistructured schedules, the interviewer has considerable latitude.

In contrasting the unstructured clinical interview with the schedules that have now been developed, Spitzer and Endicott (1975) noted that "although valuable information can be obtained from the usual, relatively unstructured clinical interview, attempts have been made during recent years to improve the research value of a psychiatric interview by standardizing the interview techniques so that the variability associated with differences in interviewing methods and coverage is reduced. Interview schedules have been developed which combine the flexibility and rapport that are inherent in a clinical interview with the completeness of coverage and comparability of interviewing method that result from using a structured interview procedure" (p. 224). Structured and semistructured interview schedules, because of their greater precision than the unstructured interviews, have also enhanced the likelihood of interstudy comparisons for diagnostic research and treatment trials.

SPECIFIC TECHNIQUES

If the final objective of the interview is to establish a formal diagnosis, some very specific material will have to be covered. Information of relevance would include but not be limited to: (1) mental status; (2) presenting complaints; (3) psychiatric history; (4) psychiatric history of close relatives, if relevant; (5) medical history; (6) social history; (7) educational and/or military history; (8) work history; (9) dating or marital history; (10) alcohol or drug history; (11) vegetative functioning including sexual history; (12) interpersonal relationships; (13) legal history, if applicable; and (14) leisure-time activities.

One of us (Hersen), in teaching interviewing to sophomore medical students, recalls presenting these 14 points to his class, emphasizing that they tended to be covered in a good diagnostic interview. In literal response to such emphasis, one of the medical students proceeded to conduct a practice interview, with the 14 points listed on a sheet in front of him. Moreover, he followed each of the 14 points in sequence, irrespective of the flow of the patient's information.

We all know, of course, that all the 14 points can be dealt with in an interview without adhering to a rigid format as our sophomore medical student did. Indeed, the experienced interviewer, through skillful manipulation, generally is able to weave in the 14 points within the 60–90 minutes available. Specifically how this is done is certainly of considerable interest. Again, we wish to underscore that the type of patient and his or her responsiveness will dictate whether the interview is directed or free-floating and whether open-ended questions or closed-ended questions predominate.

We can remember starting one interview rather existentially by asking our young schizophrenic patient: "How did you get here?" He responded in a most literal fashion: "By taxicab, doctor." This mildly amusing anecdote makes clear that with this kind of patient, a clearer and more precise question was warranted: "What are the events that led to your being hospitalized on this psychiatric ward?" Of course, there is no guarantee that the new question would bear fruit, but at least a closer approximation of requisite historical information might emerge.

Some patients (e.g., severe obsessives, schizophrenics, and manics not controlled pharmacologically) need to be "kept on track" and periodically "retracked" during the course of the interview. Thus, if the interviewer is nondirective and uses mainly open-ended questions, the specific information being sought may never surface. Nondirective interviewing with these kinds of patients will invariably lead to circumlocution and a morass of endless and irrelevant detail. This mode of response in itself is diagnostic but does not fulfill the objective of the interview. With such patients, clear and direct questions (frequently closed-ended) are a must! Regrettably, students of many disciplines are still being taught that direct questioning techniques are unwarranted. This practice not only is a disservice to the student, but also in the long run will not prove to be of benefit to the client or the patient. Indeed, the key is for the interviewer to have a large armamentarium of interview strategies at his or her disposal, hence maximum flexibility, depending on the patient's unique presentation. By contrast, with defensive and highly suspicious patients, use of closed-ended questions will invariably result in rather terse replies (e.g., "Yes," "No,", "Maybe," "I don't know"). With these patients, it is generally better to use open-ended questions (e.g., "Tell me how things are going for you in recent weeks"). Such a strategy may be helpful, but may also fail at times. Suspicious patients may retort, "What do you mean by that?" or "I don't understand what you are saying." When this happens, it is advisable for the interviewer to reflect the patient's concerns and to discuss them openly. However, sometimes when all the techniques at hand have been tried, failure to break through the patient's defensive stance will still result.

Further, with some patients, the open-ended approach may yield unreliable or invalid information. This especially happens when interviewing alcoholics and drug addicts. Generally, we instruct our students, when interviewing suspected alcohol or drug addicts, to say the following: "Tell me, how much alcohol [or the specific drug] are you using a day?" Or, going one step further: "What is your favorite bar in your neighborhood?" This strategy, of course, obviates the silly game-playing (professionally referred to as "denial") that often occurs between the alcoholic or drug addict and the interviewer. Mild confrontation, when accomplished with skill and interviewer openness, will also prove to be beneficial in cutting through patient denial and defensiveness. However, the clinician will realize, with increasing experience, how far to push a given patient. Of course, with aggressive patients, the issue may become one of safety for the interviewer and those others in his surroundings.

A very critical element in the effective interview is the issue of timing. By timing, we mean exactly when in the interview sequence a particular question or topic is introduced. Beginning interviewers tend to be awkward in this regard, postponing questions that need to be asked earlier and, conversely, presenting topics too early in the interview sequence. Again, the nature of the interview and its relative emergency valence will determine how quickly the interviewer moves. In the emergency room situation, questions about suicide, aggressiveness, and sexual conduct cannot wait. That is not to say that the issue of suicide potential in the more leisurely paced interview can be delayed significantly. But with more time available and less pressure for decision-making, greater interviewing finesse is possible.

THERAPIST BEHAVIOR AFFECTING THE INTERVIEW

For too long, difficulties in obtaining relevant information in the interview have been attributed to patient and client characteristics. As graduate students and beginning clinicians, we would often hear such statements as these: (1) "He's being defensive and won't let his guard down. Therefore, he's not really telling you how he feels." (2) "She's lower class and not particularly verbal, so you're going to have a lot of trouble getting her to think in terms of psychological notions." (3) "His sullenness and terse replies reflect a 'negative transference' toward authority figures. You're going to have a hard time making him talk." (4) "Your adolescent patient is into drugs, is sociopathic, and is a chronic liar. Don't believe very much of what he says to you." (5) "She's hysterical and telling you all about that sexual material to keep you entertained. This is all part of her defensive structure to avoid her real problem of basic depression." (6) "He's only got an IQ of about 90 and will not be a terribly good psychotherapy candidate. He won't grasp the subtleties of what you're trying to do."

The preceding list of six items may exaggerate somewhat the commentaries of some of the supervisors we may have experienced (and others still do), but they do reflect the pervasive trend of focusing on only one aspect of the interview equation (i.e., the client's behavior). Unfortunately, this narrow-band approach does not take into consideration the complicated interpersonal interactions that are constantly occurring during the course of the interview. Irrespective of whether we are dealing with an initial interview or one later in therapy, the interviewer's behavior critically affects how the client will respond (cf. Waterhouse & Strupp, 1984). Indeed, there is an extensive research literature clearly documenting how particular strategies carried out by the interviewer will alter interviewee behavior. An excellent review of this work was provided as far back as 1972 by Matarazzo and Wiens (1972), and the interested reader is referred to that source. Although over two decades old, the meticulous work conducted by Matarazzo and Wiens holds up exceedingly well, even by today's more exacting standards.

In looking at how the therapist's behavior can affect the interview process, let us consider the role of each of the following: (1) jargon, (2) empathy, (3) self-disclosure, and (4) humor. In so doing, we will provide examples from both our clinical experience and supervisory interactions with graduate students, psychiatric residents, psychology interns, and medical students.

Jargon

Use of jargon, irrespective of theoretical persuasion, is the mark of the inexperienced and naïve interviewer. From our perspective, there is no justification for using technical language with clients at any point in the interview process. To say to a client that his or her behavior "reflects an unresolved Oedipal complex" or that she or he is "responding to a discriminative stimulus and not sufficiently reinforcing to her or his child" does not enhance the interview. First, unless the client is psychologically sophisticated, the meaning of such terminology will be lost. Second, even if the client is psychologically sophisticated and highly intelligent, the abstract nature of such jargon will interfere with the emotional understanding of the interviewer's points. Third, if the interviewer is really intent on using jargon, considerable effort will be expended in teaching the client the nature of the terms. We firmly believe that doing so represents a waste of valuable time. Moreover, it tends to inhibit the flow of a good interview.

Experience dictates that it is best for the interviewer, instead of using jargon and technical language, to use clear behavioral descriptions of what clients do and how they respond. Again, we argue that this holds true whether the interviewer proceeds from a psychoanalytic stance or a behavioral position. The interviewer may think and conceptualize psychoanalytically or behaviorally, but he or she should speak in clear English. Also, the interviewer should never speak to clients at a level beyond their comprehension, nor should he or she underestimate their intellectual capacity. Indeed, the same question may be posed in different ways to clients of varying mental capacities. Moreover, the sensitive interviewer is able to modulate his or her response according to the cultural presentation of the particular client. That is to say, people from different cultures will undoubtedly perceive the interview situation from different perspectives. Thus, sophisticated interviewers learn to modulate their approach given the unique cultural backgrounds and inherent mental capacities of their clients.

Empathy

Many an interview has gone awry because the therapist has been intent on extracting information from a client but seemingly oblivious to his or her feelings. Or the interviewer may be pursuing a line of inquiry that is inconsistent with the client's most pressing problems at the time. For example, if a therapist is treating a young women who suffers from acrophobia, and she reports having just broken up with her boyfriend, it would be most insensitive to pursue the original subject and ignore the new crisis. To the contrary, it behooves this therapist to explore the client's feelings about her recent loss and the possible resulting depressive symptomatology. Indeed, the empathic interviewer must always be in touch with how the client feels. Thus, if the interviewer is empathic, it may be necessary to shift interview or therapeutic gears. The interviewer should not only pay careful attention to what the client says, but also be especially attuned to paralinguistic features, facial expressions, gestures, and general body language. This is what Reik (1948) referred to as "listening with the third ear." On the other hand, a competent albeit empathic interviewer knows how to control the interview and prevent the patient from being diverted and engaging in a virtual flight of ideas. We are basically saying here that there should be some unifying thematic content to the interview, under the interviewer's direction.

Being empathic, of course, requires much more than being a good listener: Interviewers must communicate to clients that they understand how they feel, that they appreciate their frustrations and are fully aware of the intricacies of their lives. Researchers have now shown that empathy in the interviewer is a feature that cuts across all theoretical persuasions (cf. Bellack & Hersen, 1990; Greenwald, Kornblith, Hersen, Bellack, & Himmelhoch, 1981; Sloane, Staples, Cristol, Yorkston, & Whipple, 1975). There is no one technical strategy to communicate such empathy to the client. To the contrary, there are many, including the line of questioning that is to be pursued, the interviewer's affect and facial expressions, the timing of comments, and the reflection of feeling in the Rogerian sense. Accomplishing this rapprochement is still something of an art, but the key to doing so is that the client must experience the interviewer as genuine.

Without empathy, the therapist not only will find the interview difficult to carry out but also may very well lose the client altogether. When well-conducted taped interviews are played back, the empathic quality of the therapist is ever present. Indeed, we have found that a genuine interviewer is able to extract from the client even some of the most embarrassing material that has never been revealed in the past. If the interviewer maintains his or her empathic response but does not reflect shock at what has been heard, the client will be reassured and will continue to reveal critical information that will be useful in the diagnostic and therapeutic process.

Self-Disclosure

Early during the course of Hersen's clinical training, one of his "oldline" supervisors made the categorical statement that you never disclose any of your personal business to the patient or client. Consistent with his mentor's instruction, he maintained such distance from his clients. However, at the end of the 1-year treatment of the wife of a faculty member at the university, he "slipped" and let her know he was about to be married. One year later, he received a thank-you note from this patient for his therapeutic efforts. She apprised him that her marriage was much better and that she had just given birth to a baby girl (named Hope). She ended her note by saying that she really appreciated it when he informed her he was engaged to be married: "It made you seem more human and less remote to me."

That is not to say that a therapist should indiscreetly reveal highly personal information (e.g., one's sex life, income, illnesses, fears, frustrations) to clients. But the occasional sharing of information, timed just right, certainly can have a facilitative effect on the interview process. A recent example that comes to mind is a client who was complaining about her 8-year-old stepson who needed to be "entertained" and "kept busy" on weekends. The interviewer commiserated: "I can remember when my son was 8 and what that was like."

Again, we would like to underscore that self-disclosure, used sporadically and well placed, is useful to enhance the flow of the interview and to communicate empathic understanding to the client. But, like sweets, too much may not be a good thing. Thus, the interviewer must walk the proverbial fine line. The caution is that the interviewer should be friendly, but not a friend in the traditional sense of the word.

Humor

Use of humor (or bantering with the patient) is yet another one of the bugaboos of the old-line supervision that some of us received in the 1960s and 1970s. Somehow the notion was perpetrated that psychotherapy was serious business and that you were never to crack a smile. This idea undoubtedly is a holdover from psychoanalysis, in which the therapist was often conceptualized as a blank mirror in which the patient was reflected. However, during the course of our practices and supervision of students, we have found that humorless interviewing and therapy are not effective. Even in the most difficult and trying situations, the perceptive patient and therapist can identify some humorous elements. We recall a very well-educated patient who was in his third marriage, and it too seemed to be headed for failure. When asked about how he might deal with the ensuing loneliness of possible separation, he replied, "Well, you know, the first one was hard; the second was a bit easier; this one should hurt even less."

There can be no doubt that some of the lighter therapeutic exchanges in the interview can have a beneficial effect. That is, they serve to release tension (for both the therapist and the client) from some of the more difficult material previously tackled. Humor can also be used to direct attention to desired behavioral change from one session to the next. When some of our patients ask, "When is my next appointment?," we often reply "Next week, same day, same time, same station, but a different story!"

As in the case of self-disclosure, humor has its place. It too should be used sparingly and must be timed properly. Moreover, the key is that one laughs, not *at*, but *with* the client. We would argue that well-timed humor in the form of bantering has a positive humanizing effect in the interview that by no means invalidates the notion that the client is dealing with serious problems that will require well-thought-out solutions.

SPECIAL POPULATIONS

In the previous sections, we have outlined some general guidelines that apply to the interviewing of a large variety of diagnostic categories. However, there are a number of diagnostic groupings for whom additional guidelines should prove useful, particularly for the beginning interviewer with less broad exposure to special populations. Many of our recommendations are of a common sense nature, but unfortunately may be overlooked at times. Therefore, we will briefly comment on interviewing patients who are (1) intellectually deficient, (2) aggressive, (3) psychotic, (4) physically disabled, or (5) in pain.

When interviewing individuals who suffer from mental retardation, it is critical that the therapist ensure that questions posed have been clearly understood. That is, language used by the interviewer should be consistent with the retarded individual's level of comprehension. However, the interviewer should also be warned that he or she can go too far in the opposite direction. Thus, it is important to avoid a line of questioning that is condescending and patronizing. One strategy to ensure that this type of client has understood the question is to have him or her rephrase it or explain what is required. Furthermore, the sensitive interviewer should be aware that people with mental retardation do have feelings and are subject to the same types of psychopathological responses as nonretarded individuals.

With highly aggressive individuals (who may be psychotic, organically impaired, or deranged as a function of illicit drug use), the interviewer's safety may be of concern. We definitely do not recommend that the patient be interviewed when in a highly agitated state. An interview conducted under such circumstances never proves to be productive in any way. However, when such individuals are sufficiently sedated or have run the course of an explosive episode, then interviewing may be attempted. For the interviewer secure in his or her abilities, the interview will then proceed without incident. If, however, the interviewee should evince signs of aggressivity, he or she needs to be warned that such behavior will not be tolerated. When the patient becomes visibly agitated, it is advisable to terminate questioning. Also, the sensitive interviewer will word questions in such a way that they will evoke minimal arousal. There are times, however, when ideal interview conditions will not be possible, such as in the emergency room situation. Under these circumstances, the presence of a security officer will serve to reassure both the patient and the interviewer, especially if handled in a non-threatening and matter-of-fact manner.

With highly psychotic patients, the interview process frequently proves to be difficult and tedious. The problem is that the interviewer must extract bizarre material without attempting to reinforce it and prolong its discussion (e.g., delusions, hallucinations). Also, an additional difficulty here is to keep the patient's responses on track and relevant. Under such circumstances, the interviewer must be fully in charge and not allow the patient to ramble and become discursive. Short, directed questioning helps, as does frequent interruption when the patient strays. As an amusing aside, Hersen remembers interviewing a 35-year-old African American in a state hospital unit. This person was of above-average intelligence but highly delusional, believing that he was Jesus Christ. Whenever he referred to being Christ, Hersen would look away and evince marked disinterest, in order to *extinguish* that verbal behavior (this was during Hersen's neophyte days as a behavior therapist). After several such incidents, the patient said: "I guess you don't like what I'm saying. Why didn't you just tell me and I would stop?" If this case vignette has any value, it certainly underscores the importance of *directness* on the interviewer's part.

Novice interviewers, when dealing with the physically disabled, often ignore their disabilities during the course of the interview. Doing so is as technically inadequate as totally focusing on the disability and ignoring psychopathology. Obviously, a proper balance needs to be achieved. In our opinion, it is important for the interviewer to acknowledge the interviewee's physical disability in the attempt to understand how psychopathology may be related to its existence. Thus, the possible interplay between the two has to be carefully evaluated. Moreover, the interviewee's attitude toward the patient's disability should be determined.

Finally, we should note that it is most difficult to interview patients who are experiencing severe *physical* pain, whether such pain is acute or chronic. In general, beyond a given pain threshold, some interviews may not be possible: The patient may be totally preoccupied with the pain and its resolution. Even when pain is not that intense, the patient may have a limited attention span for the usual methods of interviewing. Our experience dictates that such interviews, if really necessary, should be brief (no more than 15 minutes at a time) and focused. If specific information is required, it can be obtained through serial interviewing. Once again, it behooves the interviewer to be exquisitely sensitive to the patient's tolerance for diagnostic questioning. Indeed, irrespective of the possibility of the patient's being in pain, it is of critical import to have a comprehensive evaluation and understanding of his or her medical condition and how this condition impacts on the psychopathological presentation (George, 1991).

SUMMARY

In this introductory chapter, we have looked at a number of variables that contribute to conducting a successful clinical interview. In so doing, we have highlighted our discussion with examples from our own clinical experience in a variety of inpatient and outpatient settings. In considering clinical issues in the interview setting, we have looked at the impact of the setting on the type of interview that is conducted in emergency diagnostic centers, outpatient settings, and medical settings. Furthermore, we have carefully delineated the issues when interviewing clients whose backgrounds are different from that of the interviewer.

Irrespective of the setting, however, the importance of confidentiality has been underscored. Also, it is clear that the astute interviewer takes into consideration the critical impact of racial and ethnic variables of the interviewee. These variables certainly can affect the interview process and the ultimate diagnosis that is reached.

We then considered the various methods of obtaining information, including use of structured and semistructured schedules. Examples of difficult patients to interview were presented for illustration.

Next, we discussed how the therapist's behavior can affect the interview process. We talked about the use of jargon, development of empathy in the interview, self-disclosure, and humor. The final section was devoted to a discussion of interviews with specific populations, such those with mentally retarded, aggressive, and psychotic patients, patients with physical disabilities, and patients suffering from physical pain.

REFERENCES

Adebimpe, V. (1982). Psychiatric symptoms in black patients. In S. M. Turner & R. T. Jones (Eds.), *Behavior modification in black populations: Psychological issues and empirical findings* (pp. 57–69). New York: Plenum Press.

American Psychological Association (1992). *Ethical principles of psychologists and code of conduct*. Washington, DC: Author.

Ammerman, R. T., Hersen, M., Van Hasselt, V. B., Lubetsky, M. J., & Sieck, W. R. (in press). Maltreatment in psychiatrically hospitalized children and adolescents with developmental disabilities. *Journal of the Academy of Child and Adolescent Psychiatry*.

Banks, B., Berenson, B. G., & Carkhuff, R. R. (1967). The effects of counselor race upon counseling process with Negro clients in initial interview. *Journal of Clinical Psychology, 23*, 70–72.

Banks, W. M. (1971). The differential effects of race and social class in helping. *Journal of Clinical Psychology, 28*, 90–92.

Bell, C. C., Dixie-Bell, D. D., & Thompson, B. (1986). Further studies on the prevalence of isolated sleep paralysis in black subjects. *Journal of the National Medical Association, 75*, 649–656.

Bellack, A. S., & Hersen, M., (Eds.). (1990). *Handbook of comparative treatments of adult disorders*. New York: John Wiley.

Bennett, B. E., Bryant, B. K., Vandenbos, G. R., & Greenwood, A. (1990). Professional liability and risk management. Washington, DC: American Psychological Association.

Bettelheim, B. (1960). *The informed heart: Autonomy in a mass age.* Glencoe, IL: Free Press.

Block, C. B. (1984). Diagnostic and treatment issues for black patients. *The Clinical Psychologist, 37,* 52–54.

Boyd-Franklin, H. (1984). Issues in family therapy with black families. *The Clinical Psychologist, 37,* 54–57.

Burrell, L., & Rayder, N. F. (1971). Black and white students' attitudes toward white counselors. *Journal of Negro Education, 40,* 48–52.

Carkhuff, R. R., & Pierce, R. (1967). Differential effects of therapist race and social class upon patient depth of self-exploration in the initial clinical interview. *Journal of Counseling Psychology, 31,* 632–634.

Carter, J. H. (1974). Recording symptoms in black Americans. *Geriatrics, 29,* 97–99.

Casciani, J. M. (1978). Influence of model's race and sex on interviewers' self-disclosure. *Journal of Counseling Psychology, 25,* 435–440.

Chambers, W. J., Puig-Antich, J., Hirsch, M., Paez, P., Ambrosini, P. J., Tabrizi, M. A., & Davies, M. (1985). The assessment of affective disorders in children and adolescents by semistructured interview: Test–retest reliability of the K-SADS-P. *Archives of General Psychiatry, 42,* 696–702.

Comas-Diaz, L., & Griffith, E. E. H. (Eds.) (1988). *Clinical guidelines in cross cultural mental health.* New York: Wiley.

Endicott, J., & Spitzer, R. L. (1978). A diagnostic interview: The Schedule for Affective Disorders and Schizophrenia. *Archives of General Psychiatry, 35,* 837–844.

Frankl, V. J. (1963). *Man's search for meaning: An introduction to logotherapy.* Boston: Beacon Press.

George, A. (1991). Medical assessment. In M. Hersen, A. E. Kazdin, & A. S. Bellack (Eds.), *The clinical psychology handbook* (2nd ed., pp. 491–505). New York: Pergamon Press.

Greenwald, D. P., Kornblith, S. J., Hersen, M., Bellack, A. S., & Himmelhoch, J. M. (1981). Differences between social skill therapists and psychotherapists in treating depression. *Journal of Consulting and Clinical Psychology, 49,* 757–759.

Hamilton, M. (1960). A rating scale for depression. *Journal of Neurology, Neurosurgery, and Psychiatry, 23,* 56–61.

Hodges, K., McKnew, D., Cytryn, L., Stern, L., & Klein, J. (1982). The Child Assessment Schedule (CAS) diagnostic interview: A report of reliability and validity. *Journal of the American Academy of Child Psychiatry, 21,* 468–473.

Jenkins, C. D. (1977). Epidemiological studies of the psychosomatic aspects of coronary heart disease: A review. In S. Kasl & F. Reichsman (Eds.), *Advances in psychosomatic medicine,* Vol. 9 (pp. 1–19). New York: Karger.

Jones, A., & Seagull, A. (1977). Dimensions of the relationship between the black client and the white therapist: A theoretical overview. *American Psychologist, 32,* 850–855.

Jones, B. E., & Gray, B. A. (1986). Problems in diagnosing schizophrenia and affective disorders among blacks. *Hospital and Community Psychiatry, 37,* 61–65.

Jones, E. E. (1984). Some reflections on the black patient and psychotherapy. *The Clinical Psychologist, 37,* 62–65.

Jones, E. E., & Korchin, S. J. (1982). *Minority mental health.* New York: Praeger.

Jones, J. M., & Block, C. B. (1984). Black cultural perspectives. *The Clinical Psychologist, 37,* 58–62.

Klosko, J. S., DiNardo, P. A., & Barlow, D. H. (1988). Anxiety Disorders Interview Schedule—Revised. In M. Hersen & A. S. Bellack (Eds.), *Dictionary of behavioral assessment techniques* (pp. 31–32). New York: Pergamon Press.

Kovacs, M. (1983). The Interviewing Schedule for Children (ISC): Form C, and the follow-up form. University of Pittsburgh: Unpublished manuscript.

Lopez, S. R., & Hernandez, P. (1986). How culture is considered in evaluations of psychopathology. *The Journal of Nervous and Mental Diseases, 176,* 598–606.

Loring, M., & Powell, B. (1988). Gender, race, and DSM-III: A study of the objectivity of psychiatric diagnostic behavior. *Journal of Health and Social Behavior, 29,* 1–22.

Matarazzo, J. D., & Wiens, A. N. (1972). *The interview: Research on its anatomy and structure.* New York: Aldine-Atherton.

Maultsby, M. C., Jr. (1982). A historical view of blacks' distrust of psychiatry. In S. M. Turner & R. T. Jones (Eds.), *Behavior modification in black populations: Psychological issues and empirical findings* (pp. 39–53). New York: Plenum Press.

Mayo, J. A. (1981). The concept of masked anxiety in young adult black males. In D. F. Klein & J. Rabkin (Eds.), *Anxiety: New research and changing concepts.* New York: Raven Press.

Mitchell, A. C. (1978). Barriers to therapeutic communication with black clients. *Nursing Outlook, 6,* 109–112.

Murphy, H. B. M. (1974a). Differences between mental disorders of French Canadians and British Canadians. *Canadian Psychiatric Association Journal, 19,* 247–257.

Murphy, H. B. M. (1974b). Psychopharmacologie et variations ethnoculturelles. *Confrontation Psychiatrique, 9,* 163–185. Abstracted in English in *Transcultural Psychiatric Research Review, 11,* 28–31.

Neal, A., & Turner, S. M. (1991). Anxiety disorders research with African Americans: Current status. *Psychological Bulletin, 190,* 400–410.

Neighbors, H. W., Jackson, J. J., Campbell, L., & Williams, D. (1989). The influence of racial factors on psychiatric diagnosis: A review and suggestions for research. *Community Mental Health Journal, 25,* 301–311.

Reik, T. (1948). *Listening with the third ear.* New York: Groner Press.

Schwab, J. J. (1975). Amitriptyline in the management of depression and depression associated with physical illness. In *Amitriptyline in the management of depression* (pp. 61–85). Rahway, NJ: Merck, Sharp, & Dohme.

Singer, B. D. (1977). *Racial factors in psychiatric intervention.* San Francisco: R. E. Research Associates; Cambridge, MA: Harvard University Press.

Sloane, B. R., Staples, F. R., Cristol, A. H., Yorkston, J. J., & Whipple, K. (1975). *Psychotherapy versus behavior therapy.* Cambridge, MA: Harvard University Press.

Spewack, S., & Spewack, B. (1953). *My three angels.* New York: Random House.

Spitzer, R. L., & Endicott, J. (1975). Assessment of outcome by independent clinical evaluators. In I. E. Waskow & M. B. Parloff (Eds.), *Psychotherapy change measures* (pp. 222–232). Rockville, MD: National Institute of Mental Health.

Stewart, E. D. (1981). Cultural sensitivities in counseling. In P. P. Pederson, J. C. Draguns, & J. E. Trimble (Eds.), *Counseling across cultures.* Honolulu: University Press of Hawaii.

Stromberg, C. D., Haggarty, D. J., Leibenluft, R. F., McMillian, M. H., Mishkin, B., Rubin, B. L., & Trilling, H. R. (of the law firm of Hogart and Hartson). (1988). *The psychologist's legal handbook.* Washington, DC: The Council for the National Register of Health Service Providers in Psychology.

Stromberg, C., Schneider, J., & Joondeph, B. (1993). *The Psychologists Update Number 2 (August).* Washington, DC: National Register of Health Service Providers in Psychology.

Thomas, C. S., & Lindenthal, J. J. (1975). The depression of the oppressed. *Mental health: A publication of the Mental Health Association,* Summer, 13–14.

Turner, S. M., Beidel, D. C., Hersen, M., & Bellack, A. S. (1984). Effects of race on rating of social skill. *Journal of Consulting and Clinical psychology, 52,* 474–475.

Turner, S. M., & Jones, R. T. (Eds.) (1982). *Behavior modification in black populations: Psychological issues and empirical findings.* New York: Plenum Press.

Waterhouse, G. J., & Strupp, H. H. (1984). The patient–therapist relationship: Research from the psychodynamic perspective. *Clinical Psychology Review, 4,* 77–92.

Wing, J. K., Birley, J. T., Cooper, J. E., Graham, P., &Isaacs, A. D. (1967). Reliability of a procedure for measuring and classifying "present psychiatric state." *British Journal of Psychiatry, 13,* 499–515.

2

Mental Status Examination
The Art and Science of the Clinical Interview

HAGOP S. AKISKAL AND KAREEN AKISKAL

INTRODUCTION

The mental status examination represents the most important step in the clinical evaluation of individuals suffering from or suspected of having mental disorders. The evaluation is based on observations of a patient's overt and verbal behavior as well as on his or her subjective experiences. Patients' presenting problems dictate both the types of questions asked and the depth of inquiry necessary for a relevant and complete assessment of the mental status. In general, the more deviant and severely disturbed the patient, the more probing the mental status examination should be.

Some individuals who present for outpatient counseling can be viewed as having "problems of living," officially categorized as adjustment disorders. In these cases, the relevant mental status information can be largely gleaned from a well-conducted history-taking or intake interview; the task is largely one of organizing the information gained in the interview into the structure and terminology used to report a patient's mental status. On the other hand, if the patient appears to be suffering from significant disturbance of mood, perception, thinking, or memory, a formal mental status examination is in order (Kraepelin, 1904). Such an examination is almost always required with psychiatric inpatients and with medical patients whose mental functioning is cause for concern. Thus, although much can be learned about a patient's mental status from general observations made during a standard interview, specific probes are often needed to gain essential information about pathology that goes beyond adjustment reactions.

In the past, some psychologists tended to frown on the "medical" conceptualization of mental disorders; furthermore, they felt that a clinical approach based on

HAGOP S. AKISKAL AND KAREEN AKISKAL • Department of Psychiatry, University of California at San Diego, La Jolla, California 92093-0603.

Diagnostic Interviewing (Second Edition), edited by Michel Hersen and Samuel M. Turner. Plenum Press, New York, 1994.

evaluation of signs and symptoms and the subsequent formulation of a clinical diagnosis were both unreliable and invalid. Recent data-based clinical research on the psychopathology, diagnosis, and classification of mental disorders (Akiskal, 1989)—areas in which psychologists have made important contributions (Hersen & Turner, 1991; Willerman & Cohen, 1990)—have effectively countered such criticism. Moreover, in light of current research on the biological underpinnings of normal psychic life (Groves & Rebec, 1992) and mental disorders (Taylor, 1993), the contribution of cerebral dysfunction to the origin or maintenance of major mental disorders can no longer be discounted. Thus, the concept of illness has been extended beyond the traditional organic mental disorders[1] (e.g., delirium and dementia) to include what were once considered to be "functional" disorders, notably the schizophrenias and mood disorders, as well as obsessive–compulsive disorders and selected anxiety and personality disorders.

For patients suspected of suffering from these conditions, an in-depth mental status examination represents the foundation of the clinical evaluation. Only after such a systematic examination is it possible to weigh the relative contribution of social, psychological, and biological factors in the origin of a given patient's mental disturbance. At a more general level, mental health research today is less concerned about either/or questions of etiology, and more interested in how psychosocial and biological factors interact in a specific mental disorder. There should no longer be a conceptual gulf between social behavior, individual psychology, and physiology (McGuire & Troisi, 1987; Benjamin, 1993). This is true whether one is considering variations of normative behavior, or abnormalities in the realm of personality, anxiety, and mood states (den Boer & Ad Sitsen, 1994; Zuckerman, 1991).

Psychologists are often front-line evaluators, particularly in community mental health settings where many of these cases are seen in their milder and prodromal forms. Psychologists are also present in increasing numbers in medical settings, where they are called on to evaluate patients with known physical diseases and to collaborate with other professionals in the treatment process (e.g., stress reduction or promoting compliance with medical regimens). Many physical diseases are accompanied by mental symptoms (Lishman, 1987) that may result from the direct impact of the disease process on the neural substrates of mood and cognition (e.g., endocrine disease or brain tumor), from the use of medications that affect mood or cognitive capacity (e.g., antihypertensive medications or narcotics), or from their personally disabling psychosocial consequences. Familiarity with mental status terminology enables the psychologist to communicate more effectively with psychiatrists and other medical specialists, who have been trained to organize their findings in this fashion. The systematic nature of the mental status examination also forces the examiner to document findings with factual examples and to move from global impressions to specific observations; this process, in turn,

---

[1]The designation *organic mental disorders*, while admittedly awkward, is used in this chapter for conditions in which abnormal mental or behavioral states can be traced to known structural lesions and/or metabolic, toxic, and otherwise well-established or demonstrable physiochemical pathology. This designation is not meant to imply that other mental conditions are "nonorganic," but simply to convey a lesser certitude of organic lesions specific to them at the present stage of our knowledge. The DSM-IV terminology "due to a general medical condition" is too vague.

permits formulation of a working diagnosis, preparing the ground for a more coherent and focused treatment plan. The mental status examination is also of great relevance to the increasing number of psychologists who are embracing research careers to investigate the causes of major mental disorders; in such research, intimate knowledge of descriptive psychopathology and phenomenology is mandatory.

AREAS OF THE MENTAL STATUS EXAMINATION

A systematic examination of the mental status covers several major areas that are outlined in Table 1 and discussed throughout this chapter. The interviewer begins by noting the date, time, and setting of (or reason for) the interview. The interview proper then follows, broken down into each of the areas examined.

Appearance and Behavior

Although appearance and behavior constitute the first item in a mental status examination, relevant data on appearance and behavior are gathered throughout the interview. Attire, posture, facial expression, mannerisms, and level of grooming are described in such a way that the person reading or listening to this narration can visualize the patient's physical appearance at the time of the examination, much as if the clinician had taken a photograph. The setting of the interview is also briefly described in this section.

In some cases, little will be revealed about the mental status by these observations, beyond the fact that the patient's physical appearance was unremarkable, failing to distinguish him or her from other people of the same age, educational level, and socioeconomic background. In other instances, this initial section may already provide some important clues about the patient's personality, mood, thoughts, awareness of social convention, and ability to function adequately in society at the time of the evaluation. Some examples will illustrate the value of this initial paragraph of the mental status examination.

TABLE 1.   Proposed Outline of
Mental Status Examination

Date, time, and setting of (or reason for) interview
General appearance and interview behavior
Attitude toward interviewer
Psychomotor activity
Affect and mood (emotional state)
Speech and thought
Perceptual disturbances
Sensorium: orientation, attention, concentration
Memory
Intelligence and fund of knowledge
Reliability, judgment, and insight

> This 20-year-old, self-referred single, Chinese-American student was interviewed in the
> student counseling center. She is a petite, frail-looking woman appearing much younger
> than her stated age. She wore no makeup, and was dressed in simple attire consisting of a
> blue button-down boy's shirt, a pair of cutoff blue jeans, woolen knee stockings, and
> penny loafers. She carried a knapsack full of books that she held closely on her lap.
> Throughout the interview, her hands were tightly clasped around her knapsack. Her
> fingernails were bitten down to the quick.

The description of this patient's appearance gives us clues about a moderate level of anxiety and tension, clues that should be pursued during the remainder of the examination. The next example illustrates a more disturbed patient.

> This divorced white woman was brought to the county mental health center by her
> distraught son and daughter-in-law because she had become increasingly hostile and
> combative at home and was staying up all night. She was restless during the interview,
> rising frequently from her chair, looking at every diploma on the walls, making comments
> about each of them, doing essentially all the talking during the interview. She looked her
> stated age of 53, but her clothes would have been appropriate only for a much younger
> person: Although quite obese, she wore orange "hot pants" and a halter top that showed a
> bare midriff. Her legs had prominent varicose veins. She wore old wooden beach sandals
> with high spike heels. Her general level of grooming was very poor: Her short gray hair
> was matted on both sides of an irregular part. Her fingernails were long and yellowed
> from nicotine; her toenails were also very long, each painted a different color.

The general appearance of this patient suggests a psychotic level of disorder and raises hypotheses of much different nature from those generated by our first patient, necessitating further inquiry along the lines of a manic disorder.

The general appearance of our third patient suggests entirely different diagnostic possibilities;

> A 25-year-old single white engineer was seen in a private office. He was impeccably
> dressed in a three-piece gray pinstripe suit and matching dress shoes. His hair and
> mustache were carefully groomed. The secretary noted that when he signed his name on
> the admission form, his hands were visibly tremulous. He generally appeared uneasy and
> glanced furtively about the room, paying special attention to electrical outlets, air-
> conditioning vents, and, most especially, the security camera.

Inquiry along the lines of a delusional disorder is suggested by this patient's general appearance, and differential diagnosis should consider such conditions as amphetamine psychosis and paranoid schizophrenia.

Psychotic patients may display extreme forms of inappropriate behavior (e.g., exposing intimate parts of their bodies) or maintain bizarre and uncomfortable postures for long periods of time (e.g., standing on tiptoes). All such gross deviations in behavior should be carefully recorded.

Attitude toward the Interviewer

Attitude toward the interviewer is available by observation, without specific inquiry. Some patients may relate easily, be cooperative and open, and reveal information freely. Other patients may be suspicious and guarded, requiring frequent reassurance that the content of the session is confidential. Still other patients are hostile, engaging in one-upsmanship, and trying to embarrass or humiliate the examiner. This type of patient might make snide remarks about the interviewer's age or credentials, such as, "How old are you, anyway?" or "I want to talk to a *real* doctor." In extreme cases, the patient may refuse to talk altogether. Some patients are manipulative and obsequious, trying to get the interviewer on their side, often by emphasizing how much better and more competent and more likable the examiner is than "all those other doctors who don't seem to care." Other patients might exhibit seductive behavior toward the interviewer.

Whatever the quality of the interaction, the examiner must document with specific examples how the reported conclusions were reached. For instance, the statement that a patient was "covertly hostile" can be documented by observing that after waiting 15 minutes to be seen, the patient remarked to the examiner, "I thought you had died and . . . gone to heaven." This patient can also be said to be exhibiting some *ambivalence*, having both negative and positive feelings toward the interviewer.

Psychomotor Activity

A patient who displays *psychomotor agitation* moves around constantly, appearing to have difficulty sitting still; there may be hand-wringing, food-shuffling, crossing and uncrossing of knees, picking on scabs, scratching, nail-biting, hair-twisting, or even hair-pulling. In more severe illness, the patient may get up from the chair or bed, wander around the room, and engage in behaviors inappropriate to the context of the interview, such as trying to move furniture. Agitation should be distinguished from *psychomotor acceleration*, which simply refers to great rapidity of activity and thought processes. This, in turn, is to be contrasted with *psychomotor retardation*, characterized by a general slowing of movement, speech, and thought: The patient will sit quietly, moving very little; the speech will be soft and slow, accompanied by minimal, if any, gestures; the facial expression can be immobile; talking seems to be an effort, with frequent periods of silence, and questions are answered after a prolonged latency. That agitation and retardation are not opposites is suggested by the fact that in some disorders, such as mixed bipolar psychoses (in which manic and depressive phases are mixed rather than being independent attacks), psychomotor agitation and retardation may coexist (e.g., the patient may be physically restless and mentally slowed down). Precise description of psychomotor retardation is now possible through the use of the Salpêtrière Retardation Scale (Widlöcher, 1983). If neither psychomotor agitation, acceleration, nor retardation is observed, the patient's psychomotor activity is judged as "normal." This designation would be the case in the majority of patients who seek counseling for milder mental disturbances. Abnormal psychomotor activity, observed on repeated examination, tends to be indicative of a major psychiatric disorder.[2]

---

[2]It is beyond the scope of this chapter to provide a detailed description of various motor disturbances—such as *tics, stereotypies, chorea, ataxia, mitmachen*, and *mitgehen*—seen in neuropsychiatric disorders. The interested reader is referred to Fish's *Clinical Psychopathology* (Hamilton, 1974). It is also beyond the scope of this chapter to describe the various neuroleptic-induced movement disorders (Taylor, 1993). Of theses, *akathisia* is one that beginning students of psychopathology should distinguish from agitation: The latter refers to a generalized dysphoric restlessness, while the former refers to inability to sit down and an urge to move not secondary to an affective state.

Stupor consists of almost total arrest of all motor activity (including speech), with little or no response to external stimuli. Thus, stupor represents an extreme degree of psychomotor retardation and mutism combined. The condition has been observed on the battlefront and in civilian catastrophes as "paralysis by fear," and in catatonic schizophrenia and stuporous depression. However, stupor can also be a sign of severe and life-threatening physical illness, and the first order of business is to rule out brain or systemic disease or drug-induced states (even if one were to find psychologically "plausible" reasons to explain the patient's condition).

Affect and Mood

Affect refers to the prevailing emotional expression during the interview as observed by the clinician. A "normal" patient will show a range of affect, laughing when something is funny and looking somber when sad or painful issues are discussed. In other words, affect will be congruent with the content of the conversation.

Commonly observed disturbances in affect include *hostility* (a predominantly argumentative and antagonistic stance toward the interviewer and others) and *lability* (rapid shifts from happiness to sadness, often accompanied by giggling and laughing or sobbing and weeping; these shifts may cover the whole gamut of emotion in the course of an interview).

Inappropriate affect is observed when the patient's emotional expression is grossly incongruent with the content of the conversation (e.g., giggling while relating the gory details of an accident that maimed a large number of people).

The patient with a *blunted affect* has minimal display of emotion, with little variation in facial expression. *Emotional flattening* is a more severe degree of emotional impoverishment and refers to the absence of all emotional reactivity.

It is important to note that cultural or subcultural variables play an important part in the interaction during the interview on which the judgment of affect is based. A frightened, insecure patient from a minority background may give the wrong impression of emotional blunting because he or she is unwilling to reveal personal information to an interviewer with whom rapport has not been established. In such situations, definite conclusions should be suspended until there has been an opportunity to unobtrusively observe the patient interacting with peers, family members, nursing staff, or others. Assessment should be carried out to determine whether there is an inability to display emotional warmth or whether the patient was responding to the social context of a threatening interview with an unfamiliar and inadvertently intimidating professional. Invoking such cultural variables to explain abnormal findings obviously presupposes a thorough knowledge of the culture in question.

Mood refers to the emotion experienced by the patient over a period of time and therefore is based on self-report. Such self-reports do not always coincide with the affect that is observed during the interview. A *euthymic* person is one who displays no marked affective disturbance during the interview. Another patient may show no facial expression of depression—may even smile—yet report deepening depression over the preceding several weeks. Such incongruities, which are commonplace in the assessment of emotion, should be specifically recorded in the mental status examination. In addition to *depressed mood* (e.g., "I am down in the dumps, and I don't seem to be able to pull myself out of it"), which is one of the common complaints in a clinical population, the clinician may hear reports of *elated* or *euphoric mood* ("I feel as high as a kite" or "I feel on Cloud 9"), *irritability* ("I am short-fused, everything seems to bother me: I yell at my kids, at my colleagues . . ."), and free-floating , diffuse, or *generalized anxiety* characterized by a sense of foreboding ("I feel kind of scared, like something bad is about to happen"). *Panic* is a crescendo buildup of anxiety, typically associated with intense autonomic arousal. *Phobias* are irrational fears of specific situations that, objectively, do not appear dangerous; avoidance of the particular situation is typical, otherwise the subject may panic. By contrast, panic attacks in panic disorder tend to occur unexpectedly. *Terror* represents an extreme degree of sustained anxiety; it may be elicited by overwhelming danger (e.g., during a natural calamity, rape or hostage experience, recall of such experiences, or cues that reawaken them); terror could also be secondary to psychotic experiences that have the force of reality for the patient. Thus, although different manifestations of anxiety are most commonly observed in primary anxiety disorders, they can also manifest in the context of mood, schizophrenic, and delirious disorders.

Speech and Thought

The patient's speech is described with regard to loudness, speed, complexity, usage of words, and ability to come to the point.

> The patient's speech was soft and slow. At times, she was barely audible and had to be asked to repeat what she said. She spoke only in response to specific questions and needed to be asked repeatedly to elaborate on her answers. Her vocabulary was limited, commensurate with her eighth-grade education. However, her speech was coherent, and her answers were appropriate.

It is important to document any deviations from what would be considered "normal" by citing relevant examples, preferably using the patient's own words. Thus, it is not sufficient to summarize one's observations by noting "Stilted verbal behavior" or "Pressure of speech." Such conclusions must be corroborated by relevant quotes or by a description of the behavior that led the examiner to arrive at them.

> His speech was contrived and stilted. He tried hard to convey that he was well-educated, using sophisticated words, often inappropriately. For example, when trying to say that things often got hectic at his job as a telephone operator, he stated that things got "exuberant."

Thought form or *thought process* refers to how and in what sequence and at what speed ideas are put together. A patient may exhibit no abnormality in speech and thought processes, in which case he or she can be described as *coherent*. On the other hand, there may be varying degrees of digression or lack of clarity or logic. *Circumstantiality* is a tendency to answer questions in tedious and unnecessary detail and circumlocution. This tendency is sometimes seen in people from a rural background. Circumstantiality is also frequent in people with extreme obsessionality who want to make sure they include all facts that might be remotely relevant to the point in question. Severe circumstantiality often goes hand in hand with other indications of low intelligence or cerebral pathology or both. The most severe degree of circumstantiality is known as *tangentiality* (oblique or totally irrelevant responses) and is observed often, though not exclusively, in schizophrenic disorders.

In *pressure of speech*, seen in anxiety states and agitated depressions, the patient feels compelled to talk. Not only do patients with *flight of ideas*, a major diagnostic sign in mania, feel pressured to talk, but also their thoughts race ahead of their ability to communicate them; they skip from one idea or theme to another. In contrast to the looseness in schizophrenia, the connection between different ideas is not entirely lost in mania, but may be tenuous, consisting of rhymes or puns (*clang associations*).

> Her speech was loud and rapid, interspersed with laughter and jokes. At times, she appeared to trip over her words, and her thoughts seemed to be racing ahead of her ability to put them into words. When asked who the president was, she replied: "Johnson, Johnathan, my son, sunshine, Einstein." [This patient entertained the belief that her son was smarter than Einstein and would become the next president.]

In the extreme, it may be difficult to draw the line between flight of ideas and *looseness of associations* (Andreasen, 1979b). In the latter, the patient's speech is derailed and, ultimately, loses any meaningful or logical sequence. Patients may actually invent words that have meaning only to them (*neologisms*). Here is an example of severe loosening of associations, interspersed with neologisms: It is the opening paragraph of a written statement presented to one of us by a patient who hoped that the statement would clarify his reasons for coming to the hospital:

> Good Day! *Natherath*. In early times man has struggled for the long *surrinel* of the human orator, the inner intestinal cavity, the lungs. It is knowledgeable that the bone structure of man is durable with tinctured calcium, skin seven epidural thick which replenishes it in the case *endergy* and mental powers. [Italicized words are reproduced as spelled by the patient.]

At times, mild loosening of associations manifests itself in a general *vagueness* of thinking; although not as disjointed as the preceding sample, very little information will be conveyed, even though many words may have been used. This disturbance, known as *poverty of thought content*, is diagnostic of schizophrenia when organic mental disorders are ruled out (Andreasen, 1979b).

In *perseveration*, the patient adheres to the same words or concepts and seems unable to proceed to other topics. For instance, a patient responded to sequential questions as follows: "How many years have you been married?" "Seven." "How many children do you have?" "Seven." "How many weeks have you been out of work?" "Seven." *Echolalia* is the irrelevant echoing or repeating of words used by the interviewer ("Can you tell me what brings you here to the emergency room?" "Room, room, room.") Echolalia is often accompanied by *echopraxia*, which consists of repeating movements initiated by the examiner. These disturbances are often seen in catatonic and organic mental disorders.

Confabulation denotes fabrication of information to fill in memory gaps (seen, for instance, in the amnestic syndrome, a complication of alcoholism).

Thought block refers to the sudden stoppage of thought in the middle of a sentence. Sometimes, after a momentary pause, the patient may begin a new and unrelated thought. At other times, the patient may seem perplexed and unable to continue to talk. This experience, when mild, may be due to exhaustion, anxiety, or a retarded depression. More severe thought block is seen in schizophrenia, possibly as the observable counterpart of the subjective experience of thought withdrawal (see below).

Retardation or *inhibition of thought processes*, characteristic of bipolar depressives, consists of a slowing of thinking—subjectively experienced as poor concentration, indecision, or ruminative thoughts. Such patients may complain of "poor memory," which—together with poor performance on cognitive tests—may lead to the erroneous diagnosis of dementia in elderly subjects. These "pseudodemented depressions" should obviously be distinguished from true dementia, as the former tend to respond favorably to antidepressant medication.

Mutism is the complete loss of speech. The patient cannot be made to talk at all. It is seen in conversion disorder, catatonia, and patients suffering from midline lesions of the brain. Patients who intentionally refuse to speak to certain people are said to display *elective mutism.*

Aphonia and *dysphonia*, unless based on laryngeal pathology, are almost always due to conversion or related somatization disorders or both. In aphonia, the patient loses his or her voice; in dysphonia, he or she cannot raise it above a whisper. In aphonia—as contrasted with mutism—one observes lip movements or nonverbal attempts to communicate. Aphonia can be an "unconscious" compromise in an inhibited individual who, for example, feels like cursing but is ashamed to do so.[3]

Whereas *thought form* refers to how thoughts are communicated, *thought content* refers to what the patient communicates. Much of this information becomes apparent in the course of the interview, but it may be necessary to ask some specific questions. The nature of inquiry into thought content again depends largely on the patient's clinical picture and presenting problem.

Every mental status examination should have an explicit statement about the presence or absence of *suicidal thought content*. Approaching this topic can be difficult for the beginning clinician. There is a popular misconception that one might inadvertently put ideas into the patient's head by exploring this issue. In fact, the danger lies in failing to inquire about suicidal ideation, thereby failing to properly assess the seriousness of suicide risk and the necessity to institute appropriate interventions. A tactful way to inquire about suicidal ideas is as follows: "You have told me a lot about the painful things that have happened in your life. Have you found yourself thinking that one way to forget it all is to go to sleep and not wake up?" If the answer is affirmative, the next question should be, "Have you had the thought that you might just want to end it all by taking your

---

[3]Aphonia should be distinguished from *aphasia*, which refers to inability to understand or express language because of cerebral pathology; both of these should, in turn, be distinguished from *dysarthria*, which refers to slurred articulation (often with drooling), also of central origin (Taylor, 1993).

own life?" At this point, some patients will vigorously deny that they are considering suicide. Others will admit to suicidal ideas. It is important to find out whether these thoughts have evolved into a specific plan for action and whether there have been suicide attempts in the past. Suicidal risk is greatly increased if the patient feels truly hopeless.

Homicidal thoughts may emerge during the interview and should be carefully noted in the patient's record; when indicated (e.g., in those with history of, or imminent potential for, impulsive or aggressive behavior, or those who have made threats), the interviewer should gently and cautiously inquire about them. *Religiosity* (religious preoccupation that exceeds culturally accepted standards in the patient's religious denomination) will also probably emerge in the interview. However, *obsessions* (repetitive and irrational ideas that intrude into consciousness and cannot be shaken off) and *phobias* (specific irrational fears) may not emerge spontaneously and should be specifically inquired about. Related symptoms, which may or may not be spontaneously verbalized, include *depersonalization* (the uncanny experience that one has changed) and *derealization* (the experience that the environment has changed). Although these two experiences can occur in normal persons as isolated events (as in severe exhaustion), they happen most commonly in agoraphobia (Lader & Marks, 1971) and, less commonly, in depressive illness (Lewis, 1934). Discussed under thought content here, strictly speaking, depersonalization and derealization represent disorders in the experience of the self and its boundaries; they can result from anxiety, mood, psychotic, or organic disorders.[4]

Delusions are false, unshakable beliefs that are idiosyncratic to the individual and cannot be explained on a cultural or subcultural basis. For example, the belief that one is possessed by the devil or that one is the victim of a voodoo curse is not necessarily delusional. Neither are beliefs in unusual health practices and folk remedies. However, the judgment that one is dealing with culturally accepted phenomena must be made on the basis of thorough knowledge of the culture. In fact, in cultures in which voodoo and witchcraft are still part of daily life, delusions often consist of pathological elaborations of these beliefs that would not be endorsed or shared by the patient's kin or associates. The inexperienced examiner may fail to recognize serious pathology by being overly willing to invoke "cultural" phenomena. For this reason, it is often desirable to inquire whether other members of that culture share the beliefs in question.

Delusions are divided into primary and secondary categories. *Primary delusions* cannot be understood in terms of other psychological processes (Jaspers, 1963). They were described by Schneider (1959) as "first-rank symptoms," and they consist of ego-alien or externally imposed thought (*thought insertion*), emotion, and somatic function (*passivity feelings*), as well as experiences of *thought broadcasting* (Mellor, 1970). Primary delusions seem to arise out of the context of a "delusional mood" in which the patient is in such mental perplexity that the sense of reality is

---

[4]A temporal lobe epileptic focus is to be suspected if depersonalization and derealization coexist with a perceptual disturbance such as *déjà vu* and *déjà vécu* (the feeling that one has seen or experienced a given situation), *micropsia* (objects getting smaller and receding into space) or *macropsia* (getting larger), or smelling markedly offensive odors.

impaired and false beliefs are easily formed. For example, neutral percepts (such as a black car) may acquire special personal significance of delusional proportion (e.g., the end of the world is imminent); this phenomenon is known as *delusional perception*. The presence of several of these first-rank symptoms is suggestive of schizophrenia, although one should first rule out amphetamine (or cocaine) psychosis, temporal lobe (complex partial) seizures, and alcoholic hallucinosis. Finally, these first-rank symptoms can be incidental findings in the affective psychoses (Andreasen & Akiskal, 1983).

Secondary delusions arise from concurrent or preexisting psychopathological experiences (Jaspers, 1963); i.e., they are explanatory elaborations of other psychological themes. Examples of secondary delusions include:

1. Delusions based on hallucinations. For example, a patient who hears machinelike noises may be convinced that he or she is being subjected to electrical surveillance.
2. Delusions based on other delusions. For example, a patient who believes that his or her "skin is shrinking" may ascribe it to being slowly poisoned by his or her "enemies."
3. Delusions based on morbid affective states, known as *affective delusions* (Akiskal & Puzantian, 1979). For instance, a manic patient stated that his experience of ecstasy, physical strength, and sharpened thinking was so overwhelming that there was only one explanation, namely, that he was chosen by God to serve as the new Messiah.
4. Delusions based on cognitive deficits. For example, a patient with early dementia and memory disturbances may have the delusion of having been robbed (not remembering where he left his wallet).

It may not always be easy to classify delusions into primary and secondary categories; for this reason, it is customary to describe them by content. As described by Wing, Cooper, and Sartorius (1974), delusions can be classified into the following categories: delusions of *reference* (e.g., the idea that one is being observed, talked about, or laughed at); delusions of *persecution* (e.g., that one is the target of malevolent or hostile action); delusions of *misidentification* (the belief that, for example, one's persecutors have been disguised as doctors, nurses, family members); delusions of *jealousy* (false belief in infidelity of the spouse or lover); delusions of *love* [also called *erotomania* (in which a public figure is believed to be in love with the patient)]; *grandiose delusions* (belief in unusual talents or powers, or belief that the patient has the identity of a famous person, living or historical); delusions of *assistance* (e.g., benign powers assisting the patient in his or her plans); and delusions of *ill health* (hypochondriacal delusions; the patient pleads for a cure of his or her imaginal and often bizarre "disease"); delusions of *guilt* (the belief that one has committed an unforgivable act); *nihilistic* delusions (insistence that body parts are missing); and delusions of *poverty* ("I have squandered all my money; my family will starve"). Except for the first few, these delusions are characteristic of the affective psychoses.

The clinical trainee interested in a more general exposition on delusional beliefs can consult a recent monograph on the subject (Oltmanns & Maher, 1988).

Perceptual Disturbances

A *hallucination* is a perception without an external stimulus in an awake subject (e.g., hearing voices when no one is around or seeing things that are not there). Any sensory modality can be involved: hearing, vision, taste, smell, touch, and even the vestibular sense. Certain forms of hallucinations cannot be ascribed to such discrete sensory modalities, however. For instance, patients intoxicated with psychedelic drugs may report that they can "hear colors," "smell music," and the like; this phenomenon is known as *synesthesia*.

Illusions are often described by the patient as "hallucinations." However, they are simply misperceptions of actual stimuli (e.g., mistaking a clothes tree in a dimly lit room for a person). Such experiences may result from exhaustion, anxiety, altered states of consciousness, delirium, or a functional psychosis.

Perceptual disturbances may occur in individuals who do not suffer from a mental illness. Most of us have on occasion, while waiting for an important phone call, actually "heard" the phone ring; it is not uncommon for an anxious subject to "hear" a voice calling his or her name when no one is actually there. In normal individuals, these experiences are more likely to occur in periods of high emotional arousal (as in grief) or expectancy and tend to be isolated and infrequent events.

Auditory hallucinations are classified as elementary (noises) or complete (voices or words). Both forms are most commonly found in schizophrenic disorders. They may also occur in organic mental disorders, including intoxications. For instance, alcoholic patients frequently hear voices (alcoholic hallucinosis). Voices that are continuous, making a running commentary on the patient's behavior, or argue about him or her in the third person are special categories of hallucinatory phenomena included in the first-rank symptoms listed by Schneider (1959). Another Schneiderian first-rank hallucination consists of hearing one's own thoughts spoken aloud (*écho de pensée*). Like primary delusions, these Schneiderian hallucinatory experiences are characteristic of, but not specific to, schizophrenia (Andreasen & Akiskal, 1983).

Auditory hallucinations occur not only in schizophrenic and organic mental disorders but also in depressive and manic psychoses. The term *affective hallucination* is used to describe hallucinatory experiences based on, or understandable in terms of, a prevailing morbid affective state. The voice may tell the patient that he or she is "a sinner" or "a masturbator" and should be punished by death. A striking example of affective hallucinations in mania was reported by Akiskal and Puzantian (1979, p. 429):

> A 28-year-old female heard "motors" and believed that this perception represented the noise of carriages that were specially sent to transport her, her children, and the entire household into heaven.

When perceptual disturbances occur in mood disorders, they tend to be transient, usually occurring at the height of mania (or stage III mania) (Carlson & Goodwin, 1973), or the depth of depression, or during the unstable neurophysiological transition from depression to mania or vice versa (switch process). They can also appear as organic complications secondary to exhaustion, dehydration, or the superimposed drug or alcohol abuse that is often comorbid with mood disorders.

Visual hallucinations are characteristic of organic mental disorders, specifically the acute delirious states (Lipowski, 1990); they tend to involve figures or scenes less than life-size ("Lilliputian"), may coexist with auditory hallucinations, and are often frightening in nature. They are common complications of sensory deprivation (e.g., cataract surgery). Psychedelic experiences with drugs can be pleasant or frightening depending on mental set. Visual hallucinations are uncommon in schizophrenia but occur in normal grief (visions of a dead relative) and in depressive illness (e.g., seeing oneself in one's casket), as well as in brief reactive psychoses.

Olfactory hallucinations are difficult to distinguish from illusions of smell. (The same is true of *hallucinations of taste*.) Some delusional female patients, for instance, are always conscious of their vaginal odor and tend to misinterpret neutral gestures made by other people as indicative of olfactory disgust. In temporal lobe epilepsy, hallucinations of burning paint or rubber present as auras.

Hallucinations of touch, or *haptic hallucinations*, usually take the form of insects crawling on one's skin and characteristically occur in cocaine intoxication, amphetamine psychosis, and delirium tremens. When they occur in a schizophrenic disorder, they may take such bizarre forms as orgasms imposed by an imaginary phallus.

Vestibular hallucinations (e.g., those of flying) are most commonly seen in substance-induced or withdrawal states such as delirium tremens and LSD psychosis. Patients with such misperceptions have been known to sustain serious injuries or even death by trying to fly out of windows.

In *hallucinations of presence*, experienced by schizophrenic, histrionic, and delirious patients, the presence of another individual is somehow sensed. In *extracampine hallucinations*, the patient visualizes objects outside his or her sensory field (e.g., seeing the devil standing behind him or her when he or she is looking straight ahead). In *autoscopy*, the patient sees himself or herself in full figure without the benefit of a mirror; this experience, which can occur in epileptic, histrionic, depressive, and schizophrenic disorders, it also known as seeing one's *doppelgänger*, or double. It is artfully portrayed in Dostoevski's novel *The Double*.

Other varieties of hallucinations include visual experiences that occur in the twilight state between wakefulness and sleeping (*hypnagogic*) or sleep and awakening (*hypnopompic*). Although their occasional occurrence is normal, repeated experiences suggest narcolepsy. Some narcoleptic subjects may actually have difficulty distinguishing vivid dreams from reality. It must be kept in mind, however, that patients with histrionic personalities may also give flamboyant accounts of hallucinations: They may actually "perceive" objects or events that fit their fantasies, and they may, in addition, dramatize the occurrence of such normal experiences as dreams in an attention-seeking manner.

Sensorium: Orientation, Attention, and Concentration

Under the term *sensorium* are subsumed the related higher mental functions of orientation, attention, and concentration, which all depend on an optimal level of arousal and vigilance

Orientation is conceptualized in four spheres: orientation to *time* (day, week, month, and year), *place* (location of interview, name of city), *person* (identity of self and interviewer), and *situation* (interview as opposed to, for example, inquisition or trial). A patient who is oriented in all spheres is noted to have a *clear sensorium*.

Patients with signs and symptoms of psychosis may or may not be oriented in all spheres. Those with affective and schizophrenic psychoses are not typically disoriented, whereas patients suffering from delirium or dementia are characteristically disoriented. They are described as having a *clouded sensorium* or as being *confused*. In delirious states, the sensorium tends to fluctuate; in a hospital setting, these patients often show remarkable changes depending on time of day, with worsening orientation at night (known as *sundown syndrome*). The symptomatic picture in drug intoxication often closely resembles acute psychoses of "functional" origin (schizophreniform and manic psychoses). Whether the patient is disoriented and whether his or her mental status fluctuates are therefore important diagnostic clues.

Some specific questions that should be asked are as follows:

Orientation to time: "Can you tell me what day of the week it is today?" "Do you know what day of the month it is?" "And what month?" "What year is it?"

Orientation to place: "Tell me your name." "Do you know who I am?" (If the patient cannot be expected to know the examiner's name, one should make sure that one's name tag is legible.) "Can you tell me what I am doing here?"

Orientation to situation: "Tell me what this is all about?" "Why are you here?" "What is the purpose of this visit to the clinic?"

If the patient is not able to answer these questions, the examiner should provide answers and clarification, in a reassuring and supportive manner. At a later point, the patient can be asked the same questions again. Whether he or she is able to retain this information will give important clues regarding short-term memory.

Obviously, it is not necessary to inquire formally about orientation items in every patient. A student with the chief complaint of fear of public speaking need not be examined in depth about his or her orientation, which will be evident from his or her general demeanor and life situation.

To test properly for orientation, the interviewing clinician must make sure that he or she has the patient's attention. A patient with deficits in *attention* has trouble achieving the appropriate set that would permit the interview to proceed. He or she may fall asleep as you talk; may practically ignore you, being distracted by television, telephone, and other irrelevant stimuli; cannot filter relevant from irrelevant stimuli as they pertain to the interview situation. Care must be taken to distinguish between deficits in attention, which are involuntary, and lack of cooperation or oppositional behavior, which is a purposeful attempt to obstruct the interview process. An example of the latter would be a patient who pointedly leafs through a magazine while you are trying to talk to him or her.

A patient with deficits in *concentration* may be able to achieve the set required for a successful interview, but has trouble maintaining it: The interviewer will have to repeat questions, and the patient will commonly make complaints such as, "My mind is not working." This is a nonspecific finding and can occur in anxious, depressed, or psychotic patients, as well as those with cerebral disease. Some patients with *poor concentration* also complain of easy *distractibility* of their thinking process; this disturbance can also exist without poor concentration, as in mania. Patients with severe mental disorders, typically at the psychotic level, also evidence emotional or intellectual *perplexity*; these patients are not able to comprehend what is going on around them. Such disturbances of attention and concentration often result from high levels of emotional arousal. The clinical examiner must also note that reduced arousal due to drug intoxication, metabolic disease, cerebral infection, or trauma can also lead to fleeting attention and poor concentration. Such patients are described as being in a *twilight state* between the awake and dreaming states.[5]

Memory

Much has recently been learned about the basic and neuropsychological aspects of memory (Squires, 1987). The purpose of the discussion here is to provide the beginning clinical student with a framework for understanding the types of disturbances that are encountered in general psychiatric patients. Patients with specific neuropsychiatric disorders or those seen in neurological and neurosurgical units will need a more advanced approach.

Memory disturbances can be classified on the basis of cause as psychogenic or organic and on the basis of functional impairment as *dysamnesia* (distortion of memory) and *amnesia* (loss of memory). Distortions of memory include several phenomena. In *retrospective falsification*, the patient modifies his or her memories in line with emotional needs. Thus, the depressed patient views all his past as failure; so-called "borderline" patients tend to view relationships with significant others in either idealized or extremely negative terms. As noted previously, the *confabulating* patient fills extensive gaps in memory with details that never took place; this falsification could be due not only to organic factors (such as alcohol), but also to schizophrenic illness wherein fantastic events are fabricated to justify delusional claims (such as the claim to a throne). *Pathological lying* (or *pseudologia fantastica*) is observed in psychopathic individuals, who invent stories to impress other people. A related condition is the *Münchausen syndrome*, which consists of fantastic tales of adventure and misadventure, as well as fabricated medical histories (leading to unnecessary hospitalizations, medical tests, or procedures).

As for amnesias, they can be secondary to severe anxiety or dissociative states in which there is partial or complete loss of memory or identity. In the extreme, this manifests as a wandering or *fugue state*. Psychological mechanisms are believed to play an important role in the foregoing amnesias. Organic factors are generally deemed more important in the *retrograde* and *anterograde* amnesias, which, respectively, precede and follow insults to the head (such as in a car accident or boxing match).

---

[5]It is obviously impossible to conduct a proper mental status examination in patients who have even greater compromises in arousal such as those in *stupor* and *coma*. Curiously, some stuporous patients— those with affective and schizophrenic psychoses—may on awakening from their stupor recall vividly all that happened while in stupor even if at the time they could not respond.

Memory deficits can also be classified on the basis of the span of time involved in the loss of function: *immediate* (the patient cannot repeat things he or she has just been told), *short-term* (the patient cannot retain information for 5 minutes or so), *long-term* (the patient is unable to remember the events of the past months or years), and *remote* (concerning events many years in the past).

Impairment in immediate and short-term memory may actually reflect inability to concentrate, a distinction that is not always easy to make. The patient whose deficits arise from difficulty concentrating will appear preoccupied and anxious and will have problems following the clinician's instructions. On the other hand, the patient with memory deficits will try his or her best and will understand what he or she is supposed to do but be unable to perform. Anxiety may also be present, but will be more of a response to the patient's realization that his or her mind is not functioning properly. A supportive and reassuring stance on the part of the examiner is essential.

Sometimes the examiner may actually decide to "coach" a patient with memory deficits: Severely depressed patients often display concentration disturbances that result in poor performance on cognitive tests (*depressive pseudodementia*). With encouragement and reassurance, these patients often find the correct answers. However, such coaching does not work in true dementia, in which random answers are given, despite proper coaching.

Some specific tasks that can be used in assessing memory and concentration are as follows:

Street address: "Now I am going to give you an address that I want you to remember for me. I will ask you again in about 5 minutes what this address is. The address is 1625 Cedar Street. Can you repeat this for me? [Let the patient repeat the address.] O.K. I'll ask you about it in 5 minutes. Now let's go on and talk some more about the other things we were discussing." After 5 minutes, most patients without organic impairments will be able to recall the address correctly, or almost correctly.

Digits forward and digits backward: "Now I am going to ask you to repeat some numbers for me. I will say the numbers, and when I am done, you say them after me. Now I will start: 1-4-5. Can you repeat these for me?" One then goes on to increasing numbers of digits. When the patient has reached the maximum number of digits he or she can recall, the process can be repeated with the instruction to recall digits backward, starting with two numbers, and going on to longer strings. Most patients with normal intelligence and without organic impairment can repeat six digits forward and as many as four in reverse. For this exercise to be useful, the clinician should *not* try to make up the numbers but should read them off a table, in an even cadence (lest he or she forget them!).

Memory for three objects: "Now I am going to ask you to remember three things for me. I will ask you again in about 5 minutes, and you tell me what they are. Here are the three things: The color *red*; the word *pencil*, and the number *17*. Repeat these for me. O.K., try to hang onto these three things, and I'll ask you again, in about 5 minutes."

Serial subtraction: This is more specifically a test of concentration. Ask the patient to subtract 3 from 100, then 3 from that number (which it is hoped will be 97), then 3 again, and so forth. If this poses no problem for a few rounds, ask the patient to subtract 7 from 100, from 93, and so forth. Educational level and calculating ability must be taken into consideration.

Recall of recent events: By asking a patient about verifiable events that occurred in the past days, one can assess mental functioning in an unobtrusive way. These questions can include what the patient ate for lunch, the current issues in the TV news (if the patient reports having watched the news), and the like. It is important that the answers can be verified, because patients with organic brain dysfunction often *confabulate* their answers (e.g., they invent plausible responses in order to avoid the painful realization that they cannot remember). Intellectual functioning can also be unobtrusively assessed in this way, by asking the patient about current events and his or her understanding of their implications.

Remote memory: Such memory function is often well preserved, even in patients who suffer from significant organic impairment. It can be checked by getting patients to talk about their childhood and adolescence, places where they have lived, military service, occupations, and (most verifiably) by assessing recollections of important historical or well-publicized events and their impact (e.g., Pearl Harbor, the Great Depression, who was president during those times). Some specific questions may include "Who was Martin Luther King?" "Cleopatra?" "What happened to them?" "What was Sputnik?" "Watergate?" (Make sure to ask one question at a time, leaving sufficient time for answers.)

Intelligence

One can get a general estimate of a patient's intelligence simply by talking to him or her. Specifically, the patient's *vocabulary* will give clues about intelligence, especially if considered in view of educational level. A college graduate can be expected to have a good vocabulary, but if a janitor with a third-grade education shows evidence of a rich vocabulary, one may conclude that his intelligence is much above his level of scholastic achievement.

Abstraction ability is another indicator of intellectual functioning. Some specific questions will help in this assessment: The "similarities" section of the Wechsler Adult Intelligence Scale lends itself to use in a mental status examination. One may wish to set the stage for this line of questioning by giving an example: "Now I am going to ask you a few more questions. They have to do with how some things are like other things. Here is an example: A hammer and a screwdriver are like each other in that they both are tools. Now, can you tell me how an apple and an orange are like each other?" "A table and a chair?" "A coat and a dress?" (Again, it is important not to bombard the patient with such questions, leaving ample time between them.)

Concrete answers are more likely to reflect lack of education than intellectual impairment. However, the answers to these questions can be revealing at both ends of the spectrum. A patient with minimal schooling who shows a high level of abstraction ability can be assumed to have good intelligence. A patient with a doctoral degree whose answers are concrete (an apple and an orange both have peels; a table and a chair both have four legs . . .) should be further tested neuropsychiatrically to determine the causes of such mediocre intellectual functioning. The implications of such concrete, or literal, thinking are discussed in more detail below.

Another way to test abstraction ability is by asking the patient to interpret proverbs. However, knowledge of the patient's sociocultural background is essential because one cannot assume that the patient has ever heard or understood the proverbs that we take for granted. Proverb interpretation can be approached as follows: "Now I am going to give you a few sayings, and I want you to tell me what they mean. Have you ever heard the saying, 'Don't cry over spilt milk'?" If the patient says "Yes," ask him or her to interpret. If he or she says "No," interpret the saying: "It means that there is no use worrying about something bad that has happened and that can't be fixed. Now let's try another one: Can you tell me what could be meant by 'A stitch in time saves nine'?" Literal interpretations should be evaluated in the same way as concreteness in "similarities."

Reliability, Judgment, and Insight

The interviewer must decide whether the patient can be deemed to be a *reliable* informant. This decision will depend largely on an estimate of the patient's intellectual functioning and on the clinician's impression of the patient's honesty, attention to detail, and motivation. For example, a patient who comes to treatment under family duress may give a very self-serving story that cannot be judged as reliable. A very histrionic patient may believe his or her own reports, but they may be colored by exaggeration, retrospective falsification, and wishful thinking. A patient with sociopathic traits may tell bald-faced lies to get out of legal trouble, and a patient with limited intelligence may simply make up facts to avoid embarrassment and to get the doctor "off his back." Psychotic patients and patients with organic mental disorders are often unreliable informants. Whether or not the patient is deemed reliable must be stated explicitly.

Unreliability due to carelessness, poor memory, or psychosis should not be confused with *talking past the point* or *vorbeireden*. First described in prisoners (and labeled *Ganser syndrome* after the psychiatrist who observed it), it consists of giving deliberately wrong answers in a fashion that indicates that the question was understood. For example: "Who is the president?" "George Clinton." "Who was president before him?" "Bill Bush." Such patients, typically sociopathic, are either malingering to appear insane or, in the case of schizophrenic individuals, are simply amused by the question–answer sequence. Because in most instances the impression given is one of dementia, the condition is also described as *hysterical pseudodementia* (Hamilton, 1974).

Judgment must be evaluated clinically in light of the entire history. Many patients who have normal intellectual functioning suffer from notoriously poor judgment in organizing their personal lives. This information can be gleaned from the facts obtained during the interview; evidence of poor judgment should, again, be documented with specific examples. For instance, walking around city streets wearing a bikini is poor judgment (in most places!), as is a history of repeated suicidal gestures or of impulsive job changes. Judgment can, if necessary, be assessed more specifically by using items from the Wechsler Adult Intelligence

Scale, such as the well-known "What would you do if you were the first one in a movie house to see smoke and fire?" or "What would you do if you found a sealed letter that has an address and a stamp on it?" The examiner may wish to improvise, by creating situations commensurate to the patient's age, social background, and sophistication.

The clinician has to assess whether the patient has adequate awareness that he or she has a problem and, if so, offer possible causes and reasonable solutions. This is known as *insight* and can be poor or absent (as in a psychotic illness), partial (some cognizance of the emotional nature of the problem), or good (understanding of the emotional roots of the problems). Insight usually depends on adequate intellectual functioning, but the converse is not true; that is, many highly intelligent people may be sorely lacking in insight.

COMMONLY MISUSED TERMS AND THEIR DIAGNOSTIC SIGNIFICANCE

Beginning clinicians often find it difficult to distinguish between *apathetic*, *depressed*, and *flat* affect (Andreasen, 1979a). Apathy can sometimes be due to severe physical illness wherein the patient simply feels too ill and too weak to engage in a conversation. Apathy can also be encountered in chronic schizophrenia and organic mental states.

A patient with *depressed* affect is best described as being in a state of mental anguish or pain (James, 1902). The patient will not be cheered up by reassurance or jokes, or will be unable to imagine a time when he or she will not be suffering the pain of depression. This is typically a phasic disturbance and tends to fluctuate with episodes of the disorder. In severe depression, there may be loss of emotional resonance whereby the patient cannot experience normal emotions such as grief and love. This inability to feel—especially inability to experience positive feelings for loved ones—is itself painful and typically associated with guilt.

On the other hand, *blunted* or *flat* affect refers to emotional impoverishment. It is characteristic of schizophrenia and tends to go hand in hand with formal thought disorder, and is often present throughout the course of the illness in patients with so-called "negative schizophrenia" (Andreasen, 1979a).

Apart from referring to the patient's history, differentiation of depression and emotional flatness on a mental status examination can be accomplished by observation and empathy. The facial expression of the chronic schizophrenic is typically vacant; that of the depressed patient is one of gloom, pain, and dejection. The interviewer usually has difficulty empathizing with the schizophrenic (known as *praecox feeling*) except on an intellectual level ("How this person must suffer inside!"), but the depressed person's dejection and pain tend to be communicated to the clinician and elicit emotional as well as intellectual empathy. Admittedly, this criterion is subjective, but it is invaluable in the hands of experienced clinicians.

Another difficult distinction is that between a *labile* effect (which changes quickly, often from one extreme to the other) and an *incongruent* affect (which is inappropriate to the thought content or the context). Both labile and incongruent affect should be differentiated from *affective incontinence*, in which the patient laughs or cries for extended periods with little or no provocation (i.e., the patient loses control over emotional expression). Lability may be encountered in character disorders such as histrionic personalities; in manic and mixed states, wherein emotions can shift easily from elation to irritability to panic and sobbing; and in delirious states, wherein the affect can quickly change from anxiety to terror. By contrast, incongruent affect (e.g., laughing while relating the gory details of a fatal accident) should raise the suspicion of schizophrenia. Emotional incontinence occurs most commonly in organic mental states such as multi-infarct dementia and multiple sclerosis.

Euphoria and *elation*, although characteristic of manic states, can also occur in organic mental disorders such as those resulting from systemic lupus erythematosus, multiple sclerosis, and liver cirrhosis. The euphoria seen in mania has warmth that is communicated to the observer, although, in the extreme, the manic patient can be cantankerous, obnoxious, and alienating. A silly kind of euphoria occurs in chronic schizophrenia and frontal lobe lesions; this sign is known as *Witzelsucht* and consists of the patient's relating patently silly jokes. Manic euphoria tends to be contagious or infectious—the clinician cannot help but enjoy the patient and laugh along with him or her. This is not the case with the silly euphoria found in schizophrenic and organic states. Again, these are not entirely reliable judgments but seem to carry diagnostic weight in the hands of experienced clinicians.

The term *paranoid* refers to psychotic conditions in which delusions predominate (e.g., paranoid schizophrenia and delusional disorder). Thus, the term *paranoid delusion* is redundant and should be replaced in the psychiatric vocabulary by more precise phrases such as *persecutory delusions, delusions of reference,* or *delusions of jealousy*.

Delusions should be distinguished from *overvalued ideas*, which refer to fanatically maintained notions such as the superiority of one sex, nation, race, or of one school of thought, philosophical approach, or artistic endeavor over others. Finally, delusions should be differentiated from *pseudologia fantastica*. This disorder, observed in attention-seeking (i.e., histrionic) psychopaths, consists of fantastic storytelling wherein the individual eventually loses track of which statements are true and which are false.

Thought disorder is a rather nebulous term and should not be used without qualification. One should always distinguish between *formal thought disorder* and *disorder of content*. Thus, the presence of delusions is not necessarily indicative of formal thought disorder; as already discussed, delusions can arise from affective and memory disturbances. Furthermore, in paranoid schizophrenia, delusions can exist in the absence of gross disturbances in the formal aspects of thought.

Formal thought disorder is a disorder in associations whereby thoughts are dissociated, disconnected, or rambling. It is also known as *derailment* (thoughts that are off the track). If mild, it leaves the impression of vagueness; if extremely severe, the patient makes no sense at all and is often said to exhibit *word salad*. The phrase "loose associations" is used for an intermediate degree of severity wherein one finds fragments of thoughts that seem totally illogical. Nevertheless, such thinking may have some symbolic significance—a highly personalized meaning that derives from "primary process" or "unconscious" associations; for that reason, it has been referred to as "autistic thinking," a thought form that is entirely related to the self, the inner world, and divorced from reality (Bleuler, 1950). Autistic patients invent neologisms to convey highly personalized concepts or meanings for which they find conventional language inadequate. The incoherence that one observes in the thinking of patients suffering from dementia is qualitatively different from formal thought disorder in that it lacks symbolism and the autistic quality. It is sometimes difficult to assess whether a patient whose answers are vague and rambling is intellectually dull or has trouble focusing. In the absence of intellectual impairment (e.g., if the patient has completed college), the hypothesis of a thought process disorder should be entertained. Beginning clinicians may be overly eager to give such patients the benefit of the doubt, supplying in their interview accounts connections and logical transitions that the patient did not supply. This favoritism is especially likely when the patient is intelligent and shares other characteristics of the examiner, thereby making it threatening for the examiner to recognize the patient's pathology.

The converse can also occur. Some clinicians who have a broad concept of schizophrenia tend to diagnose schizophrenia with "soft" evidence. This tendency is often based on proverb interpretation. The work of Andreasen (1977) has shown proverbs to be generally unreliable in diagnosing schizophrenia. Yet it is often erroneously assumed that inability to abstract on proverbs or similarities (i.e., *concrete thinking*) carries major diagnostic weight for schizophrenia. If a patient does not exhibit gross loosening of associations and displays concreteness on proverbs, he or she is sometimes labeled as having "subtle thinking disorder." There is little scientific rationale for this type of practice because concreteness correlates best with poor intellectual endowment, cultural impoverishment, and organic mental impairment. All three circumstance frequently coexist with schizophrenia, and to this extent schizophrenic patients will have impaired ability in abstraction. Indeed, schizophrenic patients are often annoyed by proverbs. In the authors' opinion, it is best to avoid direct testing of abstracting ability, unless one suspects organicity or mental retardation. The main value of the proverbs test in schizophrenia lies not in the degree of concreteness of responses (which may be due to low intelligence and social impoverishment) but in the patient's tendency to give bizarre and idiosyncratic responses.

In its severe manifestations, somatization disorder may mimic major mood illness, schizophrenia, and even organic mental disorders. The histrionic patient may transiently display (or report to have experienced) a plethora of severe symptoms suggestive of a major psychotic disorder. There can be repeated, bizarre, and florid symptoms; such symptomatology is often reported with an affect known as *la belle indifférence*, (i.e., a remarkable lack of concern for what to others would seem heartrending problems). This attitude is often mistaken for flat affect and the flighty and disorganized verbal accounts for formal thought disorder. Whenever feasible, it is almost always prudent to reexamine patients with confusing clinical presentations. It is finally imperative for beginning clinical trainees to keep in mind that no single sign or symptom carries major diagnostic weight in the pathognomonic sense. A specific mental disorder can be diagnosed only on the basis of a constellation of signs and symptoms with a characteristic course pattern (Kraepelin, 1904). For some patients, especially young psychotic patients, hospitalization often provides the best opportunity for direct repeated examination and proper medical workup to rule out organic contributions (Slater & Roth, 1977).

ILLUSTRATIVE MENTAL STATUS REPORTS

In this section, we will provide samples of mental status examinations performed in different settings.

Case 1

Mrs. A., a 38-year-old Hispanic-American woman, married, mother of three teenagers, was referred by her gynecologist because gynecological examination had failed to elucidate the cause of her decline in sexual interest. She was a tall, slender woman, impeccably dressed and groomed. Her hair was carefully styled. She wore makeup, conscientiously applied, and expensive-looking jewelry. She was cooperative and appeared to answer all questions to the best of her ability. She sat at the front of her armchair, appearing very "edgy." Her predominant facial expression was one of worry. She was oriented in all spheres. She engaged in considerable hand-wringing when she talked about her troubles and often picked nervously at her clothes, removing tiny specks of lint. She exhibited several instances of nervous laughter when relating painful events.

She described her mood as dysphoric and worried, "like I feel something bad is going to happen, and I have no control in the matter." In response to the direct probe, "Do you feel down?" she said she was not sure, but had decided to seek help because of some reduction of her enjoyments of things, and that she wept at times, feeling she might be unable to pull herself back together. No history of discrete panic attacks was elicited, nor did she have specific obsessions or compulsions. She admitted to worrying with the "teenage problems" of her kids. While discussing these, she stated that she felt worse in the mornings, which was the time her husband wanted to engage in sex; she said she could be more receptive sexually at night, though she had been anorgasmic then as well. There had been no change in appetite, but she had difficulty falling asleep.

Her attention appeared good, but she had trouble concentrating and often had to be brought "back on track"; she had a tendency to get lost in the details of her story. She asked several times, "What was it we were talking about?" Her memory for events appeared normal, but she complained that she had "trouble remembering things." For example, she almost had a fire at home last week because she forgot to unplug her iron; she often came home from the store without items she had intended to buy. She said this was not like her; she always prided herself in being conscientious and well organized. She stated, "I guess I just have too much on my mind."

Her intelligence was above average, commensurate with her education (a master's degree in education). She expressed herself well and stated the nature of her problems in immaculate English.

Her report is considered reliable. There was no abnormality in her thought form or content. She stated that she was concerned that she was about to "really lose it" when, a few days ago, she heard the doorbell ring, and nobody was there. She described no other instances of perceptual disturbances. She vigorously denied suicidal thoughts, stating that her faith [Catholic] would keep her from even considering such acts because she feared "eternal damnation." Although she freely verbalized anger toward her husband, children, and friends who had sometimes "let her down," there was no evidence of homicidal ideation. Indeed, she expressed guilt for feeling angry. Her judgment and insight were good, as she realized the emotional nature of her presenting problem. She felt that her main problem was her inability to communicate it properly to her husband.

This mental status is compatible with a generalized anxiety disorder, major depression, or both, a differential diagnosis that should be resolved on the basis of present illness, past psychiatric and medical history, and family history.

Case 2

Mr. B. was a 21-year-old white male who was brought into the emergency room by the police after he had disrupted a funeral at a local cemetery. He was pale and disheveled. His clothes were dirty. Although it was summer, he wore two woolen hats and a long muffler. He was oriented to time and place. However, he stated with a silly grin that he was the "Antichrist" and the examiner [a male] was "the Virgin Mary." He was restless during the interview and often stood up from his chair. He seemed bewildered and was reluctant to talk. When asked who had brought him to the hospital, he stated: "The police! Inquisition! Ha! Ha! Armageddon!" He was reluctantly and superficially cooperative, asking repeatedly, "Done now? Let me go!" His affect was silly. He giggled inappropriately, often after saying "Quiet!," at which time he seemed to be listening to voices. When asked about them, he said he received instructions from "above," but refused to elaborate. He denied other Schneiderian first-rank symptoms. He stated his mood was "wonderful." His attention and concentration were impaired, possibly by distraction from inner stimuli or thoughts. He refused to try serial subtractions and cursed at the examiner, stating, "Don't you ever mess with the Antichrist no more." His intelligence could not be assessed. His educational level is unknown. He claimed he has a "Ph.D. and Ed.D. and an M.D. degree." When asked about what it meant to be the Antichrist, he said, "If you don't know that by now, you never will." After this, he refused to communicate any further and stared quietly into space for the remainder of the session. For this reason, suicidal or homicidal thoughts, or specific delusions, could not be assessed. His judgment and insight are considered to be nil.

This mental status raises differential diagnostic possibilities ranging from schizophrenic to manic and drug-induced psychoses. Historical, familial, and laboratory (e.g., urinary drug screen) evaluations are necessary to differentiate between these alternatives.

Case 3

Ms. C. was seen for consultation on the medical service of a community hospital where she was hospitalized following a large overdose of alprazolam, which she had stolen from her mother's medicine cabinet. She sat propped up in her bed, dressed in a hospital gown. She is a slim white woman who looked younger than her stated age of 24. Her hair was braided in corn rows and slightly disheveled, but she was otherwise neat and clean. She states with a smile that she knew the examiner thought she was a "real mental case" but that she had taken the pills following an argument with her "fiancé" and had had no intention to die. She just thought he "needed to be taught a lesson." Her psychomotor activity was normal, and she was oriented in all spheres. Her affect appeared shallow. She said she "had been depressed, but not any longer" and that "all is well now": the gentleman in question had "come around" to her way of thinking, and there were not going to be "any more problems." When asked how the future looked to her, she said "Perfect." Upon further query, she admitted to "tense moments" with him. She denied discrete panic attacks, as well as phobic behavior.

Her attention, concentration, and memory appeared normal. Her intelligence and vocabulary seemed commensurate with her educational level [10th grade]. Her account of what led up to her overdose seemed reliable, but her judgment was immature. There was no evidence of formal thought disorder, and her speech was normal in flow and content. She denied any hallucinations, stating, "You really think I'm a nut!" Her insight is deemed to be poor, but she has no suicidal or homicidal ideas at the present time.

This mental status, which fails to reveal the presence of a major Axis I disorder, is suggestive of a personality disorder, the nature of which should be explored in future sessions of individual or, preferably, group therapy (assuming, of course, that the patient is wiling to follow through).

Case 4

Mrs. D., a 57-year-old African American, widowed former schoolteacher, was seen in consultation on the gastroenterology service. According to the referring physician, her mental status on admission was "unremarkable." On the fifth day in the hospital, she became visibly anxious and her condition worsened during the night. The night shift nurse reported that she refused to stay in her room and was found wandering the halls in the nude on two occasions. The nurse on the morning shift described the patient as "a sweet lady who has gone bonkers on us!" In retrospect, the nurse recalled that the patient had complained of insomnia and nightmares beginning with the second night of hospitalization. However, her request for a hypnotic had not been granted by her physician.

When Mrs. D. was seen by the consultant the following morning, she wore only her pajama bottoms and had a towel twisted around her head like a turban. She mumbled to herself and displayed considerable restlessness, getting up and wandering around her room, picking invisible objects off her chest and arms. Her hands showed a coarse, irregular tremor. She was marginally cooperative, agreeing to put on her pajama top and following simple directions such as "Can you stick out your tongue?" "Would you turn your head to the left?" and the like. However, her attention span appeared very impaired, and she seemed to be distracted by visual and auditory hallucinations. She stated, with irritation, that she could not sleep because "these Jehovah's Witnesses were singing hymns in my room all night long." She also complained that the nurses had put a half gallon of vanilla ice cream on her night table where it was "melting and dripping away." [There had never been any ice cream.] Her affect was labile, alternating from pleasant cooperation to irritability. Her orientation was marginal. She stated that she was in a hospital but seemed genuinely puzzled about why she was there. She knew her name and home address. She was disoriented to time. There was no gross loosening of associations; rather, she proved to be extremely distractible and often drifted off the subject, mumbling to herself. At one point, she announced she needed to go now because she was tired of hearing "Big Mama" call her for a "bologna sandwich." Her memory and concentration were extremely poor. She was unable to perform any of the relevant tasks [serial sevens, three objects, digits forward and backward]. There was no evidence of systematized delusions. Her insight and judgment were nil.

This patient exemplifies a delirious state. Further history revealed that she had been taking various types of minor tranquilizers since her husband's death a year ago to help her sleep. Enforced abstinence in the hospital had resulted in drug-withdrawal delirium, similar to that seen in alcohol withdrawal states, but occurring much later than the 2- to 3-day latency from abstinence typical for delirium tremens. This is due to the longer half-life of minor tranquilizers.

SUMMARY

Current evidence indicates that despite overlapping manifestations, discrete categories of mental disorders do exist. The diagnosis of these disorders requires systematic history-taking and interviewing. Eliciting the various signs and symptoms described in this chapter not only is necessary to support differential diagnostic decisions, but also serves the important task of communicating with other colleagues, as well as objective documentation of current difficulties for future reference.

A carefully conducted mental status examination is the cornerstone of good clinical work and research in psychopathology. In addition to presenting a general psychopathological framework pertinent to all mental health professionals who come into contact with the mentally ill, this chapter has emphasized situations and concerns particularly relevant to psychologists. The art and science of interviewing mentally ill patients goes beyond mere description of signs and symptoms. It requires an empathic understanding of the *phenomenology* of the psychopathology as experienced by the patient (Jaspers, 1963). This undertaking, which attempts to depict the patient's experience in as faithful a manner as possible, has a long European tradition (Wing et al., 1974) that is, in the authors' view, insufficiently appreciated in the United States. DSM-IV is a reliable framework, but instruments based on it or its predecessors do not necessarily provide valid diagnoses. A diagnosis is formulated by a clinician after all the relevant facts about a patient are known. Thus, a diagnosis is a clinical phenomenon and must ultimately be judged by its utility for clinical prediction.

Although a multitude of structured psychopathological interview schedules are now available for clinical research, the evaluation of mentally ill patients is still very much an art that depends on experience and clinical judgment. A semistructured interview—which follows a systematic outline while permitting patients to use their own words in describing their experiences—represents the best compromise between the traditional open-ended mental status examination and the more recently developed ultrastructured computerized schedules. A user-friendly schedule—which nonetheless utilizes sophisticated psychopathological concepts in a flexible format—is the one developed by the World Health Organization (1992) as a companion neuropsychiatric assessment instrument for its section on mental and behavioral disorders. The interested reader can adapt parts of this schedule—and its specific interview probes—to suit his or her clinical interview or research needs. Above all, the best schooling in psychopathology is acquired by interviewing patients in a variety of clinical settings.

Acknowledgments.   An earlier version of this chapter published in the first edition of this book resulted from collaboration between the first author (HSA) and Renate Rosenthal, Ph.D., at the University of Tennessee, Memphis; her contributions, especially to the parts dealing with cognitive testing, are gratefully acknowledged. Other areas of the Mental Status Examination covered in this second edition were extensively revised when the present authors (HSA and KA) served as consultants to the University of Tennessee–affiliated Mood Disorders Program at the Charter Lakeside Hospital, Memphis, where they interviewed a consecutive series of over 300 psychiatric inpatients and outpatients. The final draft of this version was completed when the first author was on leave at the National Institute of Mental Health, Rockville, Maryland. The opinions expressed in this chapter are the authors', and do not necessarily reflect those of the Institute.

References

Akiskal, H. S. (1989). The classification of mental disorders. In H. I. Kaplan & B. J. Sadock (Eds.), *Comprehensive Textbook of Psychiatry*, 5th ed. (pp. 583–598). Baltimore: Williams & Wilkins.

Akiskal, H. S., & Puzantian, V. R. (1979). Psychotic forms of depression and mania. *Psychiatric Clinics of North America, 2,* 419–439.

Andreasen, N. C. (1977). Reliability and validity of proverb interpretation to assess mental status. *Comprehensive Psychiatry, 18,* 465–472.

Andreasen, N. C. (1979a). Affective flattening and the criteria for schizophrenia. *American Journal of Psychiatry, 136,* 944–947.

Andreasen, N. C. (1979b). Thought, language, and communication disorders. I. Clinical assessment, definition of terms, and evaluation of their reliability. *Archives of General Psychiatry, 36,* 1315–1321.

Andreasen, N. C., & Akiskal, H. S. (1983). The specificity of Bleulerian and Schneiderian symptoms: A critical reevaluation. *Psychiatric Clinics of North America, 6,* 41–54.

Benjamin, L. (1993). *Interpersonal diagnosis and treatment of personality disorders.* New York: Guilford Press.

Bleuler, E. (1950). *Dementia praecox, or the group of schizophrenias* (J. Zinkin, Trans.). New York: International Universities Press.

Carlson, G. A., & Goodwin, F. K. (1973). The stages of mania: A longitudinal analysis of the manic episode. *Archives of General Psychiatry, 28,* 221–228.

den Boer, J. A., & Ad Sitsen, J. M. (1994). *Handbook of depression and anxiety.* New York: Marcel Dekker.

Groves, P. U., & Rebec, G. V. (1992). *Introduction to biological psychology,* 4th ed. Dubuque, IA: Wm. C. Brown Publishers.

Hamilton, M. (Ed.). (1974). *Fish's clinical psychopathology: Signs and symptoms in psychiatry.* Bristol: John Wright.

Hersen, M., & Turner, S. M. (1991). *Adult psychopathology and diagnosis,* 2nd ed. New York: John Wiley.

James, W. (1902). *The varieties of religious experience.* New York: Random House.

Jaspers, K. (1963). *General psychopathology* (J. Hoenig & M. H. Hamilton, Trans.). Manchester: Manchester University Press.

Kraepelin, E. (1904). *Lectures on clinical psychiatry.* London: Balliere, Tindall & Cox.

Lader, M., & Marks, I. M. (1971). *Clinical anxiety.* New York: Grune & Stratton.

Lewis, A. J. (1934). Melancholia: A clinical survey of depressive states. *Journal of Mental Science, 80,* 277–378.

Lipowski, Z. J. (1990). *Delirium: Acute confusional states.* New York: Oxford University Press.

Lishman, W. A. (1987). *Organic psychiatry: The psychological consequences of cerebral disorder.* Oxford: Blackwell.

McGuire, M. T., & Troisi, A. (1987). Physiological regulation–deregulation. Part I. General theory and methods. *Ethology and Sociobiology, 8,* 9s–25s.

Mellor, C. S. (1970). First rank symptoms of schizophrenia. I. The frequency in schizophrenics on admission to hospital. II. Differences between individual first rank symptoms. *British Journal of Psychiatry, 117*, 15–23.

Oltmanns, T. F., & Maher, B. A. (1988). *Delusional beliefs.* New York: John Wiley.

Schneider, K. (1959). *Clinical psychopathology.* New York: Grune & Stratton.

Slater, E., & Roth, M. (1977). *Mayer-Gross' clinical psychiatry,* 3rd ed., revised. Baltimore: Williams & Wilkins.

Squires, L. (1987). *Memory and brain.* New York: Oxford University Press.

Taylor, M. A. (1993). *The neuropsychiatric guide to modern everyday psychiatry.* New York: Free Press.

Widlöcher, D. J. (1983). Psychomotor retardation: Clinical, theoretical, and psychometric aspects, *Psychiatric Clinics of North America, 6*, 27–40.

Willerman, L., & Cohen, D. B. (1990). *Psychopathology.* New York: McGraw-Hill.

Wing, J. K., Cooper, J. E., & Sartorius, N. (1974). *The measurement and classification of psychiatric symptoms.* Cambridge: Cambridge University Press.

World Health Organization (1992). *The ICD-10 classification of mental and behavioral disorders.* Geneva: WHO.

Zuckerman, M. (1991). *Psychobiology of personality.* Cambridge, UK: Cambridge University Press.

II

Psychiatric Disorders

3

Anxiety Disorders

DEBORAH C. BEIDEL

DESCRIPTION OF THE DISORDERS

The *anxiety disorders* are the second most common group of psychiatric disorders (after substance abuse), with 6-month prevalence rates ranging from 6.6% to 14.8% of the general adult population (Robins et al., 1984). Complaints of anxiety are common in general practitioners' offices as well as in mental health clinics (e.g., Marsland, Wood, & Mayo, 1976). In addition, anxiety is often a component of other psychiatric disorders, such as affective disorders (Barlow, DiNardo, Vermilyea, Vermilyea, & Blanchard, 1986; Breier, Charney, & Heninger, 1984; Dealy, Ishiki, Avery, Wilson, & Dunner, 1981; Lesser et al., 1988; Uhde et al., 1985; Van Valkenberg, Akiskal, Puzantian, & Rosenthal, 1984) and substance abuse disorders (Kushner, Sher, & Beitman, 1990). Furthermore, anxiety is often only one facet of a more pervasive condition, including personality disorders (American Psychiatric Association, 1987). Given the ubiquitous nature of anxiety, it is likely that most clinicians will encounter patients seeking treatment for this disorder.

Anxiety patients present with a myriad of symptoms, including physical complaints, intrusive thoughts, dysphoria, and behavioral avoidance. Although most clinicians are familiar with the tripartite model of anxiety (Lang, 1977), a thorough assessment involves much more than simply an evaluation of the specific anxiety complaints. Factors such as family history, conditioning experiences, medical status, and developmental history are among the areas that must be included in a comprehensive assessment. Although the results of many clinical trials have demonstrated that some pharmacological and many behavioral treatments are effective in reducing anxious symptomatology, certain disorders appear to be more or less amenable to specific interventions. Thus, because treatment implications follow naturally from the overall symptom picture, proper diagnosis is necessary to provide the most appropriate intervention. In this chapter, guidelines for interviewing patients with anxiety disorders will be presented.

DEBORAH C. BEIDEL • Department of Psychiatry and Behavioral Sciences, Medical University of South Carolina, Charleston, South Carolina 29407-7274.

Diagnostic Interviewing (Second Edition), edited by Michel Hersen and Samuel M. Turner. Plenum Press, New York, 1994.

There are seven anxiety disorders listed in the *Diagnostic and Statistical Manual of Mental Disorders*, third edition, revised (DSM-III-R) (APA, 1987). The features of each of these disorders will be elucidated briefly. However, prior to that discussion, a comment about the changing conceptualization of panic attacks is necessary.

One of the major changes to occur in DSM-IV (American Psychiatric Association, 1993) is the removal of the definition of "panic attack" from the diagnostic criteria of any one particular disorder (i.e., panic disorder). Instead, preceding the description of the particular disorders, the section on anxiety disorders begins with a discussion of panic attacks and their relationship to certain situational triggers. Essentially, the relationship can be one of three types. *Unexpected* (uncued) panic attacks are not associated with an obvious trigger. *Situationally bound* (cued) attacks occur immediately on exposure to, or in anticipation of, the situation. Finally, there are *situationally predisposed* attacks, which are more likely to be but are not invariably associated with a particular cue. The description of panic attacks, separate from any one particular disorder, is an important advancement for DSM-IV. It recognizes that panic attacks can occur as part of any anxiety disorder, rather than being specific to or biologically predisposed to any one particular disorder.

The primary characteristic of *panic disorder* (with or without agoraphobia) is the occurrence of "spontaneous" panic attacks that appear unexpectedly and are not triggered by situations in which the person was the focus of attention by others. An attack is characterized by a myriad of physical and cognitive symptoms, of which the attack must manifest a minimum of four in order to be considered a panic attack. If fewer than four symptoms are present, the individual is considered to have limited symptom attacks. To meet diagnostic criteria, the person must have experienced four attacks in a 4-week period or one attack with worry (about the occurrence of another attack) that lasts for 1 month. In DSM-IV (APA, 1993), the diagnostic criteria are essentially unchanged. However, the requirement of having four attacks in a 4-week period has been dropped. Instead, the impairment criteria are defined as "at least one of the attacks has been followed by a month (or more) of: (a) persistent concern about having additional attacks; (b) worry about the implications of the attack or its consequences (e.g., losing control, having a heart attack, 'going crazy'); or (c) a significant change in behavior related to the attacks" (p. K:2).

In certain individuals, the panic attacks are coupled with *agoraphobia*, a fear of situations in which escape is perceived to be difficult or help unavailable. Situations often avoided or feared include crowded places, such as theaters, shopping malls, restaurants, and churches. In addition, the individual often avoids activities such as driving on limited access roads, through tunnels, or over bridges; traveling alone; or being "too far" from home. Some panic-disordered patients do not appear to develop extensive patterns of avoidance, although careful assessment often reveals aspects of a restricted life-style, even in patients who deny situational avoidance (Turner, Beidel, & Jacob, 1988).

Agoraphobia without history of panic disorder is used to refer to those individuals who exhibit behavioral avoidance consistent with a diagnosis of agoraphobia but who have never met criteria for panic disorder. Like patients with panic disorder with agoraphobia, these patients fear being trapped in situations in which escape might be difficult or help unavailable. Rather than panic attacks, the fear is of the development of a specific symptom, such as dizziness or falling, depersonalization or derealization, loss of bladder or bowel control, vomiting, or cardiac distress. There are no changes in the proposed diagnostic criteria for DSM-IV.

Although the Epidemiological Catchment Area (ECA) data indicate that agoraphobia without history of panic disorder is present in the general population (2.9%), it is very rarely seen in anxiety disorder specialty clinics (Beidel & Turner, 1991). In an effort to resolve this discrepancy, Jacob and Turner (1988) noted that among those individuals in the ECA study who were diagnosed with agoraphobia without panic, 47% had a history of panic symptoms but of insufficient severity to meet DSM-III criteria. Of the remaining 53%, approximately 40% had another anxiety disorder, usually depression. When these factors were considered, the prevalence rate for agoraphobia without panic dropped to approximately 1%. Recently, Beidel and Bulik (1990) proposed that although the specific behavioral pattern may be consistent with agoraphobia, other aspects of the clinical presentation indicate that consideration must be given to conceptualizing this disorder as falling within the obsessional spectrum.

Social phobia is a persistent fear of situations in which the individual is open to possible scrutiny by others or fears that he or she may do something that will be embarrassing or humiliating (APA, 1987). Public speaking is the most common situation feared by individuals with social phobia (Turner, Beidel, Borden, Stanley, & Jacob, 1991). Although many individuals will present for treatment of a circumscribed fear such as public speaking, only rarely is the social phobic's distress limited to one specific situation (Turner et al., 1991). Recently, there has been much empirical attention given to the issue of social phobia subtypes (specific vs. generalized) and the association of this disorder with avoidant personality disorder (Herbert, Hope, & Bellack, 1992; Holt, Heimberg, & Hope, 1992; Turner, Beidel, & Townsley, 1992), but the exact nature of these relationships remains unclear. However, the severity of the disorder does appear to have significant treatment implications, and thus careful attention to the specific clinical presentation is necessary. In addition, impairment as a result of the fear must be carefully determined, because many individuals will endorse public speaking concerns or consider themselves to be "shy."

In DSM-IV, social phobia will also be known as *social anxiety disorder* (APA, 1993). In addition, there is recognition that the distress may take the form of situationally bound or situationally predisposed panic attacks, and specific descriptions about the manifestation of this disorder in children are included. The generalized subtype distinction remains in the proposed criteria.

Fears that do not concern public scrutiny, being trapped and unable to receive help, or panic attacks are termed *simple phobias*. Although they appear to be common in the general population, only rarely does an individual present at an anxiety clinic with an isolated simple phobia. Rather, the fear is often accompanied by other psychiatric complaints, or the simple phobia presents as co-occurring with another anxiety disorder (Sanderson, Rapee, & Barlow, 1987). The most commonly occurring simple phobias include fears of animals, blood–injury, heights, and enclosed spaces (Agras, Sylvester, & Oliveau, 1969; APA, 1987), although in clinics the most common complaints are claustrophobia and acrophobia (Emmelkamp, 1988). It is interesting that although there are numerous studies of college students selected on the basis of severe fear of a certain object or situation, studies of anxiety patients seeking treatment for simple phobia are exceedingly rare (Borden, 1992).

Simple phobia is renamed *specific phobia* in DSM-IV (APA, 1993), a designation that more accurately reflects the fact that these phobias are rarely simple (Sanderson et al., 1987). Like those for social phobia, descriptors of the manifestation of specific phobia in children are included in the new criteria. In addition, the following types of specific phobia are now listed in the DSM-IV: animal type, natural environment type (e.g., heights, storms, and water), blood, injection, injury type, situational type (e.g., planes, elevators, or enclosed places), other type. A biphasic cardiovascular response to blood, injection, or injuries appears to differentiate this type from other specific phobia (Connolly, Hallam, & Marks, 1976), but it currently is unclear whether the classification of other phobias into specific types has any clinical or scientific utility.

Obsessive–compulsive disorder consists of (1) recurrent and persistent thoughts, ideas, or impulses (obsessions) that are experienced as intrusive or senseless and (2) repetitive, purposeful, and intentional behaviors (compulsions) that are performed in response to an obsession, according to certain rules, or in a stereotyped fashion (APA, 1987). The description of the clinical phenomenology remains essentially unchanged in DSM-IV (APA, 1993). One difference is that the diagnostic criteria now require the presence of obsessions *or* compulsions, rather than both. Also included is a poor-insight type for which the criterion is that for most of the time during the current episode, the person does not recognize that the obsessions and compulsions are excessive or unreasonable.

Patients with obsessive–compulsive disorder will attempt (unsuccessfully) to suppress or ignore the thoughts or impulses. Furthermore, they recognize that these thoughts are products of their own minds. Common content for obsessional thoughts includes dirt and contamination, aggression, inanimate–interpersonal features (e.g., locks, bolts), sex, and religion (Akhtar, Wig, Verna, Pershad, & Verna, 1975). The compulsive behaviors are usually considered to have a neutralizing or preventative function, but the behaviors are clearly excessive. Common compulsive rituals include hand-washing and bathing, cleaning, checking, counting, and ordering (Akhtar et al., 1975). In certain cases, the repetitive behavior may appear to be totally unconnected to the potential frightening events or obsessions, a fact that most patients clearly acknowledge.

Although the word "stress" is a common part of our vocabulary, *posttraumatic stress disorder* (PTSD) refers to a constellation of symptoms that occur after the experience of an event that is outside the range of usual experience and would be distressing to almost anyone (APA, 1987). Such situations include: (1) serious threats to one's life, bodily integrity, relatives, or friends; (2) sudden destruction of one's home or community; or (3) witnessing another being killed or seriously injured as a result of an accident or physical violence. In DSM-IV (APA, 1993), a second necessary criterion has been added: The person's response involves intense fear, helplessness, or horror (p. K:8).

The event is persistently reexperienced through recurrent and intrusive recollections or dreams, acting or feeling as if the event were recurring, and intense psychological distress at exposure to events that symbolize or resemble an aspect of the traumatic event. In addition, there is avoidance of stimuli associated with the trauma or numbing of general responsiveness and persistent symptoms of increased arousal. The disturbance can have an immediate or a delayed onset. The onset is characterized as delayed if the symptoms occur at least 6 months after the trauma. Finally, the disorder is specified as *acute* if symptom duration is 3 months or less or *chronic* if symptom duration is 3 months or more.

DSM-IV (APA, 1993) introduces a new diagnostic category called *acute stress disorder*. Essentially, the diagnostic criteria are the same as those for PTSD. The difference is in symptom duration and onset. In acute stress disorder, the minimum symptom duration is 2 days and maximum duration is 4 weeks. Furthermore, the onset of symptoms occurs within 4 weeks of the traumatic event.

Generalized anxiety disorder (GAD) is characterized by unrealistic or excessive worry about at least two different life circumstances (e.g., one's own physical health or that of a family member, personal finances). The worry must be consistent for a period of at least 6 months and bother the person more days than it does not. The worry is unrelated to any other Axis I disorder (e.g., the individual is not worrying about public speaking or the occurrence of panic attacks) and does not occur only during the course of a mood disorder. Such worry is accompanied by symptoms of motor tension, autonomic hyperactivity, and vigilance and scanning. Previously considered to be a "wastebasket" classification, the diagnostic criteria were refined with the publication of DSM-III-R. Thus, to some extent there is a smaller body of empirical data for GAD than for many of the other anxiety disorders.

Changes in the diagnostic criteria for DSM-IV include a change in the title indicating that GAD now *includes overanxious disorder of childhood*. Furthermore, there is a statement that "the person finds it difficult to control the worry."

New categories introduced in DSM-IV include *anxiety disorder due to a general medical condition* and *substance-induced anxiety disorder*. These disorders refer to the presence of prominent anxiety, panic attacks, obsessions, or compulsions that are secondary to a medical condition or substance abuse. Treatment of these disorders must take into account the treatment of the precipitating condition. Because of these complicating factors, these disorders will not be addressed in this chapter.

As discussed below, there are certain associated features that accompany many of the diagnostic categories previously described, and attention to these factors is necessary in order to derive an accurate diagnosis. The next section presents an assessment of the dimensions necessary to ensure diagnostic accuracy.

Procedures for Gathering Information

As noted, a proper assessment of anxiety requires attention to many different clinical features. Table 1 lists specific domains that should be addressed in the

TABLE 1. Domains to be Included in an Anxiety Disorders Diagnostic Interview

1. Characteristics of the presenting complaint (behavioral, cognitive, and somatic components; situational determinants).
2. Existence of other Axis I disorders that may account for or alter the presentation of the symptomatology or that may affect the treatment outcome.
3. Existence of Axis II disorders that may account more fully for the presenting symptomatology or that may alter or influence the treatment outcome.
4. Existence of medical conditions that may produce, contribute to, or augment the presenting symptomatology.
5. Environmental influences such as conditioning experiences, stressful events, or familial factors that may contribute to or maintain the current clinical picture.
6. Developmental history factors that may have produced, contributed to, or augmented the current symptom picture.
7. Assessment of prior treatment history that may assist in clarifying issues of primary vs. secondary symptomatology.

evaluation process. Obviously, this list is not exhaustive, but it is meant to confer a sense of the elements that need to be addressed in order to understand the patient's clinical condition.

First, the characteristics of the presenting complaint need to be carefully delineated. The most often addressed components, assessment of overt behavior, subjective distress, and somatic response, are only a small part of the total symptom picture. For example, although most panic patients assume that their panic attacks come "out of the blue," several studies have indicated that these attacks are related to the presence of stressful life events or negative affective states (Turner et al., 1988). Similarly, patients with obsessive–compulsive disorder will often report that panic attacks occur, but usually only when they come into contact with fearful stimuli. Barlow (1988) reported that a patient who initially presented with a "fear of knives" was determined, on evaluation, to be suffering from obsessive–compulsive disorder. Finally, although it is true for patients with any psychiatric disorder, it is likely that the anxiety patient's conceptualization of the presenting complaint may be more circumscribed than the actual clinical presentation. For example, social phobia patients, knowingly or unknowingly, often minimize the extent of their complaints or may not recognize that specific behaviors (e.g., avoidance) serve an anxiety-reducing function (Turner & Beidel, 1989). The same holds true for patients suffering from any of the anxiety disorders.

Second, many individuals suffer from more than one anxiety disorder (Sanderson et al., 1987). In addition, depression is a common complaint of those with panic disorder (Barlow et al., 1986; Breier, et al., 1984; Lesser et al., 1988), obsessive–compulsive disorder (Barlow et al., 1986; Insel, Zahn, & Murphy, 1985), and, to a lesser extent, social phobia (Turner et al., 1992) and generalized anxiety disorder (Barlow et al., 1986). In general, there is a high degree of comorbidity among all these disorders. Boyd et al. (1984) reported an 18.8-fold increased risk of panic disorder and a 15.3-fold increased risk of agoraphobia given a primary diagnosis of major depression. If the individual had a primary diagnosis of agoraphobia, there was an 18-fold increased risk of panic disorder, and there was a

4.3-fold increased risk of alcohol abuse given panic disorder. Co-occurring substance abuse is fairly common among a variety of anxiety patients (Keyl & Eaton, 1990; Kushner et al., 1990), and the existence of any of these additional disorders obviously serves to complicate both the case conceptualization and the consideration of treatment strategies.

Third, personality disorders are commonly found among those with Axis I anxiety disorders (Mavissakalian & Hammen, 1986, 1988; Reich & Noyes, 1987; Turner & Beidel, 1989) and, similar to co-occurring Axis I disorders, serve to complicate the diagnostic presentation and the consideration of treatment outcome (Jenike, Baer, Minichiello, Schwartz, & Carey, 1986; Stanley, Turner, & Borden, 1990).

Fourth, many medical conditions have been associated with the presence of anxiety disorders. Certain conditions such as thyroid disease can mimic panic disorder (Stein, 1986). Others, such as mitral valve prolapse, vestibular dysfunction, and seizure activity, have been associated with panic disorder, although the exact nature of these relationships and their association with the anxiety disorder have yet to be fully determined (Crowe, Pauls, Slymen, & Noyes, 1980; Gorman, Fyer, Glicklich, King, & Klein, 1981; Jacob, Moller, Turner, & Wall, 1985; Kathol et al., 1980; Shear, Devereaux, Kranier-Fox, Mann, & Frances, 1984; Stein, 1986). Neurochemical imbalances have also been reported to be associated with several anxiety disorders. For example, results of lactate infusion studies initially suggested that the neurochemical functioning of panic disorder patients might be different from that of normal controls and of patients with other types of anxiety disorders (Gorman et al., 1983; Liebowitz et al., 1984; Liebowitz, Fyer et al., 1985; Liebowitz, Gorman et al., 1985). However, these results are open to alternative interpretations, including the influence of situational context at the time of the laboratory assessments (Margraf, Ehlers, & Roth, 1986; Turner et al., 1988; van der Molen & van den Hout, 1988).

In addition, current diagnostic practice dictates that in some instances, the presence of certain medical conditions precludes an anxiety disorder diagnosis. For example, DSM-III-R (APA, 1987) states that if an individual's social concerns are due to the presence of a physical condition, such as stuttering or Parkinson's disease, then a diagnosis of social phobia is not assigned. In practice, however, simply excluding these patients from receiving a diagnosis is open to debate. There are some individuals with these physical conditions who appear to express concern about negative evaluation that far exceeds that which one would expect based solely on their impairment. In such cases, a diagnosis of social phobia might still be warranted (see the "Do's and Don't's" section in this chapter). Nonetheless, because some medical conditions may mimic symptoms most commonly associated with panic disorder or generalized anxiety disorder, assessment of the patient's medical status is necessary.

Fifth, environmental factors, such as traumatic events, specific conditioning experiences, and familial factors, may play a role in the development or maintenance of the anxiety disorders (Keyl & Eaton, 1990). With respect to etiology, a study by Öst (1987) indicated that specific or traumatic events accounted for the onset of 76.7–84% of panic/agoraphobias, 58% of social phobias, and 45–68.4% of simple phobias. Thus, although a significant proportion of anxiety patients can recall a specific traumatic event associated with the onset of their fears, not all patients can do so. In addition, environmental factors other than direct conditioning experiences may also contribute to the onset of a disorder. In the study cited above, Öst (1987) noted that a substantial proportion of anxiety patients acquired their fear through information or social learning (modeling). Furthermore, for other patients, the onset of their disorder was not necessarily associated with a specific incident, but nonetheless occurred during the context of a major life event. For example, Klein (1964) reported that for some women, the onset of panic disorder occurred after the birth of a child. Although he attributed the onset of the disorder to the hormonal changes accompanying childbirth, there are alternative non-biological explanations as well. For example, depression or a major grief episode has been associated with the onset of panic attacks (Keyl & Eaton, 1990). Similarly, Turner and Beidel (1988) reported that the onset of obsessive–compulsive disorder is often associated with life-events, such as getting married, purchasing a home, birth of a child, or death of a close relative. Furthermore, these disorders are often exacerbated by ongoing environmental tensions, such as dysfunctional marriages or hostile parent–child relationships (Turner & Beidel, 1988). To summarize, many factors may be associated with the onset of anxiety, and an understanding of the contributory effect of environmental events must be broader than a simple conceptualization of direct conditioning experiences.

Sixth, developmental history is also an important area of diagnostic interviewing. One caveat, however, is that a patient's recall of past events may be colored by the presence of current psychopathology. Nonetheless, family history is an important consideration in making a diagnostic assessment. Although family history data are often interpreted as evidence of biological etiology, other equally important factors must be considered. For example, significantly higher familial rates of a disorder in a family may demonstrate the powerful impact of modeling (as noted above). In addition, Kagan, Reznick, and Snidman (1988) have shown that children considered to be behaviorally inhibited at an early age can become less inhibited if their parents make a concerted effort to expose the children to peer social interactions. Thus, parenting may play a significant role in the remediation or continuation of anxious symptomatology. Furthermore, a study by Messer and Beidel (in press) indicated that parental and familial variables, such as the father's psychopathology and the family environment (anxious children have family environments that significantly restrict the children's independence), have significant predictive validity in discriminating anxious and nonanxious children. Even if these factors are reactive rather than causal, it is likely that a restrictive family environment may serve to maintain anxious symptomatology. Thus, although the specific role of these developmental factors is unclear, it is apparent that an assessment of these factors is necessary.

Seventh, prior treatment history may be an important factor, particularly when attempting to determine primacy of depression or anxiety symptoms. For example, for patients whose depression is secondary to their obsessive-compulsive disorder (OCD), traditional antidepressants improve their mood but have little or no effect on their obsessions and compulsions (Turner & Beidel, 1988). Thus, prior treatment with antidepressants that results in significantly improved mood and also eliminates obsessional thinking may indicate the primacy of an affective, rather than an anxiety, disorder. One note of caution is in order, however. The assessment of the OCD symptomatology is critical, and the clinician must carefully assess changes in specific frequency and severity of the obsessions and compulsions, rather than just changes in general estimates of mood and OCD symptoms.

This volume is dedicated to diagnostic interviewing and, indeed, the interview is the cornerstone of clinical assessment. In recent years, there has been an increase in the use of structured and semistructured interview schedules designed to assist in the diagnostic process. Among those geared specifically to DSM-III-R criteria, some, such as the Structured Clinical Interview for DSM-III-R (SCID) (Spitzer, Williams, Gibbon, & First, 1988) and the Diagnostic Interview Schedule (DIS) (Robins et al., 1984), assess psychopathology across a range of diagnostic categories, including the anxiety disorders. The DIS is a structured interview developed for use in epidemiological studies. The interview is administered by lay interviewers, and diagnoses are derived by computer algorithm. This procedure means that although the final diagnostic decision is taken out of the lay interviewer's hands, that interviewer is still responsible for evaluating the clinical significance of the interviewee's responses. Thus, the administrators still need a significant degree of training in order to make judgments of clinical significance. Studies of interrater reliability and validity using the DIS suggest that this scale has only low to moderate reliability and validity coefficients for anxiety disorders categories (Anthony et al., 1985; Helzer et al., 1985; Robins, 1985).

The SCID is a semistructured interview designed to be used by trained clinicians to assist in deriving Axis I diagnoses. In contrast to structured interviews, semistructured interviews provide some basic interviewing questions but allow latitude for clinicians to use their clinical judgment to ask additional follow-up questions. In addition, the interviewer uses his or her judgment to assign a diagnosis. Because of the need to make a clinical judgment, semistructured interviews are not appropriate for use by lay interviewers or those insufficiently trained in psychopathology. Although formal reliability data on the use of the SCID for the diagnosis of anxiety disorders are limited, information from our clinic suggests that with proper training, acceptable interrater reliability ($r \geq 0.90$) can be achieved.

In addition to interview schedules that cover a broad range of psychopathology, the Anxiety Disorders Interview Schedule—Revised (ADIS-R) (DiNardo et al., 1986) was developed specifically to assess DSM-III-R anxiety disorders. Since the ADIS-R is a semi-structured interview schedule, it is appropriate for administration only by an individual who has had significant clinical experience. Interrater reliability coefficients for the ADIS-R are quite high [κ coefficients range from 0.571 for generalized anxiety disorder to 0.91 for social phobia (Barlow, 1988)]. Although there is some attention to nonanxiety disorders, such as depression, this interview schedule is less comprehensive than some others and thus should be augmented by additional assessments.

In addition to clinical interviewing, comprehensive evaluation usually includes assessment via different modalities. Although self-report inventories are among the most common forms of clinical assessment, relatively few instruments have been developed specifically to address the DSM-III-R anxiety disorders categories. For example, Turner, McCann, Beidel, and Mezzich (1986) demonstrated that instruments such as the State–Trait Anxiety Inventory (Spielberger, Gorsuch, & Lushene, 1970), the Social Avoidance and Distress Scale and the Fear of Negative Evaluation Scale (Watson & Friend, 1969), and the Maudsley Obsessive–Compulsive Inventory (Hodgson & Rachman, 1977) did not discriminate among the DSM-III diagnostic groups. In contrast, the Social Phobia and Anxiety Inventory (SPAI) (Turner, Beidel, Dancu, & Stanley, 1989) was developed specifically to assess social phobia and is capable of differentiating patients with this disorder from other diagnostic groups. Nonetheless, although such instruments are useful in clarifying the extent and severity of the clinical presentation, when used to assist in the determination of a diagnosis, they should be used only in conjunction with other sources of information. Similarly, daily self-monitoring can be very helpful in the diagnostic process. Carefully constructed and completed self-monitoring can provide clarification of important elements of the diagnostic picture such as antecedent triggering events, specific negative cognitions, and engagement in maladaptive behaviors (such as substance abuse or caffeine ingestion) that could produce panic attacks. For social phobics, self-monitoring may reveal that the distress and avoidance extend to interpersonal interactions, not just public speaking situations. Thus, these paper-and-pencil measures play an important role in the diagnostic process.

Case Illustration

In order to illustrate many of the issues involved in the diagnosis of anxiety disorders discussed above, the following case example is presented. This case was selected for its diagnostic complexity and its appropriateness to illustrate many of the issues discussed above. The structure of the interview is based roughly on that found in the ADIS-R semistructured interview schedule (DiNardo et al., 1986).

The patient is a 24-year-old-single male, self-referred through a newspaper advertisement offering treatment for patients with social phobia. He described a severe fear of public speaking that had restricted his occupational choices and resulted in chronic underemployment. Currently, he was unemployed and believed that his fear prevented him from acquiring a position commensurate with his personal abilities. His girlfriend was aware of his social anxiety, but he had not discussed either his fear or his decision to seek treatment with any of his immediate family and requested that all telephone contact occur through his girlfriend. The following is a transcript of the first three interviews with the patient and begins after the initial introductions and explanation of the interview process:

T: You telephoned the clinic in response to our announcement about treatment for social phobia. Perhaps you could begin by telling me what it was about that announcement that reminded you of yourself.

P: I get very nervous whenever I have to speak in public.

T: The word "nervous" means different things to different people. Can you tell me what it means to you?

P: What I mean is that I get a rush of anxiety whenever I have to give any type of formal presentation. I worry that something is going to go wrong, that I am going to be so anxious that I won't be able to continue.

T: Can you give me an example of one time when this happened?

P: Well, the last time that it happened was when I was at an orientation session for my last job. That was two years ago. We all had to get up and say our names. I felt so nervous, like I could not breathe, like I was going to die from the anxiety. I said it, but I felt so foolish, so embarrassed. This was my *name*, that's all I had to say.

Although this patient responded to an announcement about social phobia treatment, the words "going to die" are often used by individuals with panic disorder. Therefore, a decision was made to clarify the circumstances of the first experiences with anxiety to determine whether it might be more consistent with panic disorder than with social phobia.

T: I understand your feelings of frustration at being unable to do such a simple thing comfortably, and we will discuss it in more detail in a few moments. But first, can you remember the first time that you felt this way?

P: Well, I remember when I was in junior high, around the time of puberty, feeling a little nervous when I would have to speak in class. But the first time that I remember feeling like I could not breathe was when I was a senior in high school.

T: Tell me what happened.

P: I was in current events class and I was called on to read a newspaper clipping. When I started reading, I became really anxious. The anxiety kept building to a crescendo. It came to a point where I could not talk anymore. I just quit speaking. It was very embarrassing.

The situation that the patient described was clearly one of a social nature. However, once again, some of the words used in his description, particularly his physiological state, were more reminiscent of panic disorder. Therefore, it was decided to continue pursuing the existence of panic attacks.

T: Have you ever had a time when you had a very sudden rush of anxiety, when all of a sudden you felt really anxious?

P: Yes.

T: When do these feelings happen?

P: When I am worrying about some event that may have happened that day. I worry that if I did get really anxious, would I pass out? And if I did pass out, could I get help? I worry that I would pass out and look stupid.

T: Do you worry about one of those things more than the other? What I mean is, do you think that you worry more about whether someone would help you or whether you would look stupid?

P: I think that I worry more about looking stupid. I know that if you pass out, nothing bad would really happen. Probably looking stupid is worse.

T: Do the anxiety feelings ever come out of the blue? Do they ever come when you are not in public speaking situations or worrying about public speaking situations?

P: Not just like that [snaps his fingers]. Usually, I have to be thinking about the situation at the time. Initially, I will be nervous about the speaking situation, and then it hits.

T: Does the anxiety come on in every public speaking situation?

P: Not every situation. I usually do very well in job interviews. But the nervousness happens any time I feel that I have to perform. When I feel really pressed to speak. When I feel that there is no escape.

T: When you are thinking about performance situations, how often do you feel the rush of anxiety? Is it as frequently as once a week?

P: No, it is not even as frequent as once per month.

T: What I want you to do now is think about the last time that you were in a speaking situation that made you anxious.

P: That would have been two years ago at the orientation session.

T: Fine. I am going to ask you about different physical symptoms and I want you to tell me if you experience these symptoms when you are anxious, and if so, how severe the symptoms were.

At this point, all the physical symptoms included in the DSM-III-R definition of panic disorder were reviewed. The patient endorsed severe symptoms of shortness of breath, tachycardia, trembling, moderate dizziness, mild depersonalization, and mild fear of dying.

T: Other than the incidents that we have discussed, were there any other times when you had a fear of dying?

P: Well, when I was in seventh grade, I choked on a hot dog.

T: Tell me about that.

P: I was sitting in the school cafeteria at lunch time. I was with a bunch of my friends. We were talking and laughing. I literally inhaled the hot dog. It was lodged in my windpipe and I could not get any air. I can still remember clearly thinking that I was going to die. I got up and went in search of a teacher. My gym teacher was in the cafeteria and I remember walking toward him. He did not see me and starting walking away from me. I can remember the two of us circling the cafeteria, me following behind him, like some sort of dance. I was chasing him and I finally caught him. He hit me several times on the back and the hot dog popped out. I remember thinking that everyone was looking at me at the time. After that incident, I remember that I was really worried about eating food for the next several days. My mom noticed this and gave me soft foods at first. But she was also very firm about getting me to eat other things again and would encourage me to try. After a couple of weeks, I was eating normally again, but then I started to worry about getting air. Then this led to another worry that I would not be able to hiccup. I carried throat lozenges for a time. I never used them, but they made me feel better.

It is important to note here that even during this traumatic event, the patient was aware of the scrutiny of others and probably felt embarrassed by it.

T: Do you still worry about these things?

P: Well, I still worry about not getting air, but only when I am forced to speak in formal situations. I don't worry about the hiccuping anymore. I don't carry the throat lozenges either.

T: Other than speaking, do you worry about getting air in other situations?

P: Well, if I was in a real small place, like a box, or if I was buried alive, I'd be worried about air. But it's not something that I think about.

T: What about when you are in an elevator?

P: No. I don't really worry about getting air except when I'm forced to speak.

Because the patient kept using the word "worried," it appeared to be a good opportunity to assess for generalized anxiety disorder.

T: You know, you have been using the word "worry" a lot. You worry about speaking in formal presentations, you worry about not getting air. Are there other things that you worry about?

P: Well, I worry about getting a good job. I am unemployed because of the layoffs and I keep worrying that my problem, this weakness, is keeping me from getting the job that I think I am capable of.

T: Well, what about nonsocial things? For example, do you worry a lot about your health, your future? Prior to losing your job, did you worry a lot about your financial situation? Do you worry about little things such as being late for appointments?

P: No, I'm not a worrier. [Leans forward.] But I do like to be prompt, and I expect that other people will be prompt too.

T: How about feeling tense, apparently for no reason at all?

P: No, I generally feel very comfortable.

The patient's posture and affect were consistent with his remarks. He was sprawled out quite comfortably in a chair. In addition, his affect was euthymic other than when discussing his public speaking difficulties. Therefore, further assessment of GAD symptoms was not considered necessary.

T: Fine. Let's talk about different situations that might make you uncomfortable. Tell me if any of these situations make you feel nervous or panicky or if you ever worry about feeling trapped and unable to escape if you find yourself in one of them.

Since there was still some uncertainty about whether this individual was suffering from panic disorder or social phobia, situations commonly feared by individuals with agoraphobia were reviewed. The patient denied fear in any of them, with two exceptions. The transcript surrounding these two situations is presented below.

T: What about riding on buses?

P: Well, it doesn't bother me now, but it did in the past.

T: When was that?

P: When I was in junior high, I would get really nervous riding the bus to school. It was soon after I choked on the hot dog. I think that I was really worried about not getting enough air. I never avoided the bus, but I remember that I would sit near the front.

T: Do you still sit near the front of the bus?

P: No, I don't even think about it any more. It wouldn't even have occurred to me if you hadn't mentioned it.

T: Alright. What about restaurants?

P: You know, that is really weird.

T: What is weird?

P: That you mention restaurants. I get these really strange feelings in restaurants.

T: Are you saying that you feel panicky in restaurants?

P: No, not panicky. Not even nervous. Just a very strange feeling, but definitely not fear.

T: Does it matter where you are sitting in the restaurant?

P: No, not at all.

T: Do you ever avoid restaurants?

P: No, not at all. Like I said, it is not really a fear, just a strange feeling.

The "funny feeling" in restaurants may indicate some degree of generalization related to the incident in the cafeteria. At this point, it was fairly clear that the individual was not suffering from panic disorder. He also denied the presence of any simple phobias. Therefore, a decision was made to further clarify the extent of the social fears.

T: Let's return to the social situations. When you are in a formal speaking situation, are you concerned that you might do or say something humiliating or embarrassing in front of others?

P: Well, if you are considering embarrassing myself by hyperventilating or passing out and others will see that, then the answer is yes.

T: What thoughts come into your head when you are thinking about having to be in one of these situations?

P: What if the panic comes? What will they think of me? I don't want to look stupid in front of these people.

T: Does the panic come every time?

P: Yes.

T: And do you avoid these situations now?

P: Absolutely.

T: I would like to name several different situations where individuals with fears of public speaking can also feel anxious. Just tell me if any of the situations make you feel uncomfortable.

The patient endorsed few other social situations that created distress. He did acknowledge feeling anxious in meetings if he thought that he might have to speak or any time when meeting new people. He also noted some minimal distress when speaking to authority figures and stated that in the past he had felt anxious when writing in front of others.

T: Are there certain types of people that make you feel more uncomfortable when you speak?

P: I am bothered most if the audience consists of males who are my age. My peer group, you might say. I guess I really don't want to embarrass myself in front of them. It is even embarrassing for me to talk about it here. I see it as a weakness and I am not proud that I am weak. I know that I have many abilities and that I am capable of a much better job than I have had so far. But the type of job that I want will require me to speak in meetings and I cannot do that. It is very frustrating.

T: So the fear has really limited your vocational choice and your occupational opportunities. Has it limited you academically or socially?

P: No, not really.

T: We have talked about situations that often elicit anxiety in some people. However, sometimes people have thoughts or images that come into their heads that are quite frightening. Sometimes they are described as silly or nonsensical thoughts that a person cannot stop thinking no matter how hard he or she tries. Not worrying about something, but thoughts that somehow you might have run over someone when you were driving or thoughts that you might have contracted a disease in some unusual way?

P: No, nothing like that.

T: Are there any facts or behaviors that you feel you must do repeatedly or that you must do in a certain way even if it doesn't make sense to you? But, you feel that you must do it because something bad will happen to you if you do not?

P: Well, I do like things to be done in a certain way, but I could change things if I had to.

Although the patient denied the presence of obsessions or rituals, several of his responses suggested the presence of an obsessional thinking style and some compulsive personality traits. A decision was made to delay discussion of that information in order to first finish the assessment of anxious symptomatology.

T: Have you ever had any extremely stressful or life-threatening or traumatic events that have happened to you?

P: Do you mean anything like the hot dog incident?

T: Well, that would be one. Did you ever have any others like that?

P: I do remember one thing that happened when I was young. I don't know if this is exactly what you mean, but when I was three or four years old, my father got into an argument with the neighbor who lived behind our house. I don't remember what started the fight, but I do remember the neighbor coming over to our front door. I opened the door and the man started yelling at me. My father came to the door and the two of them started yelling. Then, they stepped outside. I don't know if they were going to fight it out with their fists or if it was just to get away from me. I remember watching them. They argued for about ten minutes and then the other man left. My father came back into the house, but we never spoke about it. My bedroom window looked directly out at that man's house, and I remember that at night, when I went to bed, I would be worried that the man would come over and try to hurt me.

T: How often did you think of that?

P: Every single night.

T: How long did it last?

P: A year or two.

T: What made you stop worrying about it?

P: We moved to a new house in a different neighborhood. If we had stayed in that house, I think I still would have worried about it.

The patient was assessed for symptoms of posttraumatic stress disorder that might have accompanied this incident. He denied the presence of any of these symptoms, other than the aforementioned worry when he would see the man's house through his bedroom window. Another way to interpret this event is in the context of the individual's predominant mode of thinking, which again appeared consistent with an obsessional style.

T: Before we move to other subject matters, are there any other times that you have experienced anxiety that we have not covered?

P: Well, I was really nervous when I began going to kindergarten. For about two weeks, I would cry every time my mother left me. But then I adjusted and did fine.

T: You have mentioned both your mother and your father. Why don't we take a break from talking about anxiety and you can tell me some things about your family.

P: What would you like to know?

T: Are your parents still living? Do you have brothers and sisters?

P: My parents are both living and are still married to each other. My father is retired from a steel mill where he worked as a laborer all of his life. My mother is a housewife. There are four children in our family, but I am the only boy. I have two older sisters and one younger sister. Growing up was pretty much like "Leave It to Beaver." Very traditional. I was always close to my dad. He worried that with all those girls around, I might become a sissy. So he spent a good deal of time with me on weekends fishing, hunting, baseball. He wanted to make sure that I was tough. None of my family knows that I came here. I would be so embarrassed if they knew I had this fear. I did tell my girlfriend and she encouraged me to come here.

    I did well in school. I had a B average. Math and science were my strongest subjects. I really enjoyed school. I had lots of friends, played varsity football and baseball in high school. I went to trade school after high school and got an associate degree in electronics. There are few jobs in this area. Besides, the electronics degree was a cop-out. I should have gone to college. I wanted to, but I was afraid that I would have to speak in class.

Despite the patient's earlier denial, his social fears had impaired his academic achievement in that he chose to forgo college because of the possibility that he would have to speak in class.

T: Do you know if anyone else in the family has any problems with anxiety?

P: I think that my dad has this same fear. When I think about it, he would always disappear if speaking before a group seemed imminent. But no one else in the family that I am aware of.

His father's "disappearance" when public speaking was imminent suggests that social learning may have been a factor in the etiology of the patient's disorder. The next part of the interview was directed at an assessment of personality disorders that might be associated with social anxiety. In this case, there were several cues that the patient behaved in ways that are characteristic of individuals with obsessive–compulsive personality disorder. In the Western Psychiatric Institute and Clinic Anxiety Disorders Clinic, the SCID-II (Spitzer & Williams, 1986) was used to guide the assessment of personality disorders. The following questions are taken from the opening of the SCID-II interview.

T: Fine. Now, I want to turn the topic of our conversation away from anxiety to aspects of your behavior that are typical for you, whether or not you feel anxious. The type of behavior that I am talking about is what most people call "personality." In general terms, how would you describe yourself?

P: Well, I think I would say that I am outgoing, honest, stubborn, and impatient.

T: What words would your friends use to describe you?

P: Outgoing, honest, stubborn, impatient.

T: Pretty consistent. Who or what has been the biggest influence in your life?

P: Probably my parents. I get my stubbornness from my dad. My friend Jeff. He and I are a lot alike. I confide in him. My girlfriend. She has been a real source of support.

T: How have you gotten along with these people?

P: I have always been close with my parents. But we are not affectionate. I never have been a very affectionate person. My girlfriend complains about that sometimes. I like people but it is difficult for me to express it.

T: Has the way that you interact with people ever created difficulties for you? For example, have you lost girlfriends because they thought that you did not care or that you did not tell them how you felt?

P: Maybe. I never really thought about that. I do have difficulty when I see inequality. For example, I am not tolerant of people taking advantage of others, of friends not helping each other equally. I have been told that I really set high standards for my friends.

These behaviors suggest the presence of an obsessive–compulsive personality disorder. Therefore, a decision was made to pursue this topic further.

T: Does this sometimes cause you difficulty with your friends? Do they sometimes tell you that you are stubborn?

P: How did you know? Actually, they tell me that often. I hate to give in when I am fighting with my girlfriend, even when I know she is right. They also give me a hard time about my punctuality. I like to be on time and I get irritated if someone keeps me waiting.

T: What about expressing other types of feelings? Is it easy for you to let people know how much you care about them?

P: No, that is difficult for me. I can tell my girlfriend how I feel about her, but she is the only one. I have never told my family how much I care about them. I have tried, but I just can't get the words out.

T: What about expressing your feelings nonverbally? For example, if you see something that you know a friend or family member would really like, would you ever just buy it for that person as a gift? Just because you know that it would make someone happy?

P: Only if I knew that it was a give-and-take situation. That someday, they might do the same for me. I don't mind doing a favor for someone if I know that they will have to return one some day.

T: You mentioned being stubborn. Are you perfectionistic as well?

P: Very much so. I don't like doing things if I cannot do it well. It used to slow me down in school. My instructors would always compliment me on how well I did something, but half the time the job was completed late. I am perfectionistic about my appearance too. My girlfriend teases me that I take as much time with my appearance as a girl. It didn't interfere with my job, though. I mean, there wasn't that much to be perfectionistic about. But I am really stubborn. I've always had trouble letting others do things for me. I worry that they won't do it correctly.

T: Do you every worry about whether you have done something that is morally wrong? Do you ever worry that your friends are behaving immorally?

P: I don't think I worry about it too much, but my friends seem to think so. They will often tell me that the world is not as black and white as I see it. That sometimes people break rules for the greater good. I don't understand thinking like that. For me, a rule is a rule.

T: What about being a workaholic? Do you ever find yourself so involved with work that you forget to have fun?

P: No, I've never had a job where I could do that. I don't know if I would be that way if I had a different type of job—a more professional job, I mean. All of my jobs have required punching a clock. They were never jobs that you could stay late on or take home with you.

T: One last question—are you a pack rat? Do you save things even if you don't need them right now or they don't have some special meaning for you? Do you hold on to things just in case?

P: Only with magazines. I don't know why I keep them, but I cannot throw them away. That's the only thing that I seem to save.

The interview covered all the various personality disorder criteria, but the patient denied other symptomatology. He also denied any current medical conditions or prior psychological or psychiatric treatment. In summary, the patient's clinical presentation is similar to that of many patients seeking treatment for "fear of public speaking." As with this patient, rarely is the social anxiety limited to one specific fearful situation. Rather, careful questioning revealed a more pervasive form of the disorder. Furthermore, the clinical presentation illustrates the potential overlap between symptoms more commonly associated with panic disorder and those more commonly associated with social phobia. Nonetheless, careful questioning left little doubt that the proper diagnosis was social phobia. This patient also exemplifies the concept of anxiety-proneness. He describes numerous fearful reactions to a variety of life events, suggesting that for him, anxiety is a common response to the occurrence of stressful events. In addition, his father appears to have been an important role model, and the significant social fears that appear to be present in the father suggest the possibility that a biological predisposition coupled with environmental factors such as social learning and traumatic events contributed to the onset and maintenance of the disorder. Finally, this patient met criteria for an Axis II diagnosis of obsessive–compulsive personality disorder, which is quite common among social phobics (Turner et al., 1992). Although the etiological significance of this Axis II disorder is unclear, it is likely that individuals with rigid and perfectionistic standards for behavior would likely be concerned with others' perceptions of their social behaviors.

CRITICAL INFORMATION NECESSARY TO MAKE THE DIAGNOSIS

Much of the critical information necessary to diagnose many of the anxiety disorders has been presented above. Specifically, one needs to ascertain the presence of anxiety features and to assure that the complaints cannot be more logically subsumed under a "broader" Axis II disorder. The necessity of making this distinction cannot be overemphasized, as the application of inappropriate treatment strategies could be ineffective or lead to the exacerbation of a condition. For example, it has been observed repeatedly in our clinic that the use of flooding procedures with a patient who has elements of a paranoid personality disorder (or the paranoid "flavor" that is characteristic of some avoidant personality disorder patients) leads to an exacerbation of the paranoia often directed at the therapist. Such a patient interprets the flooding procedures as a deliberate attempt by the therapist to humiliate the patient. Careful diagnosis would alert the therapist to the fact that this patient is not suffering simply from an anxiety disorder, which realization, in turn, should profoundly affect the selection of a treatment strategy.

Among the anxiety disorders themselves information critical to a differential diagnosis often can be inferred from the presenting symptom pattern. Such information may be useful in making a distinction between agoraphobia and social phobia, for example. First, Amies, Gelder, and Shaw (1983) noted that social phobics were more likely to complain of physical symptoms, such as blushing and muscle twitching, whereas those with agoraphobia were more likely to report dizziness, difficulty breathing, weakness in limbs, fainting episodes, and buzzing or ringing in the ears. Similarly, agoraphobics fear the occurrence of their physical symptoms, whereas social phobics fear the perception of those symptoms by others. Finally, the core fear of social phobics and agoraphobics is quite different. According to Marks (1970), agoraphobics fear the crowd, whereas social phobics fear the individuals who make up the crowd. Attention to these specific factors will assist in the differentiation of these two disorders.

In summary, when diagnosing anxiety, it is necessary for the clinician to begin with a broad view of the presenting psychopathology, rather than to focus on the patient's initial presentation. In other words, when considering the patient's complaint, the clinician should use a top-down mode of information processing. That is, the clinician should think first in terms of broad diagnostic categories, such as Axis I vs. Axis II disorder, medical vs. psychological etiology, rather than simply accept the patient's initial complaint at face value (despite any striking similarity to the typical textbook presentation). These possibilities need to be eliminated prior to the consideration of a specific diagnosis.

DO'S AND DON'T'S

There are several caveats that should be observed when assessing anxiety disorders. First, *do not* discount the severity of the patient's emotional distress. For example, a higher than normal incidence of suicide has been associated with the presence of panic attacks and panic disorder (Korn et al., 1992; Weissman, Klerman, Markowitz, & Ouellette, 1989) and social phobia (Schneier, Johnson, Hornig, Liebowitz, & Weissman, 1992). However, careful examination of these data indicate that it is more likely that such attempts and ideation are accounted for by the presence of Axis II disorders rather than by the panic or social phobia per se. For example, the suicidal ideation reported by the panic-disordered patients in the study by Weissman et al. (1989) occurred prior to the onset of the panic attacks. Because the DIS (the interview used in that study) does not assess Axis II disorders, it is likely that the suicidal ideation was related to the presence of a personality disorder. Similarly, the relationship between social phobia and suicidal ideation can be accounted for largely, *but not entirely*, by the presence of a personality disorder (Schneier et al., 1992). However, the presence of suicidal ideation, even if not directly related to the presence of the anxiety disorder, should alert the clinician to conduct a thorough evaluation along both Axis I and II dimensions.

Do assess carefully for the presence of medical conditions that might be etiological or maintaining factors, but *do not* dismiss anxiety complaints as simply a manifestation of a physical condition. For example, a patient sought treatment at our anxiety disorders clinic for "shaking in public." According to the patient's primary physician, he had a "congenital tremor" of both hands, the etiology of which was unknown, and the condition was not amenable to traditional medical interventions. It was termed congenital because the patient's mother suffered from the same condition. The tremors had a profound influence on his occupational achievement, in that he had been fired once because his boss suspected the tremors were the result of a problem with alcohol. He feared that the same thing might happen in his current position, should his trembling be noticed by his superiors. In addition, following his job termination, the patient became more concerned over the possibility of trembling in front of others, particularly those who were not aware of his physical condition, and this concern, in turn, increased his tremor. Although the patient was convinced that the etiology of this tremor was biological, nonetheless he admitted that the tremors were exacerbated by social anxiety. Although it was unclear whether the cause of the tremors was biological or emotional, the patient's distress was still in excess of the ramifications of his "physical" disorder. Therefore, a diagnosis of social phobia was warranted.

In summary, although patients may present with medical conditions that seem to account for their anxiety, the clinician must carefully consider whether the patient's fears exceed what would be expected for the presence of the physical condition. In such cases, the patient's anxiety would be treated identically to the others.

Summary

The purpose of this chapter has been to discuss interviewing practices for patients who present with anxiety disorders. Due to the ubiquitous nature of anxiety, patients may present with a myriad of complaints. In addition, the anxiety may not be a singular disorder but part of a more complex picture, involving more encompassing Axis I or II disorders or both. Careful diagnostic practices are necessary, because imprecision may result in inaccurate case conceptualizations or inappropriate treatment. Although interviewing remains the primary source of information-gathering, additional strategies, such as self-report or self-monitoring practices, may be used to assist in clarifying the symptom picture. Numerous factors, as outlined in this chapter, need to be considered in order to fully understand the complexity of these disorders.

References

Agras, W. S., Sylvester, D., & Oliveau, D. (1969). The epidemiology of common fear and phobia. *Comprehensive Psychiatry, 10,* 151–156.

Akhtar, S., Wig, N. H., Verna, V. K., Pershad, D., & Verna, S. K. (1975). A phenomenological analysis of symptoms in obsessive–compulsive neuroses. *British Journal of Psychiatry, 127,* 342–348.

Amies, P. L., Gelder, M. G., & Shaw, P. M. (1983). Social phobia: A comparative clinical study. *British Journal of Psychiatry, 142,* 174–179.

American Psychiatric Association (1987). *Diagnostic and statistical manual of mental disorders,* 3rd ed., revised. Washington, DC: Author.

American Psychiatric Association (1993). *Diagnostic and statistical manual of mental disorders,* 4th ed., draft criteria. Washington, DC: Author.

Anthony, J. C., Folstein, M., Romanoski, A. J., Von Korff, M. R., Nestadt, G. R., Chahal, R., Merchant, A., Brown, C. H., Shapiro, S., Kramer, M., & Gruenberg, E. M. (1985). Comparison of the lay Diagnostic Interview Schedule and a standardized psychiatric diagnosis. *Archives of General Psychiatry, 42,* 667–675.

Barlow, D. H. (1988). *Anxiety and its disorders.* New York: Guilford Press.

Barlow, D. H., DiNardo, P. A., Vermilyea, B. B., Vermilyea, J. A., & Blanchard, E. B. (1986). Co-morbidity and depression among the anxiety disorders: Issues in diagnosis and classification. *Journal of Nervous and Mental Disease, 174,* 63–72.

Beidel, D. C., & Bulik, C. M. (1990). Flooding and response prevention as a treatment for bowel obsessions. *Journal of Anxiety Disorders, 4,* 247–256.

Beidel, D. C., & Turner, S. M. (1991). Anxiety disorders. In M. Hersen & S. M. Turner (Eds.), *Adult psychopathology and diagnosis* (2nd ed., pp. 226–278). New York: John Wiley.

Borden, J. W. (1992). Behavioral treatment of simple phobia. In S. M. Turner, K. S. Calhoun, & H. E. Adams (Eds.), *Handbook of clinical behavior therapy,* 2nd ed. (pp. 3–12). New York: John Wiley.

Boyd, J. H., Burke, J. D., Gruenberg, E., Holzer, C. E., III, Rae, D. S., George, L. K., Karno, M., Stoltzman, R., McEvoy, L., & Nestadt, G. (1984). Exclusion criteria of DSM-III: A study of co-occurrence of hierarchy-free syndromes. *Archives of General Psychiatry, 41,* 983–989.

Breier, A., Charney, D. S., & Heninger, G. R. (1984). Major depression in patients with agoraphobia and panic disorder. *Archives of General Psychiatry, 41,* 1129–1135.

Connolly, J. C., Hallam, R. S., & Marks, I. M. (1976). Selective association of fainting with blood–injury–illness fears. *Behavior Therapy, 7,* 8–13.

Crowe, R. R., Pauls, D. L., Slymen, D. J., & Noyes, R. (1980). A family study of anxiety neurosis: Morbidity risk in families of patients with and without mitral valve prolapse. *Archives of General Psychiatry, 37,* 77–79.

Dealy, R. R., Ishiki, D. M., Avery, D. H., Wilson, L. G., & Dunner, D. L. (1981). Secondary depression in anxiety disorders. *Comprehensive Psychiatry, 22,* 612–618.

DiNardo, P. A., Barlow, D. H., Cerny, J. A., Vermilya, B. B., Vermilya, J. A., Himaldi, W. G., & Waddell, M. T. (1986). *Anxiety Disorders Interview Schedule—Revised* (ADIS-R). State University of New York, Albany: Unpublished manuscript.

Emmelkamp, P. M. G. (1988). Phobic disorders. In C. G. Last & M. Hersen (Eds.), *Handbook of anxiety disorders* (pp. 66–86). New York: Pergamon Press.

Gorman, J., Fyer, A. F., Glicklich, J., King, D., & Klein, D. F. (1981). Effect of imipramine on prolapsed mitral valves of patients with panic disorder. *American Journal of Psychiatry, 138,* 977–978.

Gorman, J. M., Levy, G. F., Liebowitz, M. R., McGrath, P., Appleby, I. L., Dillon, D. J., Davies, S. O., & Klein, D. F. (1983). Effect of acute β-adrenergic blockade of lactate-induced panic. *Archives of General Psychiatry, 40,* 1079–1082.

Helzer, J. E., Robins, L. N., McEvoy, L. T., Spitznagel, E. L., Stoltzman, R. K., Farmer, A., & Brockington, I. F. (1985). A comparison of clinical and diagnostic interview schedule diagnoses. *Archives of General Psychiatry, 42,* 657–666.

Herbert, J. D., Hope, D. A., & Bellack, A. S. (1992). Validity of the distinction between generalized social phobia and avoidant personality disorder. *Journal of Abnormal Psychology, 101,* 332–338.

Hodgson, R. J., & Rachman, H. (1977). Obsessional–compulsive complaints. *Behaviour Research and Therapy, 15,* 389–395.

Holt, C. S., Heimberg, R. G., & Hope, D. A. (1992). Avoidant personality disorder and the generalized subtype of social phobia. *Journal of Abnormal Psychology, 101,* 318–325.

Insel, T. R., Zahn, T., & Murphy, D. L. (1985). Obsessive–compulsive disorder: An anxiety disorder? In A. H. Tuma & J. D. Maser (Eds.), *Anxiety and the anxiety disorders* (pp. 577–594). Hillsdale, NJ: Erlbaum.

Jacob, R. G., Moller, M. B., Turner, S. M., & Wall, C. (1985). Otoneurological examination in panic disorders and agoraphobia with panic attacks: A pilot study. *American Journal of Psychiatry, 142,* 715–720.

Jacob, R. G., & Turner, S. M. (1988). Panic disorder: Diagnosis and assessment. In A. J. Frances & R. E. Hales (Eds.), *Review of psychiatry* (Vol. 7, pp. 67–87). Washington, DC: American Psychiatric Press.

Jenike, M. A., Baer, L., Minichiello, W. E., Schwartz, C. E., & Carey, R. J., Jr. (1986). Concomitant obsessive–compulsive disorders and schizotypal personality disorder. *American Journal of Psychiatry, 143,* 530–532.

Kagan, J., Reznick, J. S., & Snidman, N. (1988). Biological bases of childhood shyness. *Science, 240,* 167–171.

Kathol, R. G., Noyes, R., Slymen, D. J., Crowe, R. R., Clancy, J., & Kerber, R. E. (1980). Propranolol in chronic anxiety disorders. *Archives of General Psychiatry, 37,* 1361–1365.

Keyl, P. M., & Eaton, W. W. (1990). Risk factors for the onset of panic disorder and other panic attacks in a prospective, population-based study. *American Journal of Epidemiology, 131,* 301–311.

Klein, D. F. (1964). Delineation of two drug responsive anxiety syndromes. *Psychopharmacologia, 5,* 397–408.

Korn, M. L., Kotler, M., Molcho, A., Botsis, A. J., Grosz, D., Chen, C., Plutchik, R., Brown, S., & van Praag, H. M. (1992). Suicide and violence associated with panic attacks. *Biological Psychiatry, 31,* 607–612.

Kushner, M. G., Sher, K. J., & Beitman, B. D. (1990). The relation between alcohol problems and the anxiety disorders. *American Journal of Psychiatry, 42,* 685–695.

Lang, P. J. (1977). Physiological assessment of anxiety and fear. In J. D. Cone & R. P. Hawkins (Eds.), *Behavioral assessment: New directions in clinical psychology* (pp. 178–195). New York: Brunner/Mazel.

Lesser, I. M., Rubin, R. T., Pecknold, J. C., Rifkin, A., Swinson, R. P., Lydiard, R. B., Burrows, G. D., Noyes, R. Jr., & DuPont, R. L. (1988). Secondary depression in panic disorder and agoraphobia. *Archives of General Psychiatry, 45,* 437–443.

Liebowitz, M. R., Fyer, A. J., Gorman, J. M., Dillon, D., Appleby, I. L., Levy, G., Anderson, S., Levitt, M., Palij, M., Davies, S. O., & Klein, D. F. (1984). Lactate provocation of panic attacks. *Archives of General Psychiatry, 41,* 764–770.

Liebowitz, M. R., Fyer, A. J., Gorman, J. M., Dillon, D., Davies, S., Stein, J. M., Cohen, B. S., & Klein, D. F. (1985). Specificity of lactate infusions in social phobia versus panic disorders. *American Journal of Psychiatry, 142,* 947–950.

Liebowitz, M. R., Gorman, J. M., Dillon, D. Levy, G., Appleby, I. L., Anderson, S., Palij, M., Davies, S. O., & Klein, D. F. (1985). Lactate provocation of panic attacks. *Archives of General Psychiatry, 42,* 709–719.

Margraf, J., Ehlers, A., & Roth, W. T. (1986). Sodium lactate infusions and panic attacks: A review and critique. *Psychosomatic Medicine, 48,* 23–51.

Marks, I. M. (1970). The classification of phobic disorders. *British Journal of Psychiatry, 116,* 377–386.

Marsland, D. W., Wood, M., & Mayo, F. (1976). Content of family practice: A data bank for patient care, curriculum, and research in family-practice—526,196 patient problems. *Journal of Family Practice, 3,* 25–68.

Mavissakalian, M., & Hamann, M. S. (1986). DSM-III personality disorder in agoraphobia. *Comprehensive Psychiatry, 27,* 471–479.

Mavissakalian, M., & Hammen, M. S. (1988). Correlates of DSM-III personality disorder in panic disorder and agoraphobia. *Comprehensive Psychiatry, 29,* 535–544.

Messer, S., & Beidel, D. C. (in press). Psychosocial and familial characteristics of anxious children. *Journal of the American Academy of Child and Adolescent Psychiatry.*

Öst, L. G. (1987). Age of onset in different phobias. *Journal of Abnormal Psychology, 96,* 223–229.

Reich, J. H., & Noyes, R., Jr. (1987). A comparison of DSM-III personality disorders in acutely ill panic and depressed patients. *Journal of Anxiety Disorders, 1,* 123–131.

Robins, L. N. (1985). Epidemiology: Reflections on testing the validity of psychiatric interviews. *Archives of General Psychiatry, 42,* 918–924.

Robins, L. N., Helzer, J. E., Weissman, M. M., Orvaschel, H., Greenberg, E., Burke, J. D., Jr., & Regier, D. A. (1984). Lifetime prevalence of specific psychiatric disorders at three sites. *Archives of General Psychiatry, 41,* 949–958.

Sanderson, W. C., Rapee, R. M., & Barlow, D. H. (1987). The DSM-III-R revised anxiety disorder categories: Descriptors and patterns of comorbidity. Presented at the annual meeting of Association for Advancement of Behavior Therapy, Boston.

Schneier, F. R., Johnson, J., Hornig, C. D., Liebowitz, M. R., & Weissman, M. M. (1992). Social phobia: Comorbidity and morbidity in an epidemiologic sample. *Archives of General Psychiatry, 49*, 282–288.

Shear, M. K., Devereaux, R. B., Kranier-Fox, R., Mann, J. J., & Frances, A. (1984). Low prevalence of mitral valve prolapse in patients with panic disorder. *American Journal of Psychiatry, 141*, 302–303.

Spielberger, C. D., Gorsuch, R. L., & Lushene, R. E. (1970). *The State–Trait Anxiety Inventory: Test manual for form X.* Palo Alto, CA: Consulting Psychologists Press.

Spitzer, R. B., & Williams, J. B. (1986). *Structured Clinical Interview for DSM-III-R, Axis II.* Unpublished manuscript, Biometrics Research Department, New York State Psychiatric Institute, New York.

Spitzer, R. L., Williams, J. B. W., Gibbon, M., & First, M. B. (1988). *Structured clinical interview for DSM-III-R.* Unpublished manuscript, Biometrics Research Department, New York State Psychiatric Institute, New York.

Stanley, M. A., Turner, S. M., & Borden, J. W. (1990). Schizotypal features in obsessive–compulsive disorder. *Comprehensive Psychiatry, 31*, 511–518.

Stein, M. B. (1986). Panic disorder and medical illness. *Psychosomatics, 27*, 833–840.

Turner, S. M., and Beidel, D. C. (1988). *Treating obsessive–compulsive disorder.* New York: Pergamon Press.

Turner, S. M., & Beidel, D. C. (1989). Social phobia: Clinical syndrome, diagnosis and comorbidity. *Clinical Psychology Review, 9*, 3–18.

Turner, S. M., Beidel, D. C., Borden, J. W., Stanley, M. A., & Jacob, R. G. (1991). Social phobia: Axis I and II correlates. *Journal of Abnormal Psychology, 100*, 102–106.

Turner, S. M., Beidel, D. C., Dancu, C. V., & Stanley, M. A. (1989). An empirically derived inventory to measure social fears and anxiety: The Social Phobia and Anxiety Inventory. *Psychological Assessment: A Journal of Consulting and Clinical Psychology, 1*, 35–40.

Turner, S. M., Beidel, D. C., & Jacob, R. G. (1988). Assessment of panic. In S. Rachman & J. D. Maser (Eds.), *Panic: Psychological perspectives* (pp. 37–50). Hillsdale, NJ: Lawrence Erlbaum.

Turner, S. M., Beidel, D. C., & Townsley, R. M. (1992). Social phobia: A comparison of specific and generalized subtypes and avoidant personality disorder. *Journal of Abnormal Psychology, 101*, 326–331.

Turner, S. M., McCann, B. S., Beidel, D. C., & Mezzich, J. B. (1986). DSM-III classification of anxiety disorders: A psychometric study. *Journal of Abnormal Psychology, 95*, 168–172.

Uhde, T. W., Boulenger, J. P., Roy-Byrne, P. P., Geraci, M. F., Vittone, B. J., & Post, R. M. (1985). Longitudinal course of panic disorder: Clinical and biological considerations. *Progress in Neuro-Psychopharmacology and Biological Psychiatry, 9*, 39–51.

van der Molen, C. G., & van den Hout, M. A. (1988). Expectancy effects on respiration during lactate infusion. *Psychosomatic Medicine, 50*, 439–443.

Van Valkenberg, C., Akiskal, H. G., Puzantian, V., & Rosenthal, T. (1984). Anxious depressions: Clinical, family history, and naturalistic outcome—comparisons with panic and major depressive disorders. *Journal of Affective Disorders, 6*, 67–82.

Watson, D., & Friend, R. (1969). Measurement of social-evaluative anxiety. *Journal of Consulting and Clinical Psychology, 33*, 448–457.

Weissman, M. M., Klerman, G. L., Markowitz, J. S., & Ouellette, R. (1989). Suicidal ideation and suicide attempts in panic disorder and attacks. *New England Journal of Medicine, 321*, 1209–1214.

4

Mood Disorders

Hagop S. Akiskal and Charles Van Valkenburg

Concepts and Terminology

Transient feelings of depression are a universal experience, and depressed mood is easy to recognize. The outward expression or affect of depression is on a continuum with normal experience, and even when a depressive state has a known organic precipitant (e.g., reserpine toxicity), the observable change in affect is usually one more of degree than of quality.

Numerous common and uncommon stimuli can precipitate depression. A partial list includes failure or defeat, unemployment, bereavement and other losses, anemia, low thyroid function, seasonal reduction in daylight, brain tumor, Parkinson's disease, subacute viral infections, antihypertensive medication, and numerous other chemicals. Because only a small proportion (typically not more than 10%) of people exposed to such stressors develop depression, these stressors cannot be considered to be truly causative; familial–hereditary and developmental–temperamental predisposition appear to be necessary substrates (Akiskal & McKinney, 1975; Kendler, Kessler, Neale, Heath, & Eaves, 1993).

No matter what the provoking factors, the constellation of signs and symptoms associated with depressed mood—the depressive syndrome—is remarkably consistent. There is often a pervasive loss of interest and the ability to experience pleasure. Appetite and sleep are usually diminished, although sometimes increased. Energy is impaired, and mental and physical functioning is slowed, although there is often restless, purposeless movement. The ability to concentrate or remember is impaired. Self-esteem is lowered, and feelings of guilt and worthlessness become painful preoccupations. Finally, there may be thoughts of

The authors collaborated at the University of Tennessee, Memphis, on an earlier version of this chapter published in the first edition of this book. The present version was extensively revised and updated during Dr. Akiskal's leave at the National Institute of Mental Health, Rockville, MD. All opinions expressed in this chapter are the authors', and do not necessarily reflect those of the Institute.

Hagop S. Akiskal • Department of Psychiatry, University of California at San Diego, La Jolla, California 92093-0603. Charles Van Valkenburg • Mental Health Clinic, Veterans Administration Hospital, El Paso, Texas 79925.

Diagnostic Interviewing (Second Edition), edited by Michel Hersen and Samuel M. Turner. Plenum Press, New York, 1994.

death or suicide, or actual suicide attempts that, tragically, lead to death in 15% of untreated or inadequately treated depressives.

Clinical depression is diagnosed when mood change is accompanied by several of these symptoms. According to the fourth edition of the *Diagnostic and Statistical Manual of Mental Disorders* (DSM-IV) (American Psychiatric Association, 1994) *major depressive disorder* refers to an illness of typically acute onset over a period of days to weeks, a syndromal depression with a minimum of five signs and symptoms, and sustained duration for at least 2 weeks. This illness can present as a single episode (usually in late life) or, more commonly, pursues its course in recurrent episodes (in which case it typically begins at a younger age). About 15% of major depressions do not recover but instead pursue a protracted course, sometimes for years. Another chronic pattern in depression is represented by *dysthymic disorder*, in which onset is insidious over many years prior to any superimposed major depressive episodes (if any); it is of low-grade intensity, i.e., subsyndromal depression with two to four symptoms, and runs an intermittent course for 2 or more years (possibly over a lifetime, if untreated). Even in community settings, dysthymia often precedes major depression (Lewinsohn, Rhode, Seeley, & Hops, 1991), leading to *double depression*, i.e., major depression superimposed on dysthymia.

As a deviation from normal mood, depression may be compared to fever, which is a deviation from normal body temperature. Like depression, fever is a syndrome with numerous associated symptoms (e.g., chills, shivering and muscular rigor, malaise, headache, and sometimes photophobia, delirium, shock, convulsions, and death). In antiquity, fever was itself considered an illness. Later, fevers became a class of illnesses, and now, except in the case of "fever of unknown origin," the syndrome is not considered a diagnosis but rather a manifestation of other diseases (e.g., influenza, malaria, pneumonia, collagen disease, or spreading cancer).

The diagnosis of major depression is generally reserved for cases in which the cause of the syndrome is unknown, like that of fever of unknown origin. This is the position taken by DSM-IV, which excludes normal bereavement (caused by death of a loved one)—as well as mood disorders due to a known physical condition or medication—from the rubric of major mood disorders. However, as pointed out, physical causes of depression, like psychosocial stressors, are often insufficient explanations for the occurrence of clinical depression. Accordingly, the authors prefer a modification of the DSM-IV schema for depression whereby phenomenological affective diagnoses—irrespective of causative factors—are noted on Axis I, personality factors on Axis II, physical contributions on Axis III, and relevant psychosocial stressors on Axis IV. This multifactorial approach, in which depression is viewed as the final common pathway of many etiologies, both psychological and biological (Akiskal & McKinney, 1975), appears most consistent with current data. However, as in the case of fever, future research may demonstrate several discrete etiologies.

From a clinical standpoint, the most validated distinction within the class of mood disorders is that between bipolar disorder and depression pursuing a unipolar course. *Bipolar disorder* in its "classic" manic–depressive form (also known as *Bipolar I*) is characterized by syndromal episodes of depression and mania. Mania is the hallmark of bipolar illness and is characterized by euphoric, irritable, or hostile mood; decreased need for sleep; psychomotor excitement; pressured speech and flight of ideas; inflated self-esteem; expansive and grandiose ideation; and poor judgment, especially with regard to excessive involvement in social, sexual, or business activities with little recognition of painful consequences. Mania is typically of psychotic proportions and often leads to hospitalization. A milder degree of excitement is known as *hypomania*. In *cyclothymic disorder*, depressive and hypomanic manifestations alternate on an attenuated (subsyndromal) plane and tend to pursue a lifelong course. Although cyclothymia may exist as a self-limited condition without superimposed episodes, major depressive or manic syndromes often complicate its course; the reverse—i.e., cyclothymia appearing for the first time after a major bipolar breakdown—is rarely if ever seen clinically. Bipolar I and cyclothymic conditions appear to be phenomenologically bridged by *Bipolar II disorder*, which refers to recurrent major depressions and infrequent and short-lived hypomanic periods. Related to this disorder are *pseudounipolar depressions*, typically recurrent depressions with bipolar family history; in this case, hypomania does not occur spontaneously but appears on pharmacological challenge with antidepressants (Akiskal, 1983a).

Another widely accepted distinction within the class of mood disorders is based on the presence of classic vegetative and related disturbances. Such depressions are now dubbed as being *melancholic* (e.g., lack of reactivity, pathological guilt, early morning awakening, depression worse in the morning, marked psychomotor disturbance and weight loss) and may or may not be *psychotic* (e.g., delusional) in depth. Both melancholic and psychotic depressions usually dictate vigorous somatic interventions, with psychosocial modalities viewed as ancillary. This is not to say that other major depressions would not respond to somatic interventions; indeed, longitudinal prospective follow-up of nonmelancholic depressions has shown melancholic, psychotic, or even bipolar outcome in at least 40% of cases (Akiskal, Bitar, Puzantian, Rosenthal, & Walker, 1978). Such findings suggest that melancholic, psychotic, and bipolar depressions often arise from the background of milder depressive reactions, although it is not always easy to prospectively predict which of these milder expressions will show such denouement. Another qualifier for depressive episodes is *atypicality*, which manifests reverse vegetative signs (i.e., weight gain, hypersomnia, worse in evening, initial insomnia) and tends to show marked reactivity (i.e., could disappear in response to positive events). *Seasonal* (fall–winter) occurrence of depression often, though not invariably, tends to be atypical. All four of the foregoing qualifiers—psychotic, atypical, seasonal, melancholic—can be used to describe both bipolar and unipolar disorders.

Investigators from Washington University (Robins & Guze, 1972) have proposed that in research studies for which homogeneous samples are needed, mood disorders occurring in the setting of preexisting psychiatric disorders should preferably be distinguished from "primary" affective disorders without such antecedents. The psychiatric disorders that are commonly complicated by depression include anxiety disorders, somatization and antisocial personality disorders, alcoholism and substance abuse, schizophrenia, and early dementia. Although mania can be secondary to physical disease or medications, bipolar illness is unlikely to be "secondary" to another disorder. When alcohol and drug abuse history chronologically precedes that of bipolar mood disorders, such abuse is probably best explained as an early manifestation of cyclothymic mood swings leading to "self-treatment" with drugs (Akiskal et al., 1985). Thus, the rubric *secondary mood disorder* almost always refers to either dysthymic or major depressive conditions.

Although the primary–secondary distinction is not made in DSM-IV, we find it useful in view of the differences in course dictated by the underlying psychiatric illness (Goodwin & Guze, 1989). As the underlying disorders are usually chronic, superimposed depressive conditions tend to run an intermittent course dictated by the vicissitudes of the underlying disorders. The primary–secondary distinction is implicit in much of the research literature on depression; indeed, most, though not all, investigators who study this illness tend to focus on primary depression. As a result, relatively little is known about secondary depressions, except that their course tends to be more protracted and unpredictable. Recent data reporting a rise in the rates of depression, especially in younger subjects (Klerman et al., 1985), might, to some extent, be due to secondary depressions. Young depressives typically have comorbid anxiety, substance and alcohol abuse histories, and personality disorders.

Description of Subtypes

It must be obvious from the foregoing discussion that the different subtypes of mood disorders incorporated into DSM-IV are distributed on a continuum of signs and symptoms and can be reliably distinguished only in the most extreme cases. Indeed, Kraepelin (1921), who provided the classic descriptions of mood disorders, believed in a continuum model (at least for hospitalized patients). When interviewing a patient, the clinician must evaluate each new bit of information that is reported or observed and must consider how this information pertains to each of the possible subtypes. In many cases, a preponderance of information will eventually point to one subtype; in others, it will not be possible to establish the classification with much certainty. For the clinician, the more important clinical differential diagnostic problems involve:

1. Deciding whether an underlying and treatable physical cause exists.
2. Depressive vs. anxiety disorders.
3. Unipolar vs. bipolar conditions.
4. Cyclothymic and related dysthymic disorders vs. nonaffective personality disorders.

The descriptions of the mood disorder subtypes in this section are meant to provide the beginning clinician with prototypes, rather than all varieties of mood disorders. A comprehensive coverage of the manifestations of depression and its subtypes can be found elsewhere (Akiskal, 1983a, 1994b; Ban, 1989; Castello, 1993);

an even more encyclopedic coverage, including bipolar subtypes, is the monograph by Goodwin and Jamison (1990).

Mood Syndromes in the Setting of Medical–Neurological Disease

It is not always easy to decide whether affective symptoms represent understandable psychological reactions to concurrent medical–neurological disorders or whether they are caused by the physiochemical impact of these disorders. However, it is the obligation of the clinician to first rule out such contributions that are potentially reversible. In general, there are no distinctive clinical features that differentiate these medical–neurological mood states from their primary counterparts. Their detection depends heavily on the clinician's index of suspicion. It is wise to insist that all affectively ill patients—especially those with first breakdowns after age 40—undergo thorough physical evaluation. Table 1 lists the medical–neurological conditions most commonly associated with depressive and manic states. Especially treacherous are occult malignancies—whether systemic or involving the brain—as well as endocrine and seizure (temporal lobe) disorders; these conditions should in particular be suspected when psychological and pharmacological interventions do not yield expected positive results within a few

TABLE 1.   Medical Factors in Depressive and Manic States[a]

Type of cause	Depressive state	Manic state
Pharmacological	Steroidal contraceptives	Corticosteroids
	Antihypertensives	L-Dopa
	Alcohol and other sedatives	Antidepressants (e.g., tricyclics, SSRIs)
	Cholinesterase inhibitor insecticides	Monoamine oxidase inhibitors
	Stimulant withdrawal	Stimulants (e.g., cocaine)
Infectious	Influenza	Influenza
	Infectious mononucleosis	St. Louis encephalitis
	Tuberculosis	Q fever
	General paresis (syphilis)	General paresis (syphilis)
	AIDS	AIDS
Endocrine	Hypothyroidism	Thyrotoxicosis
	Cushing's disease	
	Addison's disease	
Collagen	Systemic lupus erythematosus	Systemic lupus erythematosus
	Rheumatoid arthritis	Rheumatic chorea
Neurological	Stroke	Stroke
	Multiple sclerosis	Multiple sclerosis
	Cerebral tumors	Diencephalic and 3rd ventricle tumors
	Parkinson's disease	Orbitofrontal meningiomas and
	Sleep apnea	aneurysms
	Dementia	Huntington's chorea
	Complex partial seizures	
Neoplastic	(Examples: pancreatic, ovarian, lymphatic)	

[a]Updated from Akiskal (1992b).

weeks. Unfortunately, the diagnosis may sometimes come too late, as is described next.

Case 1

A 46-year-old woman presented to a mental health center with the chief complaint of lassitude, irritability, hostile outbursts, insomnia, low self-confidence, and poor concentration of insidious onset over a period of 8 weeks. It was felt at the time that this was a "reaction" to her hysterectomy (for benign fibroid tumors) a year before and the fact that her husband had been neglecting her romantically since then and was increasingly immersed in his job. Their two children were attending college in another city, and the patient had no other relatives close by. Although she had always been a rather "anxious person," past psychiatric history was negative for major psychopathology.

She was treated with individual psychotherapy with a cognitive–behavioral focus and, having made no progress within 6 weeks, was referred for psychiatric evaluation. Mental status revealed a woman who looked exhausted, having lost 20 pounds in a few weeks, and who complained of inability to think. Systems review indicated that she had had mild diarrhea for 8 weeks. Laboratory studies were ordered at this time. Thyroid tests were normal, CBC revealed a mild anemic state, and blood chemistry revealed abnormalities in protein levels. Internal medicine consultation led to referral to a surgeon who performed a laparotomy, revealing an intestinal malignancy (lymphoma). The patient died 6 months later.

Major (Melancholic) Depressions

The construct of *major depression*, as defined in recent editions of the *Diagnostic and Statistical Manual of Mental Disorders*—of which DSM-IV (APA, 1994) is the latest—is a broad category, the criteria for which are relatively easy to meet and encompass a wide range of severity and heterogeneity. For this reason, the description provided here is that of the classic melancholic form of the illness. The depression often begins insidiously with irritability and minor mood changes; as it gradually worsens, it is accompanied by insomnia, agitation manifested in pacing and hand-wringing, self-reproach, fearfulness, and, sometimes, panic attacks. In 15% of cases, depression reaches psychotic severity and is characterized by delusions of guilt, persecution, or ill health. In some cases, impairment of memory and orientation in elderly melancholics may give the false impression of a primary dementia. Premorbidly, melancholics tend to be conscientious, perfectionistic, meticulous, self-sacrificing, scrupulously honest, rigid, and frugal. Before electroconvulsive and antidepressant medication therapies became available, recovery was slow, and psychiatric wards were filled with these patients. With the advent of early diagnosis and effective treatment, this extreme form of melancholia—which was once termed *involutional melancholia*—has become relatively uncommon.

Melancholia replaced the term *endogenous* (e.g., unprecipitated) depression, because current evidence indicates that the presence of precipitants carries no diagnostic specificity (Akiskal et al., 1978). Symptomatologically, the syndrome is defined by anhedonia, pathological guilt, marked psychomotor disturbance, middle and late insomnia, and weight loss, which occur autonomously. Despite opinion to the contrary, there is no evidence for a separate major depressive subtype in which melancholic signs are minimal to absent and cognitive disturbances predominate. Indeed, low self-esteem, self-reproach, and hopelessness are characteristically pronounced in melancholias. An exhaustive description of depressive symptomatology can be found in the volume *Depression* by Beck (1967), who pioneered in the description of the cognitive disturbances of depressive illness. Whether precipitated or not, the full syndrome of melancholia, once established, tends to pursue its own course, unless specific treatments are provided. Untreated episodes, if not ended by suicide, may continue unabated for many months—rarely, years. This autonomy of the morbid process imparts to the syndrome of melancholia the attributes of a medical disease. The patient is unable to sit still or concentrate well enough to answer questions and cannot be distracted from perseverative expressions of guilt, persecution, and woe. Memory or attention may be so poor that little or no information can be elicited about the circumstances or symptoms of the illness. In these extremely sick melancholic patients, often classified under *pseudodemented depressions*, the initial difficulty is distinguishing the illness from a primary degenerative dementia. In cases in which paranoid symptoms predominate, the illness can resemble late-onset schizophrenia.

The dexamethasone suppression test (Carroll, 1982) and shortened rapid eye movement (REM) latency (Kupfer & Thase, 1983) tend to be more deviant in severe melancholia in which there is little doubt of the diagnosis. These laboratory findings tend to be less reliable in the milder forms of the illness in which the patient, instead of reporting depression, might complain of irritability, anxiety, and somatic discomfort (Akiskal, 1983a). Indeed, in some patients, the clinical picture may consist of few vegetative complaints that nonetheless can produce significant functional disruption in the patients' usual social or occupational roles (Wells et al., 1989). Such cases, subsumed under the rubic of *masked depression* because of the patient's denial of subjective depression, are prevalent in primary care settings. In more classic melancholic patients observed in psychiatric settings, somatic preoccupations may acquire delusional quality.

Case 2

A 60-year-old widow was brought to the psychiatric hospital by her children, who had obtained a court commitment order. She had been admitted to the hospital several times in previous years and had always been treated with electroconvulsive therapy (ECT). On admission, the patient was grossly agitated, seemed unable to sit or stand still to answer questions about herself, and walked away from anyone who tried to talk to her. When alone, she often walked in circles. In bed, she thrashed around or kicked her legs. Her appearance was one of anguish. At times, she would admit that she felt depressed but said that she believed that nothing could be done for her and that she should be allowed to leave or to die. At other times, she asked members of the hospital staff to poison her, to put an end to her misery. The nurses confirmed that the patient stayed awake much of the night, especially after 2:00 A.M. She believed that her bowels had completely stopped working and sometimes said that her brain was dead and not working anymore. At other times, she would speak of having cancer. When given medication, she often expressed the concern that somebody might be poisoning her for past sins. She said that she had done horrible things (which she never specified) that had ruined the lives of her family members.

Interviewing her proved difficult because she generally would not answer questions about herself and would not cooperate with the cognitive portion of the mental status examination. In naming past presidents of the United States, she was able to name only three since Franklin Roosevelt and did not name the current or immediate past presidents. It was not possible to learn much from her about the past course of her illness. Most of the information in her medical record had been obtained from her family. She had had an episode of depression when she was 38, following the birth of her youngest son. Otherwise, she had apparently been well until her late 50s, when she had gradually become depressed, agitated, and delusional, a description very similar to the current illness. She had been hospitalized four times and had never recovered without ECT. She had generally returned to her normal self for periods of up to 5 years, although recently she had had a tendency toward quick relapses.

Outside her episodes of depression, she had always been an extremely religious person, conscientious and self-sacrificing, caring for disabled members of her family at considerable inconvenience to herself, and exerting a strong role in maintaining family traditions. She had never abused alcohol or other substances. Her father had suffered from repeated bouts of the same illness and had committed suicide on his 49th birthday. Her physician had prescribed antidepressant medication, but she would not take the pills with any regularity. Antipsychotic medication diminished her agitation but did not resolve the melancholic syndrome, necessitating the use of ECT.

Melancholic depressions tend to run their course in recurrent attacks (as exemplified by Case 2). Other patients (approximately 15% of major depressives) evidence considerable residuals between episodes, so much so that, for all intents and purposes, the depression should be characterized as *chronic major depression*. Finally, in a special subgroup of major depressives (accounting for 30%), major episodes arise from a low-grade (dysthymic) substrate to which the patient returns after recovery from the melancholia. This pattern is known as a *double depressive* pattern (Keller, Lavori, Endicott, Coryell, & Klerman, 1983), and onset is characteristically at a young age than that of other major depressions.

Anxious Depressions

Anxiety and depression are often associated (Maser & Cloninger, 1990). The agitation of typical melancholia is not always easily distinguished from physically expressed anxiety; patients with the latter disorder are often troubled by some degree of depressed mood and many even develop episodes of major depression (Cassano, Perugi, Musetti, & Akiskal, 1989). Depressions that are accompanied by severe anxiety are likely to become chronic and tend to respond poorly to the usual treatments (van Valkenburg, Akiskal, Puzantian, & Rosenthal, 1984).

The most reliable indicator of anxiety disorder is the spontaneous panic attack, i.e., an episode of intense anxiety that is usually unprovoked and lasts a few minutes to an hour. Associated physical symptoms include shortness of breath, hyperventilation, palpitations, chest pain or discomfort, numbness or tingling, and a feeing or fear of physical or mental loss of control or impending death.

Between the attacks, the patient may manifest or experience nervousness and tension, worrying, apprehensiveness, overactivity of the autonomic nervous system resulting in flushed or pale skin, excessive perspiration and rapid pulse, and overarousal, with vigilant scanning of surroundings for possible danger.

To evaluate whether a depressed patient is suffering from an anxious depression, the clinician must document history of panic attacks and other anxiety symptoms such as excessive worrying, tension, depersonalization, and derealization. If these symptoms are present, it is important to learn whether they are part of a long-standing anxiety disorder or whether they have been limited to the period of the depressive episodes.

If the patient is older, the anxiety and agitation are more severe, and if there were no previous neurotic or unstable personality manifestations, the illness might be melancholia in an early stage (Akiskal, 1983b).

If the anxiety and tension had their onset with or after the depression, then major depression is the most appropriate diagnosis (Coryell et al., 1988). However, current evidence (van Valkenburg et al., 1984; Akiskal & Lemmi, 1987) indicates that depression with concurrent anxiety states may be more like panic disorders than primary depressive disorders. Further, monoamine oxidase inhibitors like phenelzine appear to be the treatment of choice for both panic disorder and anxious depression (Davidson, Miller, Turnbull, & Sullivan, 1982). In Great Britain (Sargant & Dally, 1962), these patients with anxiety–depressive states have been subclassified as *atypical depressions* by the occurrence of initial insomnia, reverse diurnal variation (feeling worse in the evening), and reverse vegetative signs (hypersomnia and hyperphagia). Why some anxious depressives complain of insomnia and others of hypersomnia is not known with certainty. However, in many anxious patients, excessive daytime fatigue and somnolence appear secondary to the nighttime insomnia so characteristic of anxiety states (Akiskal & Lemmi, 1987). In line with these considerations, the current American practice (see Rapee & Barlow, 1991) is to subsume the multitude of depressions in the setting of anxiety disorders—including those associated with longstanding generalized anxiety disorder—under anxiety disorders or *mixed anxiety–depression.*

It would therefore appear that anxious depressions most often represent secondary depressions—either major or dysthymic—superimposed on preexisting anxiety disorders.

Case 3

A 33-year-old single woman was referred to a psychiatric clinic by her psychotherapist, who thought medication might help her increasingly severe and uncontrollable depressions. She had been in psychotherapy for several years, working on problems of generalized anxiety and tension, unhappiness, and dissatisfactions with career and relationships. She reported history of anxiety and tension since her late teenage years. She was also able to identify fluctuating depression, which she could not clearly distinguish from her more frequent periods of anxious brooding, but stated that the depressed mood and pessimism had been constant and incapacitating over the past 6 weeks. Panic attacks, which had begun in the past year, were not brought on by any specific stimuli, although she felt that she was under considerable stress at these times. She reported difficulty falling asleep and feeling inadequately rested in the mornings, getting out of bed with great difficulty. Appetite and weight were not changed. She stated that her concentration was not as good as it had been, although she could not think of definitive examples of this. She volunteered that her ambition and energy level were diminished. She denied feeling guilty, but said that her chronic problems with low self-esteem and self-confidence had worsened recently. Her interest in sex was reportedly quite low; she expressed concern that her boyfriend might "dump" her. She admitted recent thoughts of suicide, but had not made any serious plans or attempted suicide. On specific questioning, she said that she had been feeling more angry and hostile toward others recently. She had also had some episodes of tearfulness associated with unpleasant memories, and she became briefly tearful as she reported this.

At the time of interview, she appeared only slightly tense and agitated. She reported that she had had two or three panic attacks in each of the past several weeks. A few of these had been extremely severe and had caused her to leave the public places in which they occurred. Most of her panic attacks began very suddenly with feelings of intense fear, shortness of breath and smothering sensations, heart palpitations, mild chest discomfort, numbness and tingling, and a subjective feeling that her skin was flushing and that she was losing control of herself and attracting the attention of others (which was not the case). In her most severe attacks, she reported a very unsettling feeling that things around her seemed to have changed and taken on an "unreal" or "eerie" quality. She stated that during the more serious attacks, she became afraid that she would die, even though she was able to tell herself on a rational level that she would not.

She was treated with alprazolam and phenelzine and continued her psychotherapy. Her panic attacks ceased soon after she began these medications. Although the level of depression was bearable now, low-grade depressive symptoms persisted and self-esteem remained low.

"Pseudounipolar" Depressions

Many otherwise normal persons are subject to bouts of depression, typically beginning in the second or third decade of life, which last a few months and then resolve spontaneously. Mood, energy, and interest in life decrease, there may be a tendency to oversleep, thought processes and activities become slowed, self-esteem diminishes and self-doubts multiply, concentration and memory are less than normal, tranquility is lost, appetite becomes disturbed, and the value of continued existence is increasingly questioned. In these early-onset retarded depressions, in contrast with the agitated depressions described earlier, family history is often positive for bipolar disorder (Akiskal, 1983a). Most of these depressions turn out to be prodromal or mild manifestations of bipolar disorder, in that long-term prospective follow-up often shows evidence of spontaneous hypomanic and manic episodes (Akiskal et al., 1983).

DSM-IV subsumes these patients under major depression because evidence for bipolarity cannot be readily evaluated on a cross-sectional basis. The authors prefer the designation *major depression, pseudounipolar type*, because this illness is phenomenologically distinct from other depressions (Akiskal & Akiskal, 1988) and has clear treatment implications: Over the long term, these patients respond poorly to tricyclic antidepressants but well to lithium carbonate (Kupfer, Pickar, Himmelhoch, & Detre, 1975).

Case 4

A 42-year-old college professor was seen in consultation on the surgical service. He had shot himself through his calf muscles and reluctantly admitted having done this "to have a legitimate excuse to be in the hospital." He felt that his colleagues would not understand that depression could be an incapacitating illness. Since his late teens, he had had "paralyzing depressions" every 2 to 3 years, lasting 3 to 4 months at a time and characterized by hopeless despair, inability to face students in the classroom, excessive sleep, preoccupation with death, and a sense of failure. These episodes were initially ascribed to romantic disappointment or job stress, but both he and his wife now recognized that no adequate explanations for these episodes could be found in recent years. Moreover, they were in sharp contrast to his habitual enthusiastic and upbeat self. His father, a successful physician, had committed suicide in his early 40s. A paternal uncle was a diagnosed manic–depressive who had been placed on lithium after he had ruined the family business during a manic episode.

After 8 days of desipramine, the patient began feeling "unusually lucid," corrected in one evening 70 exam papers that had previously seemed like an onerous task, made love to his surprised wife six times during the weekend pass, and refused to come back to the hospital, stating that a poet who was as good as "Lowell, Berryman, and Delmore Schwartz combined need not stay under some shrink's care." Fortunately, he also stopped the desipramine, and his wife reported that his pharmacologically mobilized excitement abated over a week's period.

Current clinical investigations (Cassano, Akiskal, Savino, Musetti, & Perugi, 1992) have revealed that the premorbid self of many of these pseudounipolar depressions consists of cheerful and extroverted disposition with high level of energy, optimism, and self-confidence. Such individuals are best described as *hyperthymic* (Akiskal, 1992a) because rather than having hypomanic episodes or cyclothymic oscillations in mood, they have a permanently elevated temperamental baseline. Depressive episodes here represent a reversal from their hyperthymic baseline (Akiskal & Akiskal, 1988), and if hypomanic excursions occur, they appear merely as pharmacologically facilitated returns to the premorbid hyperthymic baseline. Although DSM-IV tends to deny bipolar status to such patients, the foregoing considerations make the DSM-IV position untenable.

Bipolar II

The large subgroup of recurrent major depressives who experience spontaneous but infrequent and mild periods of elevated mood without meeting the full criteria for full-blown mania have been classified as *Bipolar II disorder* (Fieve & Dunner, 1975). In DSM-III-R, these patients were referred to as "not otherwise specified," partly because of difficulties involved in ascertainment of the elevated periods. Yet current evidence indicates that these conditions are as common as more classic bipolar disorders (Akiskal, 1981, 1983a; Cassano et al., 1992). This disorder has finally been given official status in DSM-IV (APA, 1994). Patients with these conditions have retarded depressions very similar to pseudounipolar; the major difference is that hypomanic periods occur spontaneously as discrete episodes, which are distinct from the usual self of the sufferers.

Hypomanic episodes are thus of considerable diagnostic importance in these cases and must be specifically inquired about in the diagnostic interview of all depressives. The pertinent point is a history of abnormally elevated mood, a clear departure from ordinary happiness. Typical manifestations include a degree of optimistic enthusiasm that does not seem justified by the situation, little need for sleep, sexual risk-taking that is out of character, exuberant spending sprees or drinking bouts, or energetic overachievement that might be cut short by the consequences of faulty judgment. To be classified as hypomania, there should be several symptoms at the same time, all of them plausibly attributable to elevated mood, lasting at least a few days.

As these sorts of behaviors are common in sociopathic individuals who abuse drugs, hypomania should not be considered in such individuals unless these symptoms represent a clear break from the habitual self and are preceded or followed by retarded depression. Thus, a certain degree of such uninhibited behavior can be dismissed in sociopathic individuals as not indicative of bipolar disorder, whereas in patients with episodic depressions, it may be necessary to discount denials of such past hypomanias. For example, Bipolar II patients, when depressed, have difficulty remembering that they have ever felt otherwise. The best indicator of bipolar II disorder is the *repeated* tendency to develop hypomania at the tail end of depressive episodes, between depressive episodes, or prior to depressive episodes.

If hypomanic excursions are too numerous to count, these patients are best characterized as cyclothymic depressives (Akiskal, 1994a), i.e., major depression superimposed on cyclothymic disorder (see Table 2). It is finally diagnostically useful to note that seasonality in mood swings is often present in Bipolar II.

Case 5

The patient was a 46-year-old divorced woman, with the chief complaint of "dragging" in the morning, some pessimism, and hostility toward her former husband. Her medical records indicated that she had had an almost stuporous depression with hypersomnia and psychomotor retardation, and she had been treated with electroconvulsive therapy. She had been taking an antipsychotic–tricyclic combination without interruption for 12 years. This medication had been prescribed by her GP because of a history of "lazy depressions" lasting 6 to 8 weeks at a time in early fall and midwinter months. She resisted all attempts to change her medication regimen, insisting that she always had relapsed in the past when any other medications were used. Because her relapses were so very bad—"life coming to a screeching halt"—she did not want to do anything that might bring another one on.

After a television feature on tardive dyskinesia, she stopped her medication. Following several dramatic episodes of physical symptoms, insomnia, and restarting the pills on her own, she finally managed to stop using them altogether. About this time, her moods began to become more labile. For several weeks, she was easily excitable and had restless energy. She became involved in an affair with a man she met at a singles party, marveling during her clinic visits about how wonderfully sexually compatible they were; she then broke off with him abruptly and flew to California for a weekend with a boyfriend from high school whom she had not seen for 30 years. This was followed by another retarded depression, less severe than the previous one.

Ultimately, she was successfully managed with lithium carbonate. When euthymic,[1] she recalled that the "lazy periods" in her 20s had been on a few occasions followed by episodes in the spring when she felt to energetic that she could go for 48 hours without sleep and during which she wrote passionate love letters; these periods typically abated within a week.

Bipolar I

The full-blown form of manic–depressive illness is known as *Bipolar I disorder* (Fieve & Dunner, 1975). This is more severe than Bipolar II disorder in that the excited periods in Bipolar I patients develop into full syndromal height. Thus, manic psychosis is the hallmark of the disorder. However, the distinction between hypomania and mania is one more of degree than of quality. Elevated periods become classified as manic when they last more than a week and are of such intensity that they result in disruption of the patient's social standing and employment or lead to serious financial and legal difficulties.

The patient is typically unaware of the seriousness of these difficulties, and it is the patient's friends and family who act in concert to get him or her into a psychiatric hospital. The excessive energy of these patients cannot be contained or tolerated by relatives and associates. The patients' grandiose ideas and plans strike those around them as not merely unrealistic but distinctly pathological. Most episodes of mania lead to hospitalization, making a past history of manic disorder relatively easy to document.

As the severity of manic disorder increases, the mood of euphoria typically gives way to one of irritable dysphoria. The manic energy may increasingly come to resemble purposeless psychomotor agitation and may alternate with or give way to periods of profound depression and psychomotor retardation or "catatonic" immobility; despite physical inhibition, thoughts may be racing in such patients. Indeed, the admixture of depressive and manic signs and symptoms often coexists in what is known as *mixed states*. Typically psychotic, these patients often evidence euphoria, irritability, panic, suicidal ideation, mental fatigue with physical restlessness, increased sexual desire, paranoid delusions, auditory hallucinations, and confusion (Akiskal & Puzantian, 1979). At least one third of bipolar patients pass through such episodes at one phase of their illness (Himmelhoch, Mulla, Neil, Detre, & Kupfer, 1976). In other manic patients, flight of ideas may become so severe that speech appears disorganized or incoherent. Whereas a euphoric manic might cheerfully entertain thoughts of personal divinity, the paranoid manic might be more inclined to be belligerent toward any unbelieving infidel!

As delusional and hallucinatory—even mood-incongruent experiences—are not uncommon in these patients, they can be misdiagnosed as schizophrenic. Current evidence, however, indicates that acutely psychotic, assaultive, and combative patients who give evidence for a biphasic course are likely to be manic (Akiskal & Puzantian, 1979; Goodwin & Jamison, 1990). Despite the existence of

---

[1]The term *euthymic* denotes being in a state of normal mood, as distinguished from dysphoric and hypomanic.

reliable operationalized criteria for more than two decades (Feighner et al., 1972), mania is still often misdiagnosed, especially in earlier episodes.

Case 6

A 32-year-old male was referred by the psychiatric nurse of a mental health center because he suspected manic–depressive illness even though all past records described the patient as an "acute paranoid schizophrenic." He had more recently been seen in the hospital because of accelerated speech, extreme irritability, insomnia, weight loss, crying spells alternating with euphoria, religious ideation followed by sexual advances toward the nurses, and fleeting visual hallucinations of "Jesus in the sky." This psychotic state had been attenuated with a neuroleptic, and he had been sent to the mental health clinic for aftercare.

Past history revealed that the first episode requiring psychiatric hospitalization had occurred when the patient was 23; records indicated poor sleep, physical hyperactivity, singing on the streets, disturbing the peace, and euphoria. The second episode requiring hospitalization, at age 28, involved similar behavior plus preaching the Bible and having "visions" of God. This was followed by a protracted depressive episode characterized by psychomotor retardation, lack of social initiative, feeling of being unloved, staying in bed, gloomy thoughts, and decreased sexual drive.

Between these episodes, the patient described himself as "neither depressive nor optimistic" but nervous and irritable with occasional periods of insomnia. However, at age 18, he had had a 3-month period characterized by hypersomnolence, thoughts of death, irritability, and hopelessness; at the time, a general practitioner had treated him with "vitamin shots." As a result of this illness, he had graduated 1 year late from high school. The patient had not been able to maintain jobs between episodes and hoped to find a job in the near future. Family history revealed that his father, who was a "wild man" and drank heavily, had spent 2 years in a state psychiatric hospital and had committed suicide at the age of 43. Mental status revealed the patient to be oriented in three spheres. He was pleasant and cooperative, with somewhat slow thought progression. Content of thought did not reveal delusions; he avoided talking about religion. Affect was slightly depressed; cognitive functions were intact.

The patient was advised to have a lithium workup in view of psychotic manic, retarded depressive, and mixed (the most current) episodes.

Subaffective Dysthymic and Cyclothymic Disorders

We have already noted that major depressions sometimes arise from the substrate of dysthymic or cyclothymic disorders, giving rise, respectively, to the *double depressive* and *Bipolar II* patterns. Increasingly, outpatient mental health workers are seeing milder degrees of mood swing that do not go beyond subsyndromal—i.e., cyclothymic or dysthymic—oscillations. For this reason, they are best considered as *subaffective disorders* (Akiskal, 1981).

Cyclothymic individuals seem vivacious and energetic at times, dull and lethargic at others. They might report periods of enthusiasm, decreased need for sleep, and high productivity alternating with periods of *laziness* and eating and sleeping too much. As cyclothymia has its onset by adolescence or, by the latest, by early adulthood, it can initially be mistaken for a personality disorder. Many of these patients describe their mood as "always either up or down." Counting up every symptom of elevated or depressed mood they have ever had, each part of the full syndrome of manic–depressive disease might have been present at one time or another—albeit for short periods (see Table 2). These mood swings often lead to serious personal complications such as episodic promiscuous behavior, repeated conjugal failure, dilettantism, and frequent changing of residence (Akiskal, Khani, & Scott-Strauss, 1979). A therapeutic trial of lithium carbonate might help distinguish cyclothymia from mood swings associated with primary charactero-logical disorders. However, many of these individuals neither need nor want help, perhaps because they are reluctant to jeopardize the creative talent that has been described in some cyclothymics (Andreasen & Canter, 1974; Akiskal & Akiskal, 1988).

Some patients display labile mood that is highly reactive to environmental support or adversity. This condition has been labeled as *hysteroid dysphoria* (Liebo-witz & Klein, 1979) and refers to a special variant of atypical severe depressive crash, oversleeping, overeating, and a leaden inertia that will follow any personal rejection, whereas acceptance and approval by others will bring back the usual personality, which is likely to be flamboyant, intrusive, seductive, self-centered, demanding, and preoccupied with physical attractiveness. How best to classify these patients is not an easy question. We submit that a large subgroup are related to cyclothymia (Akiskal, 1992a). While hysteroid dysphorics tend to be women, cyclothymia occurs equally in the two genders.

Case 7

This 31-year-old architect presented for outpatient care with the chief complaint of having been a "moody person" since his midteens. He had been divorced twice and was separated from his third wife, who accompanied him to the clinic to make sure he would receive appropriate care. She describe the marriage as "living on a roller coaster"; having attended lectures on manic–depressive psychosis, she felt her husband had a "miniature" form of the

TABLE 2.   Clinical Manifestations of Cyclothymia[a]

Behavioral manifestations
1. Hypersomia vs. decreased need for sleep
2. Introverted self-absorption vs. uninhibited people-seeking
3. Taciturn vs. talkative
4. Unexplained tearfulness vs. bouyant jocularity
5. Psychomotor inertia vs. restless pursuit of activites
Subjective manifestations
6. Lethargy and somatic discomfort vs. eutonia
7. Dulling of senses vs. keen perceptions
8. Slow-witted vs. sharpened thinking
9. Shaky self-esteem alternating between low self-confidence and overconfidence
10. Pessimistic brooding vs. optimism and carefree attitudes

[a]Modified from Akiskal et al. (1979).

illness. She also said, "All his family is extremely temperamental—even wild—yet charming and talented," but that she could no longer live with him unless he received psychiatric treatment. The patient admitted to periods of low mood during which he would oversleep, lack energy and motivation, and "vegetate." These periods were followed, often with a switch in the morning on waking, by high periods of 2 to 3 days when he would be energetic, overconfident, sexually active, witty, sleepless, often carrying out in one day all the backlog of postponed activity accumulated from the "down" days. Such periods were often followed by 1 or 2 days of irritable and hostile mood, heralding the transition back to depression. Thus, he typically had few euthymic periods. He admitted to the frequent use of alcohol during "up" moods to help him sleep and to occasional cocaine use during the "down" periods. Medical history was unremarkable. The patient's mother was diagnosed "paranoid schizophrenic," but history obtained from the patient was more compatible with bipolar disorder with recurrent manic episodes; for example, she had been married six times!

As exemplified by this case, relatives of manic–depressives may suffer from attenuated intermittent cyclothymic disorders (Akiskal et al., 1979). Other relatives of bipolar patients suffer from mild and intermittent depressions (Akiskal et al., 1980), which are best described as subaffective dysthymic bipolar variants. This illness has an early onset and is present long enough that it can seem to be a part of the habitual self. As is often the case in Bipolar II disease, sleep and appetite disturbances are more likely to take the form of overeating and oversleeping. These manifestations have led some to call these depressions *atypical*, whereas others reserve this term for depressions of the more anxious type (Davidson et al., 1982). Interpersonal and drug abuse problems are less likely in these patients than in primary personality disorders, but this difference is usually not sufficiently discriminating to classify individual patients. When bipolar family history has been obtained, these patients can sometimes be identified with a trial of a classical tricyclic or a serotoninergic antidepressant, which can precipitate a hypomanic state, thereby establishing the primacy of the dysthymic disorder. The subtle bipolar hints in dysthymic patients have also been noted by other investigators (e.g., Klein, Taylor, Harding, & Dickstein, 1988).

Case 8

A 24-year-old divorced female presented with the chief complaint of "I have been depressed as long as I remember." On further questioning, she dated this back to age 9, when she took an overdose of aspirin "because I was disappointed in myself—I did not make straight A's." She had always been nonassertive, introverted, and self-denigrating. Other current manifestations included hypersomnolence, decreased energy, poor concentration, inability to comprehend her low moods, and death thoughts (but no suicidal wishes). Mornings were especially difficult, as she felt "gloomy much of the time." On further probing, it was apparent that her dysphoria was not continuous but manifested in periods lasting 7 to 10 days, with intervening 2- to 3-day periods of feeling "just OK." She stated that at times she would "gradually sink into deeper states of suicidal despair." Her husband had divorced her because he could not live with her "pervasive gloominess." Her father was a known manic–depressive responding to lithium carbonate.

Accordingly, she was placed on desipramine (a tricyclic antidepressant), 50 mg twice a day, and on the 8th day she began to wake up early in the morning (5 A.M. vs. her usual rising hour of 11 A.M.), feeling an overabundance of energy, increased sexual urges, and an unexplainable feeling of well-being unknown to her. After proper medical evaluation, lithium carbonate was substituted. With lithium levels of 0.7 meq/liter, much of her gloominess was gone, and she and her ex-husband remarried.

A perusal of the symptoms in dysthymia (Table 3) will explain why a clinician faced with a dysthymic patient has difficulty diagnosing depression when "subjective" manifestations outnumber "objective" signs of depression. Indeed, many dysthymics fit a pattern of low-grade depression with anxious and social phobic traits. Furthermore, interpersonal difficulties in dysthymia are so pronounced in some patients that they are not easily distinguished from the chronic dysphoric conditions seen in primary characterological disorders to be described next.

Mood Disturbances in Nonaffective Personality Disorders

Although DSM-IV lists numerous types of personality disorders, they seem to conform to three broad categories: reclusive, odd or suspicious types, referred to as *paranoid–schizotypal*, which in some cases may represent mild forms of schizophrenia; *dependent–anxious–obsessoid* types, which often coexist with the dysthymic conditions that have just been described; and *histrionic–somatizing* or *aggressive–antisocial* types. Emotional maladjustment is a common presenting feature in the latter. *Histrionic–antisocial disorders will be detailed, not because they are representative of mood disorders, but because they are often confused with them.* Cases 9 and 10, which depict, respectively, the unstable mood of antisocial and histrionic character disorders, should be contrasted with those that depict primary affective illness. A good general description of these disorders can be found in Goodwin and Guze (1989).

Sociopathic personalities are a risk-taking, sensation-seeking, and predatory group of individuals who, in their full-blown form, seem to cause trouble at every opportunity. As children, they disrupt classes and get in trouble with authorities, whereas at home, as adolescents, they fight, steal, vandalize, and overindulge in drugs and sex. As adults, they have unstable work histories, break laws and get arrested, abuse marital partners and children, fail to pay their bills, and are given to wanderlust. On psychological tests like the MMPI, they show "the 4-9 acting out psychopath" profile. The predominant mood is one of dysphoria, which may be due to the constant level of trouble and turmoil in their lives or may result from

TABLE 3.   Clinical Symptomatology
in Dysthymia[a]

Mood: gloomy, morose, brooding, anhedonic
Psychomotor: inertia, lethargy, social withdrawal
Cognitive: low self-esteem, guilty ruminations,
    pessimistic outlook, thoughts of death

[a]According to Akiskal (1983c).

their frequent abuse of alcohol and other substances. Such abuse also gives rise to psychomotor excitement, leading to difficulties in clinical differentiation from the chronic mild variants of manic–depressive disease. However, the longitudinal pattern of early-onset antisocial record in a variety of areas (DSM-IV) will provide discrimination from cyclothymia, in which antisocial record is sporadic or absent (Akiskal et al., 1979).

Case 9

A 38-year-old divorced man was seen in a public mental health clinic for a renewal of his prescription for "depression." He had been taking amitriptyline at bedtime for sleep and during the day to calm his "nerves." He made it quite clear that he would prefer a medication that would better relieve his general nervousness and muscle tension and named several benezodiazepines and other sedatives. His medical record indicated that he had abused and probably been physically dependent on at least two of these drugs in the past. When specifically asked, he admitted this, although he denied that he had ever had a problem with alcohol or with other types of drugs. He had taken amphetamines before and said that they helped him when he drove trucks (which is how he supported himself intermittently).

He said that he had been "depressed" much of his life, particularly since his early teenage years, and that he had had occasional panic attacks in the past but they were no longer a problem. He also reported fears of animals, particularly police dogs. He thought that a lot of his dysphoria had to do with his frequently unfavorable life circumstances. He had been in prison after having been apprehended in what was, by his account, the only major crime he ever committed (selling drugs). However, past records indicated that he had, on numerous occasions, falsified signatures of his sisters and girlfriends on checks.

He said that prison had been particularly depressing. His medical records indicated that while in prison he had received negative medical workups for headaches, a buzzing sensation in one ear, spells of unconsciousness associated with urinary and fecal incontinence but without seizurelike shaking, abdominal gas pains associated with nausea and numerous food intolerances, and chronic low-back pain and pains in the hips and knees, and that he had sought treatment or had been prescribed medication for many other minor ailments. He had been briefly married four times and had two children whom he neglected financially and did not wish to visit. Although he denied that he had ever been aggressive or violent and said that he had never physically harmed anyone, past records indicated he had physically abused each one of the women he had married.

Although multiple somatization is not uncommon in those with sociopathic life-styles, it is even more characteristic of somatization disorder. Indeed, a lifelong tendency to develop physical or mental symptoms that bring them special favors from others is the hallmark of those with this disorder. In some cases, particularly in men, the goal may be obvious—to obtain money or free services, to escape legal judgments or incarceration, or to avoid military service. In others, the "secondary gains" may be less obvious—perhaps increased attention and consideration from a spouse or an excuse to avoid usual obligations. The natural tendency of people to accord preferential "sick-role" status to those who are disabled by illness may be regarded by manipulative or predatory individuals as a natural resource to be exploited.

As clinicians, we cannot reliably determine the somatizing individuals' true motivation; therefore, somatization disorder is identified not by its presumed etiology but by its pattern of symptoms. The somatizers who can be identified with a high degree of reliability are those who have had so many physical and emotional symptoms over the years that no other diagnosis or combination of diagnoses can plausibly account for them all. DSM-IV requires different symptoms affecting several systems (neurological, digestive, genitourinary, and pain), associated with a lifelong pattern of "sickliness." Antisocial behavior is also common in these patients; so is fluctuating dysphoria. It should be noted that patients with mood disorder also often become hypochondriacal but typically lack such preoccupation before the onset of depression; because they may not remember this absence of preoccupation when they are depressed, the past history should be obtained from a reliable informant. Some patients with somatization disorder will give themselves away by admitting to multiple past pseudoneurological conversion symptoms, but many have become too smart for that. Some will still show *la belle indifférence* toward their symptoms or seem to be enjoying themselves too much for their reported symptoms to be credible. A history of juvenile or adult antisocial symptoms also tips the diagnosis toward somatization disorder.

Because of their tempestuous life histories and rapid mood shifts, this group can be easily confused with cyclothymic conditions. But a detailed history, as exemplified in the next case, would suggest otherwise.

Case 10

The patient, a 31-year-old divorced woman, was admitted through the emergency room at night because of urges to kill herself. She reported that she had been feeling "depressed and suicidal" for 2 weeks because of conflicts at work. On being questioned, she said that her energy had been low and she had lost a few pounds, that she had "lost all interest" in social activities, that she was feeling "very guilty" and "worthless," but that her sleep had not been disturbed. She said that she had been feeling hopeless, pessimistic, worried, irritable, hostile, and suspicious. She had been "worrying" about her health and reported nausea and vomiting and a general increase in aches and panic and "bad sensations" in her body. Her medical records indicated that she had recently had an extensive evaluation for "intractable seizures," yet no evidence of seizure disorder had been found. When asked about other neurological symptoms, she said that she had at various times had loss of all sensation in parts of her body, had lost her voice, and had experienced difficulty walking, paralysis, loss of consciousness, and double vision. She denied episodes of blindness or deafness. She reported past serious problems with dysmenorrhea. She said she had never climaxed during sex with men. She reported being bothered by visual hallucinations—typically of insects crawling on her. When specifically asked, she said she had felt that others were talking about her and harassing her. She denied sustained periods of elevated mood, but did report short periods (4 to 5 hours at a time) of unusually irritable and dysphoric mood, associated with hyperactivity, uninhibited behavior, and uncontrollable anger. In response to specific questions, she said she had been having "panic attacks" for the past 6 months. On closer scrutiny, the symptom pattern was revealed to be faintness, shakiness, restlessness, and hot flashes. She also reported general anxiety for the past 2 months and long-standing fear of crowds with some avoidance, which she said had not particularly interfered with her functioning.

She admitted past problems with alcohol, including memory blackouts, and objections of friends to her drinking. Her heavy drinking had begun at age 17 and ended by her mid-20s. She said she had not abused street drugs but had once been addicted to oxazepam. When specifically asked, she reported that she had several juvenile antisocial problems, beginning at age 10 or 12, including truancy, running away from home, and shoplifting.

She was specifically asked about each adult antisocial symptom in DSM-IV and denied them all. She had been divorced twice and said she had had pelvic inflammatory disease once, though she said this could not have been sexually transmitted as she claimed she had never had any sexual contact before its onset.

Despite the extreme number of symptoms she reported, she did not look particularly disturbed; one could describe her as "drowsy" and "dissatisfied." In the hospital, she twice signed requests for discharge against medical advice, but withdrew them after long talks with a doctor. She also requested and received several hours of supportive psychotherapy from various nurses. In spite of her threats to leave the hospital and kill herself, she resisted transfer to a locked ward. Within the next few days, the told another of her doctors that she had just remembered that she had been raped when she was 14. She said she had previously totally suppressed this, but the questions regarding her gynecological history (which included pelvic inflammatory disease) brought it all back.

At this stage, both her family and employer had telephoned to warn that she was "an extremely convincing and shameless liar." She had worked for a medical clinic and had just been fired for stealing confidential patient records, tranquilizers, uniforms, and equipment. Her family said that she had been writing many "bad checks" and, to the best of their knowledge, had neither been raped nor had pelvic inflammatory disease. She had been a very troublesome child and had been taken to various specialists for "incorrigibility" since before age 10 and had been hospitalized for a year as a juvenile because of these behaviors.

She was an avid reader of psychology and medical texts, and tended to "catch" diseases she read about, most recently bulimia and premenstrual tension. She also wondered if she was a "lesbian" as she believed the female psychiatric resident entrusted to her care was "making passes" at her. Despite her negative seizure evaluation, she had told the examining psychiatrist that the exam had in fact been positive for four different kinds of "amnestic seizures" that were all very rare in that there was no electroencephalographic evidence of seizures except during the actual seizures. She had vaguely indicated that during her periods of amnesia she did bad things—such as "unnatural sex acts"—that others later told her about. She had also begun to talk about there being two people in her, a "good one" and "a bad one," who were fighting. Her mother said that when told of things she had done, she very convincingly denied all memory of them, but when pressed with evidence, would give good indications that she actually did remember and would then lose her temper, "go berserk," or run away.

Cases 9 and 10 are presented to illustrate the fact that a chief complaint of mood disturbance does not necessarily reflect a primary mood disorder. Labeling patients with such complaints "borderline personality" does not clarify the situation either.

Reliability and Validity

Structured interview schedules for mood disorders—of which the best known is the Schedule for the Affective Disorders and Schizophrenia based on the Research Diagnostic Criteria (Spitzer, Endicott, & Robins, 1979)—were designed to provide instruments for investigating the psychopathology and nosology of affective disorders and their differentiation from boundary conditions. Such instruments have achieved acceptable reliability in the hands of relatively inexperienced clinicians who have undergone training in their rigorous application, making them suitable for use in clinical research. However, at this writing, these instruments are best regarded as exploratory tools. Their main limitations are as follows:

1. The validity of the nosological concepts that they embody is uncertain.
2. Questions are asked in a more or less "standard" manner, which would preclude delving into phenomenological subtleties.
3. They do not incorporate—or are not sufficiently detailed regarding—many categories commonly encountered in clinical work, e.g., anxious depressions, chronic mood disorder subtypes, and milder forms in the bipolar spectrum.
4. Rare but treatable forms of mood disorder—i.e., those due to a specific toxin or physical disease—are not specifically inquired about.
5. Such an interview cannot be conducted in severe forms of mood disorders, or when the patient is uncooperative.

For these reasons, the authors prefer semistructured interviews, in which there is adherence to rigorous diagnostic criteria but greater freedom for the patient and the interviewer to express or inquire about subtleties of affective experience and behavior. We have developed such a schedule—the Mood Clinic Data Questionnaire (MCDQ)—that is particularly suitable for ambulatory mood disorders (Akiskal et al., 1978). The use of this instrument requires phenomenological sophistication; it should therefore be administered by a psychiatrist, a clinical psychologist, or a social worker with clinical experience. Its intercenter reliability and utility for transnational clinical research have been shown in Italian adaptation on over 1000 patients studied in Pisa (Cassano et al., 1992).

The beginning clinician must remember that an affective diagnosis—or *any* diagnosis—is not just a collection of signs and symptoms that have reached a certain threshold of severity and duration. If this were the case, mood-rating instruments that assess severity of depression, such as the Beck Depression Inventory (Beck, 1967) or the Hamilton Rating Scale for Depression (Hamilton, 1960), would suffice, and there would be no need for diagnostic interviewing. (These instruments merely measure the *severity* of the depressive syndrome in an individual who is known to be suffering from a mood disorder.) Clinical judgment is required in assessing whether individual signs and symptoms are present; whether, *taken together*, they constitute a coherent mood disorder; and whether appropriate exclusion criteria are met. Finally, the presence of mood disorder must be validated by certain external validating strategies such as familial aggregation of illness, laboratory tests, treatment response, and course (Feighner et al., 1972).

For the clinician, the most important validation is the ability of a diagnosis to predict treatment response and course or prognosis. For the researcher, familial and laboratory markers are often more significant because they are potentially useful in construct validity. It must also be kept in mind, however, that parameters that help in construct validation may also prove useful in predicting treatment response. Further discussion of these issues is beyond the scope of this chapter, and the interested reader is referred to monographs devoted, respectively, to general diagnostic considerations and measurement of depression (Akiskal & Webb, 1978; Marsella, Hirschfeld, & Katz, 1987).

Interview Probes

Diagnostic interviewing should not be overly directive to avoid projecting symptoms onto a suggestible individual. The questions should be asked neutrally, without obvious response expectation. For instance, one should not phrase questions in a judgmental or leading manner, as, "You're not suicidal, are you?" The far more common problem is, unfortunately, not asking about such important matters at all.

If the dominant affect is one of milder depression mixed with anxiety, muscle tension, tremulousness, blushing or pallor, perspiration, mental overarousal, jumpiness, a tendency to startle easily, and fearfulness, and if frank psychomotor agitation is not evident, an *anxious depression* (major depression or dysthymia with panic attacks, phobias, or obsessive preoccupations) is the likely diagnosis. These patients are more likely to report chronic and unremitting anxiety and depressed mood, trouble falling asleep and poor quality of sleep, poor appetite or weight loss, and hypochondriacal preoccupations with their health—but typically not of delusional proportion. A subgroup of these patients display "reverse" vegetative signs—such as early insomnia, daytime or morning hypersomnolence, hyperphagia, and feeling worse in the evening—and are contrasted to those with retarded or agitated melancholia. The occurrence of panic attacks during the period of depression appears to be the best single indicator of anxious depression, but a combination of other anxiety symptoms may also help in pointing to this subtype. The cross-sectional differentiating clinical features of anxiety and depressive states are summarized in Table 4.

Table 4.   Cross-Sectional Differentiating Clinical
Features of Anxiety and Depressive States[a]

Anxiety	Depressive states
Hypervigilance	Psychomotor retardation
Severe tension and panic	Severe sadness
Perceived danger	Perceived loss
Phobic avoidance	Loss of interest—anhedonia
Doubt and uncertainty	Hopelessness—suicidal
Insecurity	Self-depreciation
Performance anxiety	Loss of libido
	Early morning awakening
	Weight loss

[a]According to Akiskal (1990).

Other patients complain of depression and anxiety, but do not look particularly anxious or depressed. Some will report "profound depression" for brief periods (hours or days), but their appearance would be one of *la belle indifférence*. This inconsistent affect suggests a personality disorder such as somatization disorder. This disorder—which can mimic every other mental and physical illness—also gives rise to depressive complaints. These patients should be asked about a variety of past physical symptoms (DSM-IV): lifelong sickliness; neurological symptoms such as past episodes of blindness, paralysis, amnesia, or seizures; abdominal pains and vomiting; menstrual symptoms; lifelong sexual dysfunction; bodily pains; headaches; and heart or breathing symptoms. In some cases, they will also report fleeting hallucinations, binge eating followed by vomiting, drug or alcohol abuse, and antisocial symptoms. What is diagnostic is a collection of ominous sounding symptoms without the signs that would normally accompany them if a known physical disease were present. Usually, these patients will report "continuous" anxiety and depression, but collateral information will rarely provide objective evidence for such moods. They tend to be vain, egocentric, flamboyant, and theatrical, characteristics that are distinguished from those of hypomania in that they denote a lack of emotional warmth. These patients should be asked about their relationships, which are likely to have been troubled and marked by overdependence, manipulativeness, and aggressive behavior. Any history of more flagrant antisocial behavior leading to arrests is more reliably obtained from records, since such individuals categorically deny such behavior.

The major differential diagnosis of depressions in somatizing and antisocial types is from anxious depressions, dysthymic disorder, and cyclothymia. Often, individuals with severe personality disorder abuse substances that can, during withdrawal, produce a mixture of anxiety and depressive symptoms. In addition, they invite life situations that can augment their dysphoric states. By contrast, in cyclothymic and dysthymic disorders, the personality disturbances are secondary to subsyndromal affective instability (Akiskal et al., 1977; Akiskal, 1983, 1994a). A careful longitudinal history will reveal that mood swing may have begun much earlier than the interpersonal difficulties. Some of these patients meet the DSM-IV criteria for borderline personality disorder, which further clouds differential diagnosis. However, current data indicate that a significant proportion of these patients represent variants of mood disorder, most commonly dysthymic or cyclothymic disorders or protracted mixed states (Akiskal, 1981; Akiskal, Yerevanian, Davis, King, & Lemmi, 1985b; Stone, 1979); dysphoric restlessness or *irritability* is a common thread that runs through these conditions, many of which seem to be on the border of bipolar illness. The most important distinctions from nonaffective personality disorders are that the course is different, in that affective manifestations preceded the personality difficulties, though this chronology is not always easy to document; that affective manifestations are sustained from a few days to a week, rather than just hours; and that affective symptoms often come "out of the blue," cannot be accounted for by substance abuse, and typically do not disappear when social rewards are provided. The self-report inventory by Depue et al. (1981) has been used in research studies for identifying cyclothymic individuals, but its utility for clinical diagnostic workup remains uncertain.

Related to cyclothymia—and likewise confused with personality disorder—are patients with the Bipolar II disorder (Akiskal, 1981, 1994a). The tempestuous biographies of these individuals are superimposed on a pattern of recurrent retarded depressive episodes of relatively short duration (4–12 weeks) and mild hypomanic periods of brief duration (2–7 days). In other words, these patients overlap with cyclothymics except that the depressive episodes are clinically disabling due to the fact that they are of full syndromal depth and tend to last weeks to months. Because hypomania in these patients is often pleasant and adaptive, they do not complain about it or seek help during such times. Thus, the presence of hypomania is ascertained typically by history and requires skilled interviewing. Table 5 summarizes criteria developed in our mood clinic for distinguishing hypomania from normal happiness (Akiskal, 1983b). Most important, hypomania—which constitutes a defining characteristic of bipolar II disorder—is a recurrent condition; happiness is not!

Because bipolar patients often deny past psychopathology, the history of past retarded depression or excited periods is best obtained from someone who has known the patient for a long time. Regarding current mania and hypomania, it is useful to ask about sleep, i.e., whether there has been a recent change and whether less sleep than usual is needed. Expansive grandiosity is best assessed by asking questions about indirect indicators—whether there has been a recent increase in spending, newly developed great plans for the future, a dramatic change in sexual appetite and prowess, or a recent increase in drinking without the usual degree of impairment. Again, most reliable information regarding such behavior comes from significant others. The affect of frank mania is easy to recognize. The infectious exuberant energy of these patients is qualitatively different from anything seen in ordinary human beings or those with primary characterological disorders.

Mania is more difficult to recognize when it progresses to a psychotic stage or a mixed episode, in which irritability, dysphoria, and hostility often replace euphoria; delusions, hallucinations, and thinking disturbances are likely to be observed (Akiskal & Puzantian, 1979). In some patients at the height of mania, as well as those during mixed bipolar states, both mood-congruent and mood-incongruent delusions and hallucinations can dominate the clinical picture (see Chapter 2). These patients can be difficult to differentiate cross-sectionally from those with acute exacerbations of schizophrenia. Their frenzied activity actually makes them seem more psychotic than patients with schizophrenia (Goodwin & Jamison, 1990). These irritable paranoid or delusional manics—who often meet the criteria of a *mixed* or *dysphoric manic* episode—can become assaultive with minimal

---

TABLE 5.   Setting the Threshold for Clinical Hypomania[a]

1. Has a "driven" quality.
2. Tends to be labile.
3. Tends to impair social judgment.
4. Is often preceded or followed by retarded depression.
5. Typically springs from familial background for bipolar disorder.

[a]Modified from Akiskal (1983b).

provocation and are best interviewed briefly and in the presence of assistants trained in physical restraint of the mentally ill.

Thus, the definitive diagnosis of primary bipolar mood disorder is established by obtaining an outside history—from family, friends, or old psychiatric records—for an episodic course of illness with periods of recovery from psychotic symptoms, by a past history of more typical episodes of mania and depression, and by a lack of psychotic symptoms during periods when neither mania nor depression was present.

SUMMARY

Although recent approaches using psychometric, family history, pharmacological-response, neuroendocrine, and neurophysiological techniques have provided new and provocative ways to supplement the diagnostic process, phenomenological diagnosis remains the solid foundation of the clinical and research endeavor. Diagnosis of depression and mania and their subtypes is based on observed signs and reported symptoms. The core signs and symptoms of depression are depressed mood and appetite and sleep changes; loss of interest, energy, self-esteem, memory, and concentration; thoughts of death or suicide; and psychomotor agitation or retardation. Additional features or a preponderance of certain features will suggest a particular subtype of depression. Anxiety often coexists with depression and creates problems in differential diagnosis. Mania is characterized by euphoric or irritable mood, increased energy, hyperactivity, racing thoughts, pressured speech, flight of ideas, grandiosity, decreased need for sleep, and disinhibited behavior. Subtypes of bipolar disorder—in which depression and mania alternate or coexist—are identified by severity and by associated psychotic symptoms. As interpersonal disturbances commonly occur in the setting of depressive and bipolar disorders, differentiating them from primary characterological disorders is often problematic.

This chapter has elaborated on the distinction between primary mood disorders and depressive states that are secondary to, or represent complications of, anxiety and personality disorders. Such differentiation is important for reasons of predictive and construct validity. In brief, the clinician must distinguish between affective subtypes because of differential treatment implications, whereas the clinical investigator must specify the subtype that he or she wishes to examine for hypothesis testing. Unfortunately, many researchers testing etiological hypotheses or the efficacy of various treatment approaches in depression do not always specify whether their study populations conform to primary mood disorder or represent depressive states in the setting of nonaffective disorders. In particular, the DSM-IV construct of "major depression" is too broad, too easy to meet, and rather heterogeneous. Future research in mood disorders should pay greater attention to validate specific major depressive subtypes. The evidence reviewed in this chapter indicates that some major depressions are related to bipolar illness, whereas others are related to anxiety disorders. In still a third group, mood disturbances are woven into the habitual self of the patient in the form of cyclothymic and dysthymic temperaments. This problematic boundary with personality disorders represents one of the principal challenges for future clinical research in the field of mood disorders.

One of the paradoxes of current clinical conceptualization of mood disorders (e.g., that reflected in DSM-IV) is the assumption that personality disorder is distinct from the affective dimension. This distinction is usually meant to imply that patients with "primitive" personality disorders—e.g., borderline, histrionic, and sociopathic—do not suffer from affective disorders or, worse, that they don't suffer at all (but make others suffer). By contrast, anxious–obsessoid, dysthymic, and cyclothymic types are accorded some or full affective status. It should be nonetheless obvious to the reader that this convention creates many paradoxes, especially as it pertains to the subclassification of nonpsychotic, nonmelancholic, and other than manic–depressive depressions. This leaves us with the large universe of anxious, atypical, and soft bipolar patients with varying degrees and types of personality or temperamental pathology. One of the authors has argued elsewhere (Akiskal, 1990, 1992a,b, 1994a) that these largely outpatient major depressives can most profitably be defined jointly by temperamental–personality traits and associated phenomenological features, providing distinct longitudinal patterns (which, with the exception of "double depressions," are quite distinct from the proposed DSM-IV longitudinal patterns):

- Dysthymic traits: Double depressions
- Anxious–phobic traits: Anxious depressions
- Cyclothymic traits: Bipolar II
- Hyperthymic traits: Pseudounipolar depressions
- Irritable traits: Hostile depressions

These longitudinal patterns, which represent suggestions for future research, are presented here to make sense in areas in which the DSM-IV schema is relatively inarticulate. The specific personality disorders listed on the Axis II of DSM-IV have not been particularly useful in the subclassification of depressions (Akiskal, 1992a). The foregoing schema is constructed on the basis of longitudinal prospective research in mood disorders that suggests that subaffective and major affective manifestations often occur on a continuum in the same individual. Among the potential benefits of such a schema is its ability to accommodate both psychological and biological levels of conceptualization.

It would be instructive in this regard to consider clinical depression arising from antecedent dysthymia and hyperthymia. Biological disturbances reflected in vegetative and limbic–diencephalic dysfunction (Akiskal & McKinney, 1975; Goodwin & Jamison, 1990) largely characterize major depressive states; contrary to clinical lore, the more familial of these disorders tend to arise from a dysthymic base, supported by recent research that has shown major depressions with the "double-depressive" pattern to be more familial (Akiskal & Weise, 1992). As for attributional biases (Abramson, Seligman, & Teasdale, 1978) reflected in a depressive cognitive set, they seem to characterize the dysthymic phase of the illness and exacerbate further during major episodes. The "brooding" or "ruminative" cognitive style, which is more commonly observed among females (Perugi et al., 1990;

Nolen-Hoeksema, Morrow, & Frederickson, 1993) and which seems to be a correlate of dysthymia, might in part explain the higher incidence of depression in women; it might be even more relevant in explaining why women recover more slowly from depression (Frank, Carpenter, & Kupfer, 1988) and thereby spend more time in depression (this being one of the possible mechanisms for the higher prevalence of depression in women). By contrast, males, who tend to use more "active" or "hyperthymic" styles of dealing with their depressions (Perugi et al., 1990; Nolen-Hoeksema et al., 1993), might spend less time in depression (possibly accounting for the lower incidence and prevalence of depression in men).

Much research needs to be conducted to validate such formulations. They have been presented here to argue for the heuristic value of subclassifying depressions on the basis of subaffective traits. Obviously, the eager student interested in understanding depressive behavior should first learn the more objective descriptive paradigm presented in the chapter at large.

References

Abramson, L. Y., Seligman, M. E., & Teasdale, J. D. (1978). Learned helplessness in humans: Critique and reformulation. *Journal of Abnormal Psychology, 87*, 49–74.

Akiskal, H. S. (1981). Subaffective disorders: Dysthymic, cyclothymic, and bipolar II disorders in the borderline "realm." *Psychiatric Clinics of North America, 4*, 25–46.

Akiskal, H. S. (1983a). The bipolar spectrum: New concepts in classification and diagnosis. In L. Grinspoon (Ed.), *Psychiatry update: The American Psychiatric Association annual review* (pp. 271–292). Washington, DC: American Psychiatric Press.

Akiskal, H. S. (1983b). Diagnosis and classification of affective disorders: New insights from clinical and laboratory approaches. *Psychiatric Developments, 1*, 123–160.

Akiskal, H. S. (1983c). Dysthymic disorder: Psychopathology of proposed chronic depressive subtypes. *American Journal of Psychiatry, 140*, 11–20.

Akiskal, H. S. (1990). Toward a clinical understanding of the relationship of anxiety and depressive disorders. In J. Maser & R. Cloninger (Eds.), *Comorbidity in anxiety and mood disorders*. Washington, DC: American Psychiatric Press.

Akiskal, H. S. (1992a). Delineating irritable and hyperthymic variants of the cyclothymic temperament. *Journal of Personality Disorders, 6*, 326–342.

Akiskal, H. S. (1992b). Mood disorders. In R. Berkow (Ed.), *Merck manual of diagnosis and therapy* (pp. 1592–1614). Rahway, NJ: Merck, Sharp, & Dohme Research Laboratories.

Akiskal, H. S. (1994a). Dysthymic and cyclothymic depressions: Therapeutic considerations. *Journal of Clinical Psychiatry, 55* (4 suppl.), 46–52.

Akiskal, H. S. (1994b). Mood disturbances. In G. Winokur & P. Clayton (Eds.), *Medical basis of psychiatry* (pp. 365–379). Philadelphia: W.B. Saunders.

Akiskal, H. S., & Akiskal, K. (1988). Re-assessing the prevalence of bipolar disorders: Clinical significance and artistic creativity. *Psychiatrie et Psychobiologie, 3*, 29s–36s.

Akiskal, H. S., Bitar, A. H., Puzantian, V. R., Rosenthal, T. L., & Walker, P. W. (1978). The nosological status of neurotic depression: A prospective three- to four-year follow-up examination in light of the primary–secondary and unipolar–bipolar dichotomies. *Archives of General Psychiatry, 35*, 756–766.

Akiskal, H. S., Djenderedjian, A. H., Rosenthal, R. H., & Khani, M. K. (1977). Cyclothymic disorder: Validating criteria for inclusion in the bipolar affective group. *American Journal of Psychiatry, 134*, 1227–1233.

Akiskal, H. S., Downs, J., Jordan, P., Watson, S., Daugherty, D., & Pruitt, D. B. (1985). Affective disorders in referred children and younger siblings of manic–depressives: Mode of onset and prospective course. *Archives of General Psychiatry, 42*, 996–1003.

Akiskal, H. S., Khani, M. K., & Scott-Strauss, A. (1979). Cyclothymic temperamental disorders. *Psychiatric Clinics of North America*, 2, 527–554.

Akiskal, H. S., & Lemmi, H. (1987). Sleep EEG findings bearing on the relationship of anxiety and depressive disorders. In G. Racagani & I. Smeraldi (Eds.), *Anxious depression: Assessment and treatment* (pp. 153–159). New York: Raven Press.

Akiskal, H. S., & McKinney, W. T., Jr. (1975). Overview of recent research in depression: Integration of ten conceptual models into a comprehensive clinical frame. *Archives of General Psychiatry*, 32, 285–305.

Akiskal, H. S., & Puzantian, V. R. (1979). Psychotic forms of depression and mania. *Psychiatric Clinics of North American*, 2, 419–439.

Akiskal, H. S., Rosenthal, T. L., Haykal, R. F., Lemmi, H., Rosenthal, R. H., & Scott-Strauss, A. (1980). Characterological depressions: Clinical and sleep EEG findings separating "subaffective dysthymias" from "character spectrum disorders." *Archives of General Psychiatry*, 37, 777–783.

Akiskal, H. S., Walker, P., Puzantian, V. R., King, D., Rosenthal, T. L., & Dranon, M. (1983). Bipolar outcome in the course of depressive illness: Phenomenologic, familial, and pharmacologic predictors. *Journal of Affective Disorders*, 5, 115–128.

Akiskal, H. S., & Webb, W. L. (Eds.) (1978). *Psychiatric diagnosis: Exploration of biological predictors*. New York: Spectrum.

Akiskal, H. S., & Weise, R. E. (1992). The clinical spectrum of so-called "minor" depression. *American Journal of Psychotherapy*, 46, 9–22.

Akiskal, H. S., Yerevanian, B. I., Davis, G. C., King, D. & Lemmi, H. (1985). The nosologic status of borderline personality: Clinical and polysomnographic study. *American Journal of Psychiatry*, 142, 192–198.

Andreasen, N. J., & Canter, A. (1974). The creative writer: Psychiatric symptoms and family history. *Comprehensive Psychiatry*, 15, 123–131.

American Psychiatric Association (1994). *Diagnostic and statistical manual of mental disorders* 4th ed. Washington, DC: Author.

Ban, T. A. (1989). *Composite diagnostic evaluation of depressive disorders*. Brentwood, TN: JM Productions.

Beck, A. T. (1967). *Depression: Clinical, experimental and theoretical aspects*. New York: Harper & Row.

Carroll, B. J. (1982). Clinical applications of the dexamethasone suppression test for endogenous depression. *Pharmacopsychiatria*, 15, 19–25.

Cassano, G. B., Akiskal, H. S., Savino, M., Musetti, L., & Perugi, G. (1992). Proposed subtypes of bipolar II and related disorders: With hypomanic episodes (or cyclothymia) and with hyperthymic temperament. *Journal of Affective Disorders*, 26, 127–140.

Cassano, G. B., Perugi, G., Musetti, L., & Akiskal, H. S. (1989). The nature of depression presenting concomitantly with panic disorder. *Comprehensive Psychiatry*, 30, 473–482.

Castello, C. G. (1993). *Symptoms of depression*. New York: John Wiley.

Coryell, W., Endicott, J., Andreasen, N. C., Keller, M. B., Clayton, P. J., Hirschfeld, R. M., Scheftner, W. A., & Winokur, G. (1988). Depression and panic attacks: The significance of overlap as reflected in follow-up and family study data. *American Journal of Psychiatry*, 145, 293–300.

Davidson, J. R., Miller, R. D., Turnbull, C. D., & Sullivan, J. L. (1982). Atypical depression. *Archives of General Psychiatry*, 39, 527–534.

Depue, R. A., Slater, J. R., Wolfsetter-Kaush, M., Klein, D., Coplerud, E., & Farr, D. (1981). A biobehavioral paradigm for identifying persons at risk for bipolar depressive disorders: A conceptual framework and five validation studies. *Journal of Abnormal Psychology Monograph*, 90, 381–437.

Feighner, J. P., Robins, E., Guze, S. B., Woodruff, R. A., Jr., Winokur, G., & Munoz, R. (1972). Diagnostic criteria for use in psychiatric research. *Archives of General Psychiatry*, 26, 57–63.

Fieve, R. R., & Dunner, D. L. (1975). Unipolar and bipolar affective states. In F. Flach & S. Draghi (Eds.), *The nature and treatment of depression* (pp. 145–160). New York: John Wiley.

Frank, E., Carpenter, L. L., & Kupfer, D. J. (1988). Sex differences in recurrent depression: Are there any that are significant? *American Journal of Psychiatry*, 145, 41–45.

Goodwin, D. W., & Guze, S. B. (1989). *Psychiatric diagnosis*, 4th ed. New York: Oxford University Press.

Goodwin, F. K., & Jamison, K. R. (1990). *Manic–depressive illness*. New York: Oxford University Press.

Hamilton, M. (1960). A rating scale for depression. *Journal of Neurology, Neurosurgery and Psychiatry*, 23, 56–62.

Himmelhoch, J. M., Mulla, D., Neil, J. F., Detre, T. P., & Kupfer, D. J (1976). Incidence and significance of mixed affective states in a bipolar population. *Archives of General Psychiatry, 33,* 1062–1066.

Keller, M. B., Lavori, P. W., Endicott, J., Coryell, W., & Klerman, G. L. (1983). "Double depression": Two-year follow-up. *American Journal of Psychiatry, 140,* 689–694.

Kendler, K. S., Kessler, R. C., Neale, M. C., Heath, A. C., & Eaves, L. J. (1993). The prediction of major depression in women: Toward an integrated etiologic model. *American Journal of Psychiatry, 150,* 1139–1148.

Klein, D. N., Taylor, E. B., Harding, K., & Dickstein, S. (1988). Double depression and episodic major depression: Demographic, clinical, familial, personality, and socioenvironmental characteristics and short-term outcome. *American Journal of Psychiatry, 145,* 1226–1231.

Klerman, G. L., Lavori, P. W., Rice, J., Reich, T., Endicott, J., Andreasen, N. C., Keller, M. B., & Hirschfeld, R. M. (1985). Birth-cohort trends in rates of major depressive disorder among relatives of patients with affective disorder. *Archives of General Psychiatry, 42,* 689–693.

Kraepelin, E. (1921). *Manic–depressive insanity and paranoia* (G. M. Robertson, Ed., & R. M. Barclay, Trans.). Edinburgh: E. S. Livingstone.

Kupfer, D J., Pickar, D., Himmelhoch, J. M., & Detre, T. P. (1975). Are there two types of unipolar depression? *Archives of General Psychiatry, 32,* 866–871.

Kupfer, D. J., & Thase, M. E. (1983). The use of the sleep laboratory in the diagnosis of affective disorders. *Psychiatric Clinics of North America, 6,* 3–25.

Lewinsohn, P. M., Rhode, P., Seeley, J. R., & Hops, H. (1991). Comorbidity of unipolar depression. I. Major depression with dysthymia. *Journal of Abnormal Psychology, 100,* 205–213.

Liebowitz, M. R., & Klein, D. F. (1979). Hysteroid dysphoria. *Psychiatric Clinics of North America, 2,* 555–575.

Marsella, A. J., Hirschfeld, R. M. A., & Katz, M. M. (Eds.) (1987). *The measurement of depression.* New York: Guilford Press.

Maser, J. D., & Cloninger, C. R. (Eds.) (1990). *Comorbidity of mood and anxiety disorders.* Washington, DC: American Psychiatric Press.

Nolen-Hoeksema, S., Morrow, J., & Fredrickson, B. L. (1993). Response styles and the duration of episodes of depressed mood. *Journal of Abnormal Psychology, 102,* 20–28.

Perugi, G., Musetti, L., Simonini, E., Piagentini, F., Cassano, G. B., & Akiskal, H. S. (1990). Gender-mediated clinical features of depressive illness: The importance of temperamental differences. *British Journal of Psychiatry, 157,* 835–841.

Rapee, R. M., & Barlow, D. H. (1991). *Chronic anxiety: Generalized anxiety disorder and mixed anxiety–depression.* New York: Guilford Press.

Robins, E., & Guze, S. B. (1972). Classification of affective disorders—The primary–secondary, the endogenous–reactive and neurotic–psychotic concepts. In T. A. Williams, M. M. Katz, & J. S. Shields (Eds.), *Recent advances in psychobiology of the depressive illnesses* (pp. 283–293). Washington, DC: U.S. Government Printing Office.

Sargant, W., & Dally, P. (1962). Treatment of anxiety states by antidepressant drugs. *British Medical Journal,* 6–9.

Spitzer, R., Endicott, J., & Robins, E. (1979). *Research diagnostic criteria (RDC) for a selected group of functional disorders,* 4th ed. New York: Biometrics Research Division, New York Psychiatric Institute.

Stone, M. H. (1979). Contemporary shift of the borderline concept from a schizophrenic disorder to subaffective disorder. *Psychiatric Clinics of North America, 3,* 517–594.

Van Valkenburg, C., Akiskal, H. S., Puzantian, V., & Rosenthal, T. (1984). Anxious depressions: Clinical, family history, and naturalistic outcome comparisons with panic and major depressive disorders. *Journal of Affective Disorders, 6,* 67–82.

Wells, K. B., Stewart, A., Hays, R. D., Burnam, M. A., Rogers, W., Daniels, M., Berry, S., Greenfield, S., & Ware, J. (1989). The functioning and well-being of depressed patients: Results from the Medical Outcomes Study. *Journal of the American Medical Association, 262,* 914–919.

5

Schizophrenia

STEVEN L. SAYERS AND KIM T. MUESER

DESCRIPTION OF THE DISORDER

Schizophrenia is a complex and confusing illness that can baffle family members, friends, the patient, and mental health professionals alike. Schizophrenia can be contrasted to psychiatric illnesses such as major depression, manic–depression, and anxiety disorders that were described long ago by Hippocrates as common behavioral disturbances. Schizophrenia has been recognized only over the past 100 years as a separate illness with its own unique pattern of onset, symptomatology, course, and treatment. The diagnosis of schizophrenia can be complicated by two important factors: First, the symptoms of the illness overlap with those of many other disorders (e.g., affective disorders, substance abuse), requiring careful attention to issues of differential diagnosis. Second, patient self-report is critical to establishing the diagnosis of schizophrenia, yet many patients deny the characteristic symptoms or are inconsistent in their report of these internal experiences. While there are difficulties inherent in the assessment of schizophrenia, accurate diagnosis has important implications for pharmacological and psychosocial intervention for the disorder. Indeed, misdiagnosis can result in ineffective treatment and a poor outcome. In order to accurately diagnose schizophrenia, the interviewer must possess an adequate fund of knowledge about the psychopathology of the illness, the relative merits of available assessment instruments, interviewing techniques, and methods for obtaining information necessary for the assessment. We begin this chapter with an overview of the nature of schizophrenia, including its prevalence, course, and outcome, followed by a review of its symptomatology and the criteria for its diagnosis.

STEVEN L. SAYERS • Medical College of Pennsylvania at Eastern Pennsylvania Psychiatric Institute, Philadelphia, Pennsylvania 19129.   KIM T. MUESER • Dartmouth Medical School, Hanover, New Hampshire 03301.

Diagnostic Interviewing (Second Edition), edited by Michel Hersen and Samuel M. Turner. Plenum Press, New York, 1994.

Basic Facts about Schizophrenia

Schizophrenia is a severe adult psychiatric illness that has pervasive effects on patients' interpersonal relationships, ability to work, and self-care skills. Evidence suggests that schizophrenia is a biological illness that can be precipitated or made worse by environmental stress. Family studies indicate that the vulnerability to developing the illness is determined partly by genetic factors, with concordance ratios of schizophrenia in monozygotic twins ranging from 15% to 75% (Walker, Downey, & Caspi, 1991). The causes of schizophrenia are not known at this time, but major theories hypothesize that symptoms are the result of an imbalance in brain neurotransmitters, structural brain anomalies, or altered blood flow and activation of specific brain regions (Buchsbaum, 1990; Crow, 1990).

The lifetime risk for developing schizophrenia is approximately 1%, which is consistent across gender, different cultures, and countries. Persons from lower socioeconomic classes appear to be at increased vulnerability to develop schizophrenia and other psychiatric disorders (Bruce, Takeuchi, & Leaf, 1991), a phenomenon that appears to reflect the effects of stress on precipitating onset of the illness (Fox, 1990). Schizophrenia usually develops gradually over a period of months, and in some cases years, between the ages of 16 and 30. Childhood onset of schizophrenia before the age of 12 is rare, as is onset after 35 years of age. Most people who develop schizophrenia do not show an obvious pattern of maladaptive behavior in childhood or adolescence before the onset of the illness. However, retrospective and prospective research indicates that subtle impairments in attentional processes (Cornblatt, Lenzenweger, Dworkin, & Erlenmeyer-Kimling, 1992), motor and interpersonal behavior (Walker & Lewine, 1990), and social and sexual adjustment (Zigler & Glick, 1986) often predate the onset of schizophrenia.

Once schizophrenia has developed, its longitudinal course is usually a chronic but episodic one, with the intensity of symptoms fluctuating over time. Patients with schizophrenia can usually be managed effectively in the community, with occasional inpatient hospitalizations required for the treatment of acute symptom exacerbations. Most schizophrenia patients are substantially disabled throughout their lives, even between symptom exacerbations, and require assistance in daily living, such as self-care, handling of financial matters, and the like. Over the individual's lifetime, the symptoms of schizophrenia gradually improve, and many patients experience total or partial remission in later life (Harding, Brooks, Ashikaga, Strauss, & Breier, 1987). Women with schizophrenia tend to have a more benign course of illness, characterized by a later age of onset, fewer hospitalizations, a higher rate of marriage, better social adjustment, and better social skills (Goldstein, 1988; Mueser, Bellack, Morrison, & Wade, 1990). Similarly, persons living in underdeveloped countries tend to have a less severe course of schizophrenia (Jablensky & Sartorius, 1975).

Antipsychotic medications are the pharmacological treatment of choice for schizophrenia and are useful for both the treatment of acute symptoms and the prevention of symptom relapses. Despite the undisputed efficacy of antipsychotics, the vast majority of patients continue to experience residual symptoms between episodes. The course of schizophrenia has been found to be improved by psychosocial interventions, namely, psychoeducational and behavioral family therapy (Mueser & Glynn, 1990) and social skills training (Liberman, DeRisi, & Mueser, 1989), although the durability of these treatments has not been established.

Psychopathology

The historical roots of the classification of schizophrenia are relatively modern, dating back primarily to the contributions of Kraepelin and Bleuler. Kraepelin (1919), more than any of his predecessors, is credited with distinguishing schizophrenia (which he termed *dementia praecox*) from manic–depressive illness and organic psychoses. According to Kraepelin, schizophrenia is characterized not only by the presence of specific psychotic symptoms in the absence of affective symptoms, but also by its chronic, deteriorating course, compared to the relatively stable episodic course of manic–depressive illness. Current diagnostic criteria for schizophrenia reflect Kraepelin's focus on descriptive psychopathology. While the course of schizophrenia is no longer assumed to be a deteriorating one, symptoms must be present for a minimum of 6 months to make the diagnosis according to DSM-IV draft criteria (American Psychiatric Association, 1993).

Bleuler (1950) theorized that delusions and hallucinations were secondary features of schizophrenia that were the result of primary disturbances in *affect* (flat or inappropriate), *associations* (loose or blocked), *autism* (preoccupation with fantasy), and *ambivalence* (rapid shifting from one idea or action to another). The focus on these more interpretative symptoms of schizophrenia influenced diagnostic practices particularly in the United States, where schizophrenia was for many years diagnosed less on the basis of specific symptoms than on the basis of the clinical interviewer's intuition. Bleuler's observations regarding impairments in affect and associations (i.e., disorganized speech) are included in the DSM-IV draft criteria, although their presence is not required for the diagnosis of schizophrenia.

The diagnostic criteria for schizophrenia according to the DSM-IV draft criteria are summarized in Table 1. If the characteristic symptoms have been present for more than 1 week but less than 6 months, then the person meets the criteria for schizophreniform disorder, which usually evolves into schizophrenia.

For descriptive purposes, the symptoms of schizophrenia can be divided into three broad categories: negative symptoms, positive symptoms, and affective disturbances (Kay & Sevy, 1990). *Negative symptoms* are defined by the *absence* or relative paucity of behaviors, cognitions (or cognitive abilities), or emotions that are ordinarily *present* in healthy individuals. Common negative symptoms include: *blunted/flattened affect* (diminished vocal and facial expressiveness), *anhedonia* (diminished ability to feel pleasure), *asociality* (lack of social drive and libido), *apathy*, *alogia* (poverty of speech or content of speech), *attentional impairment*, and *motor and psychomotor retardation*.

Positive symptoms are the opposite of negative symptoms, in that they are defined as the *presence* or excess of behaviors, cognitions, or perceptions ordinarily *absent* in healthy persons. The most common positive symptoms are *hallucinations* and *delusions*. Auditory hallucinations occur most frequently, followed by visual hallucinations, with tactile, olfactory, and gustatory hallucinations occurring less

TABLE 1.   DSM-IV Draft Criteria for the Diagnosis of Schizophrenia[a]

A. Presence of at least two of the following characteristic symptoms in the active phase for at least 1 month (unless the symptoms are successfully treated):
1. Delusions
2. Hallucinations
3. Disorganized speech (e.g., frequent derailment or incoherence)
4. Grossly disorganized or catatonic behavior
5. Negative symptoms (i.e., affect flattening, alogia, or avolition)
   Note: only one of these symptoms is required if delusions are bizarre or hallucinations consist of a voice keeping up a running commentary on the person's behavior or thoughts, or two or more voices conversing with each other.
B. Social/occupational dysfunction: For a significant proportion of the time from the onset of the disturbance, one or more areas of functioning, such as work, interpersonal relations, or self-care, is markedly below the level achieved prior to the onset (or, when the onset is in childhood or adolescence, failure to achieve expected level of interpersonal, academic, or occupational achievement).
C. Duration: Continuous signs of the disturbance persist for at least 6 months. This 6-month period must include at least 1 month of symptoms that meet criterion A (i.e., active-phase symptoms) and may include periods of prodromal or residual symptoms. During these prodromal or residual periods, the signs of the disturbance may be manifested by only negative symptoms or by two or more symptoms listed in criterion A present in an attenuated form (e.g., odd beliefs, unusual perceptual experiences).
D. Schizoaffective and mood disorders exclusion: Schizoaffective disorder and mood disorder with psychotic features have been ruled out because either (1) no major depressive or manic episodes have occurred concurrently with the active-phase symptoms or (2) if mood episodes have occurred during active-phase symptoms, their total duration has been brief relative to the duration of the active and residual periods.
E. Substance/general medical condition exclusion: The disturbance is not due to the direct effects of a substance (e.g., drugs of abuse, medication) or a general medical condition.

[a]Adapted from DSM-IV (APA, 1993).

often. Common delusions include *persecutory delusions, delusions of control* (i.e., thought insertion and withdrawal), *delusions of reference* (e.g., the television is talking to the patient), and *delusions of grandeur*. Less common positive symptoms include *loose associations, stereotypic behaviors, mannerisms and posturing,* and *word salad* (disordered syntax).

Common mood disturbances in schizophrenia include *depression, anxiety, anger,* and *hostility*. These disturbances often occur secondary to positive symptoms. For example, paranoid delusions may be accompanied by anger and hostility, whereas delusions of reference can provoke severe anxiety. Most schizophrenia patients experience depression, which often presages relapses of psychotic symptoms. Approximately 50% of schizophrenia patients attempt suicide at some during their lives, and 10% successfully commit suicide (Roy, 1986).

Schizoaffective Disorder

Schizoaffective disorder is a hybrid psychiatric diagnosis that includes symptoms of both schizophrenia and major affective disorder. The DSM-IV criteria for

TABLE 2.   DSM-IV Draft Criteria for the Diagnosis of Schizoaffective Disorder[a]

A. An uninterrupted period of illness during which at some time there is either a major depressive episode (which must include depressed mood) or manic episode concurrent with symptoms that meet criterion A of schizophrenia.
B. During the same period of illness, there have been delusions or hallucinations for at least 2 weeks in the absence of prominent mood symptoms.
C. Symptoms meeting the criteria for a mood disorder are present for a substantial portion of the total duration of the active and residual periods of the illness.
D. The disturbance is not due to the direct effects of a substance (e.g., drugs of abuse, medication) or a general medical condition.

[a]Adapted from DSM-IV (APA, 1993).

schizoaffective disorder are presented in Table 2. Inspection of Table 2 reveals that in order to meet criteria for schizoaffective disorder, the patient must have a history of schizophrenia symptoms for at least 2 weeks *in the absence of* any affective symptoms, and at some other time must have experienced an affective syndrome (either manic or depressive) accompanied by schizophrenia symptoms. That schizoaffective disorder is closely related to schizophrenia is indicated by an accumulating body of evidence, including studies of genetic vulnerability, course of illness, and response to pharmacological treatments (Kramer et al., 1989; Levinson & Levitt, 1987; Mattes & Nayak, 1984). Hence, we include schizoaffective disorder here in our discussion of clinical interviewing for the diagnosis of schizophrenia.

PROCEDURES FOR GATHERING INFORMATION

The diagnosis of schizophrenia depends most heavily on assessment of the patient's subjective experiences (e.g., delusions and hallucinations), with less emphasis placed on behavioral observation of symptoms, such as flattened affect or looseness of associations (see Table 1). Positive symptoms tend to be less stable over time than negative symptoms, in part due to their subjective quality (Lewine, 1990; Mueser, Douglas, Bellack, & Morrison, 1991). Furthermore, patients may be reluctant to admit experiencing positive symptoms for reasons such as paranoia, an awareness that these symptoms are out of the range of ordinary experience, or negative experiences with prior discussions about these symptoms (e.g., ridicule or denial by family members, attempts to hospitalize the patient). Therefore, while the interview is at the heart of diagnostic assessment, the diagnostician must utilize all available resources to determine whether the patient has schizophrenia.

The most useful sources of collateral information about patients' symptomatology include their medical records, the observations of family members, and reports of mental health professionals involved in the patients' long-term treatment. How these sources of information are utilized in conjunction with the patient interview depends on the availability of the resources and the setting of the interview. When possible, it is desirable for the interviewer to examine the patient's medical records prior to the interview in order to identify past symptoms and diagnoses. Sometimes this chart review is impossible (e.g., when the patient has no previous psychiatric hospitalizations) or impractical (e.g., when the patient is being evaluated for hospitalization in a psychiatric emergency room). In such cases, meeting with a relative or friend to briefly discuss the patient's behavior over the past several weeks and the circumstances leading up to the psychiatric evaluation can help guide the diagnostic interview.

Some diagnosticians prefer to limit the amount of information they learn about the patient before the first meeting in order to maximize their objectivity in the interview. Following the interview, the diagnostician may seek additional information from family members and professionals and, when necessary, meet again with the patient to clarify specific points. We have found that this approach provides a balance between objective assessment and the utilization of all relevant sources of information.

Case Example

A 27-year-old Catholic woman was involuntarily admitted to the hospital by her mother because of severe social withdrawal, poor personal hygiene, and increased religious preoccupation. Her chart indicated that she had had two previous psychiatric admissions and had been given diagnoses of paranoid schizophrenia and manic–depression, although the specific content of her delusions was not described. During the interview, the woman denied auditory hallucinations and, while she admitted to being religious, insisted that her beliefs were not delusional compared to those of others in the Charismatic Catholic church to which she belonged. The mother reported that her daughter had recently arranged for a priest to exorcise her and cleanse her apartment with holy water, but the patient refused to explain her actions.

The evidence from the interviews with the patient and her mother was strongly suggestive of schizophrenia, but not sufficient to establish the diagnosis. However, interviews with inpatient staff members indicated that the patient had been observed stuffing tissues into her mouth and talking downward toward the ground to "the Devil." A subsequent meeting with the patient indicated that she used the tissues to prevent the Devil from talking through her mouth, which she had experienced and found very distressing. Thus, observation of the patient's behavior provided valuable additional information that allowed the interviewer to confirm the presence of delusions and auditory hallucinations, thereby confirming a diagnosis of schizophrenia, paranoid subtype.

The diagnosis of schizophrenia requires obtaining a wide range of information from the patient during the interview, including the onset of the illness a description of events leading up to the current episode, and past and present symptomatology. As with any assessment procedure, the validity of the diagnostic interview can be threatened if it is not conducted in a relatively standardized fashion across different patients. One method for standardizing the diagnostic assessment across both patients and interviews is the use of structured interview schedules.

Structured Diagnostic Interview Instruments

Prior to the development of objectively based criteria for the diagnosis of schizophrenia in DSM-III (American Psychiatric Association, 1980), the reliability of this diagnosis was notoriously low (Matarazzo, 1983) and schizophrenia was widely overdiagnosed in the United States (Kuriansky, Deming, & Gurland, 1974). In addition to the establishment of explicit criteria for the diagnosis of schizophrenia, the use of structured clinical interviews to assess patients' history of illness and symptomatology has also improved the reliability of diagnosis. A variety of semistructured interview schedules have been developed over the past 20 years, with the most common instruments for the diagnosis of schizophrenia including the Structured Clinical Interview for DSM-III-R (SCID) (Spitzer, Williams, Gibbon, & First, 1990), the Schedule for Affective Disorders and Schizophrenia (SADS) (Endicott & Spitzer, 1978), the Present-State Examination (PSE) (Wing, 1970), and the Diagnostic Interview Schedule (DIS) (Robins, Helzer, Croughan, & Ratcliff, 1981; Robins, Helzer, Ratcliff, & Seyfried, 1982). Reliability studies of these instruments have demonstrated high sensitivity and specificity across interviewers (for a review, see Morrison, 1988). The SCID is at present the most widely used structured interview in the United States and the PSE is most widely used in England. The DIS was developed for use in epidemiological studies and designed so that it could be administered by a lay person. In general, the DIS is considered to be less precise than the other instruments.

The primary advantage of using structured interviews to diagnose schizophrenia is that they provide a standardized approach for eliciting symptoms, thereby reducing the variability of the assessment across different patients. A related advantage is that structured interview instruments provide guidelines for determining whether a specific symptom exists and for making decisions about ruling out other related disorders (e.g., manic–depressive illness). A final consideration is the availability of training in structured diagnostic interviews. Extensive training opportunities are available for all the instruments described above, including seminars, videotaped interviews, and detailed training books, and training is critical to achieving accurate diagnoses. The major pitfalls of structured interview instruments are the time required to administer them (usually about 90 minutes) and the training needed to conduct the interview reliably.

CASE ILLUSTRATIONS

Introducing the Interview

During the first meeting, it is important for the interviewer to present himself or herself in an objective, nonjudgmental, empathic manner in order to ease the patient as much as possible and convey the feeling of concern. Patients with delusions or hallucinations frequently experience severe anxiety, depression, and anger because of these psychotic symptoms.

The diagnostic interview should be introduced to the patient clearly in order to gain the greatest cooperation. The clinician may start by saying: "I am going to ask you some questions about problems and difficulties you may have. I will also ask you about difficulties you may have had in the past. As we talk, I will make some notes. Do you have any questions before we begin?"[1] It is important to give the patient an opportunity to express any misgivings about the context of the interview, such as conflicts that might have occurred immediately previous to the interview about which the clinician should be aware. Concerns about the interview should be clarified and other problems acknowledged before proceeding with the interview.

Obtaining the Overview and the History

The first stages of the diagnostic interview cover general information about the patient's age, where and with whom the patient is living, and the patient's source of income (including disability status or occupation). This gives the interviewee a warm-up phase by focusing on easy-to-answer factual questions. These items can be asked directly using questions such as: "What is your source of income?" "How do you support yourself?" "You mentioned that you receive a check—is that a disability check?" "How far did you go in school?" If the patient did not finish high school, the interview should ask what happened that prevented him or her from finishing.

In many inpatient settings, the interviewer will have access to demographic and background information. Rather than omit questions about these data, it is preferable to confirm the details with the patient in order to help establish rapport and the flow of the interview. Information can be obtained by saying: "I want to confirm a couple of details about your living situation. Previous to coming to the hospital, you lived at your mother's house at 110 South Greene Street. Do we have that correct?" "Now, who else stays with you and your mother?"

The interviewer then obtains an overview of the present episode by asking: "How did you come to be in the hospital?" or "I understand that you have been experiencing more problems with [major psychotic symptom]. Tell me what difficulties you have been having recently." Often, it is necessary to pursue a denial of problems. For example, if the patient states only that he or she has become more nervous lately, the interviewer might say, "Can you tell me a little more about that?" If the patient denies serious difficulties again, one might say, "Isn't there something else? People aren't usually admitted to psychiatric hospitals just for being nervous." It is also important to assess whether there are stressors associated with the current symptomatology. This information can be gathered by asking: "How were things going when you started having these problems?" "Were you having difficulty with your family?" "How about where you were living?" The last part of the overview of the present episode should include an assessment of medical prob-

---

[1]Where possible, we have discussed diagnostic criteria from the *Diagnostic and Statistical Manual of Mental Disorders*, 4th edition, draft criteria (APA, 1993), which is the most current manual available at the time of this writing.

lems, medications, and alcohol and drug use. Questions similar to the following will suffice: "How has your health been?" "What medications do you take?" "How much alcohol do you drink per week?" "What drugs have you taken—what about street drugs such as marijuana and cocaine?"

A brief historical overview of the patient's illness is also necessary. The interviewer can ask: "How many times before have you had the difficulties you are having now?" or "How many times have you been hospitalized for emotional or psychiatric problems?" The clinician should get a brief outline of the hospitalizations, or discrete episodes, by asking: "Let's review the first time you were hospitalized [or had difficulty]. When was that?" "What problems or symptoms were you having?" "Was it different than what you are experiencing currently?" "Where were you hospitalized?" or "Where did you go for treatment?" Each episode identified by the patient should be explored with these questions. Often, the patient is a poor reporter of the chronology of his or her disorder, so that the interviewer may wish to ask about episodes reported by friends, family, and other mental health professionals. For example, the clinician could ask: "I understand that you were in Temple Hospital for four weeks in January of 1989. Could you tell me about how you came to be in the hospital? What were some of the problems you were experiencing before being admitted?"

In all, the overview need not require more than 10 to 15 minutes. It is important that the clinician have this background so that he or she can explore the course of the disorder, the patient's important life events, and the patient's previous and current level of functioning. For many patients, this information must come from sources other than the clinical interview. However, these details must be obtained before a diagnosis can be made, and often the interview can be enhanced when the clinician has the information in advance.

Eliciting Symptoms of the Current Episode

There are two major sources of information during the interview: First, the clinician evaluates the content and the logical flow of the patient's verbalizations. The content of the patient's speech may indicate the presence of symptoms such as delusions and hallucinations, whereas the logical flow may indicate the presence of loose associations, circumstantiality, and thought blocking. Second, during the interview, the clinician uses observation of the patient's behavior and affective expressivity to detect symptoms such as blunted or inappropriate affect.

One of the most common symptoms that the interviewer should explore is hallucinations. The clinician may start by asking an open-ended question about a more general complaint. The example below illustrates this tactic with a 38-year-old patient with a 15-year history of psychiatric hospitalizations.

I: You mentioned that you were suicidal when you came to the hospital this time. What was going on that led you to be suicidal?

P: I had started to hear people talk outside of my door. I'd go outside and nobody would be there and I heard them laughing about it. Making fun of me, making me feel stupid. I started to drink because I was trying to get them to stop.

I: Where did the voices come from?

P: I don't know. I guess inside my head. I thought outside, but they weren't there. Every time I hear them I end up going to the hospital.

Delusions are also assessed by evaluating the content of the patient's verbalizations. With some patients, delusions are readily assessed because the patient is preoccupied with the theme or idea. Other patients must be engaged in a lengthier discussion before they begin to reveal much about their delusional ideas. When the interviewer successfully scratches the surface of the delusion by discussing related material, the patient may readily expound on his or her beliefs. Thus, it is helpful to find out from other sources of information (i.e., admitting records) what the possible content of the delusion may be before beginning the interview. The interviewer can start with broader questions about delusions.

I: Did it ever seem that people were talking about you or taking special notice of you?

P: I was walking down the street and a white van came up an I could hear them saying, "Let's wait 'til the next light and then jump out and grab her."

I: What did you do?

P: I stopped and stood still so they would have to continue in the traffic. I stood there about 8 or 9 hours so they couldn't get me.

I: How did that work to keep them from grabbing you?

P: I was protected while I was standing still. They couldn't get me. A trolley went by four times and the driver asked if I wanted a ride, but I said no. Where would I go, anyway?

In this excerpt, the interviewer's questions were derived largely from the patient's responses. By showing interest and concern, the clinician is able to draw out more details of the delusional system than by using rote, predetermined questions. Other types of general questions that can start this type of dialogue include the following: "Does it seem that something or someone is controlling your thoughts or your behavior?" "What about putting thoughts into your head?" "Do you have ideas or beliefs that others find difficult to believe or understand?"

While asking questions about the patient's beliefs and experiences, the clinician should take note of the logical flow of the patient's verbalizations for evidence of formal thought disorder. The severity of thought disorder can range from very mild to very severe. Mild thought disorder can be difficult to detect, but is often manifested by occasional idiosyncratic word use, neologisms, and non sequiturs in the flow of the interview. The interviewer may find that he or she has lost track of the point the patient was trying to make. This is a cue to consider whether the patient is exhibiting digressive, vague, or circumstantial speech (prodromal or residual symptoms); additionally, the patient may be exhibiting loose associations, as illustrated below. Close examination of this transcript of a diagnostic interview reveals a thread of loosely connected ideas that are difficult to follow in conversation.

I: Have you received special messages from the way things are arranged around the room, or have you received special messages from the radio or TV?

P: I like football and sports. When I was home the next-door neighbors—well they were married in '70 and they have four kids—they have a pool about the size of this room and I was the lifeguard. I did that last summer.

I: But did you receive special messages from the TV?

P: Nah. I relate to war movies, I guess. The plane is hit by the enemy—Korea and Viet Nam—and has to bail out over water and 50 states of rescue planes, PBY's, throw a life raft. Well, I did it with 50 states of ships. The face of—and 50 states of PT boats. And you build them with the San Diego Naval Base, the Brooklyn Navy Yard and you open up navy yards all—I tried to open up a navy yard where I live . . . and go to work there. I had a job application in at the Frankford Hospital but I couldn't go to work because my arms . . . I tell you, I have been trying to get strength in this arm and it won't form. I eat and eat. I'm anemic. It's blood diserialosis and I'm anemic.

CRITICAL INFORMATION FOR MAKING THE DIAGNOSIS

The essence of the diagnostic process is to decide when the threshold for a diagnostic criterion has been met. It is easy to regard diagnostic criteria as a checklist and to make these decisions superficially. However, skilled clinicians recognize the need to clarify any ambiguity in a diagnostic situation by gathering sufficient information. In the past, some of the ambiguity in the diagnostic process stemmed from the lack of *operationalized criteria* in the dominant nosological systems in use. Prior to DSM-III (APA, 1980), DSM diagnostic criteria were written to reflect hypothesized underlying psychological etiological mechanisms (e.g., rather than observable behavior). The introduction of DSM-III operationalized the criteria, vastly improving the clinician's ability to tie his or her observations to a set of criteria.

Despite these improvements in the major diagnostic systems, the clinician is asked to make a number of difficult judgments. We will discuss the critical information needed to fulfill the diagnostic criteria for several areas. First, specific symptomatic criteria, such as hallucinations and delusions, will be discussed. Second, we will discuss the information needed to establish whether the threshold of the *decrease in functioning* criterion has been met. Last, we will examine the criteria with respect to the other clinical syndromes, including affective disorders, drug abuse, and organic factors, that need to be considered and ruled out before the diagnosis is made.

Symptomatic Criteria

Some symptoms are assessed by evaluating the content of a patient's verbalizations, such as in the case of delusional beliefs. What yardstick is the clinician to use in evaluating the beliefs? To a great extent, the interviewer must rely on his or her own norms of human behavior and experience. This approach may be flawed, however, because the patient may have been raised in a subculture that supports beliefs that seem delusional in the dominant culture. Obviously, making an appropriate judgment depends on the extent of the interviewer's knowledge of beliefs in that subculture. However, more than a superficial knowledge is necessary. It is best for the interviewer to seek the consultation of a colleague who is familiar with that culture for assistance in understanding what beliefs are common and accepted.

In assessing delusions in which the person's subculture is not an issue, an interviewer may simply invite the patient to say as much as possible about the specific topic at hand. Usually, suspected delusional material will become increasingly apparent as the patient is given time to respond to questions, if the interviewer demonstrates genuine concern and interest. It is often instructive to ask a patient whether others share his or her beliefs. In addition, relatives are often available to confirm or disconfirm important aspects of the patient's beliefs. The interviewer may evaluate the internal consistency of the patient's story. Contradictions may point the interviewer to delusional material.

Changes in how bizarre delusions were handled in the DSM-III-R (APA, 1987) and current DSM-IV draft criteria (APA, 1993) for schizophrenia have caused an increase in the diagnostic importance of this symptom. As noted by Flaum, Arndt, and Andreasen (1991), it is possible to diagnose schizophrenia (in the active phase) solely on the basis of the presence of a bizarre delusion; in DSM-III (APA, 1980), an earlier edition of the DSM, bizarre delusion was only one of several classes of symptoms that could be used to diagnose schizophrenia in the active phase. Unfortunately, Flaum et al. (1991) reported that the overall reliability of judgments for bizarre delusions is poor, regardless of the rater's level of training or the definition used. The best reliability can be obtained for the bizarre delusions that illustrate the classic Schneiderian first-rank symptoms of thought broadcasting (i.e., the belief that one's thoughts can be heard by others), thought insertion (i.e., the belief that others can put thoughts into one's ind), and "made" (or imposed) volitional acts (i.e., delusion of being controlled by an external force) (see Mellor, 1970). Other types of bizarre delusions, such as somatic or grandiose delusions, lead to the lowest reliability.

These considerations suggest that the diagnostician should take great care in cases in which a patient meets criteria for schizophrenia in the active phase based solely on the presence of a bizarre delusion. Maximum effort should be made to evaluate the presence of other symptoms that might alleviate the diagnostician of the burden of depending on a symptom that cannot be reliably diagnosed. We suggest that interviewers considering the diagnosis of schizophrenia based on a sole bizarre delusion restrict the diagnosis to cases in which the delusion is one of the types found to be most reliably rated by Flaum and colleagues. Perhaps future revisions of the DSM will provide greater guidance in the evaluation of bizarre delusions.

Evaluating the presence or absence of hallucinations often requires as much detective work as the assessment of delusions. In some cases, hallucination-like experiences may occur transiently while the patient is in a semisleeping state. When this is the only time "hallucinations" occur, the phenomenon is considered a *hypnagogic experience*, rather than a true hallucination. When a patient is inconsistent about the report of hallucinations, it is useful to observe the patient for signs that he or she is responding either verbally or physically to internal stimuli that may be hallucinations. Patients are often distracted or upset by hallucinations; asking about hallucinations when the patient seems preoccupied can lead to the patient's acknowledgement that he or she is indeed hearing voices.

Criterion of Decrease in Functioning

One important criterion for the diagnosis of schizophrenia is a decrease in social functioning, occupational functioning, and self-care. How does one assess whether the patient has experienced a decline in functioning? Family and friends, and sometimes the patient, can indicate how he or she was functioning in these areas. Sometimes the patient's physical appearance indicates that his or her self-care is so poor that there is likely to have been a decrease from previous levels. A diagnostic interview that includes an overview, as discussed above, will give the interviewer some initial clues as to how the patient was functioning before the current episode. The interviewer must then ask specific questions about activities that the patient is not able to manage at this time. For example: "What activities were you able to do before your current difficulties?" "When did you last work?" "When did you last go to your day program?" For patients who have never worked outside their homes, the questions could center around household responsibilities that have been neglected recently: "Were you able to clean the house and care for your children better before your present difficulties?" "Did you begin to have problems taking care of yourself—like eating and showering?" "Did your family notice a change?" Many of the judgments must inevitably rest on subjective accounts by the patient and family members. However, greater accuracy is gained by gathering as much specific information about the patient's actual activities as possible.

Other Relevant Syndromes

The novice interviewer may consider a diagnosis of schizophrenia likely when confronted with a patient with psychotic symptoms. However, there is a myriad of psychiatric and medical conditions that are commonly characterized by psychotic symptoms. Thus, the presence of many other syndromes must be assessed and ruled out before assigning the diagnosis of schizophrenia.

Every patient receiving a psychiatric evaluation should be given a screening physical examination to rule out medical illnesses. The physical examination should include assessment of five areas: (1) vital signs, (2) autonomic system dysfunction, (3) heart and lung dysfunction, (4) neurological dysfunction and head trauma, and (5) abnormalities of the eyes (Shea, 1988). It is not necessary that the physical examination occur before the interview, but in most hospitals and psychiatric institutions the patient will be given an examination on admission.

It is important that medical and nonmedical professionals alike be familiar with many of the conditions that can commonly result in a presentation of psychotic symptoms. Examples include temporal lobe epilepsy, thyroid disorder, and meningitis. For a comprehensive list of organic causes of psychosis, consult Shea (1988).

Schizoaffective disorder and mood disorders are the disorders most commonly confused with schizophrenia by novice interviewers. It is a common misconception that the apparent predominance of psychotic symptoms vs. affective symptoms is the only consideration for differentiating between schizophrenia, schizoaffective disorder, and affective disorders. Careful consideration of the DSM-IV draft criteria for these disorders requires the clinician to uncover several crucial pieces of information, including the onset, course, and duration of each of the types of symptoms (psychotic and affective symptoms). The relative timing of psychotic and affective symptoms is crucial to establishing the correct diagnosis. For example, one patient may present as extremely paranoid and somewhat loose and rambling. He may also exhibit pressured speech, grandiosity, and irritability. If the patient were not paranoid or loose in the absence of the affective symptoms, he could not have schizophrenia or schizoaffective disorder, but would more likely have bipolar disorder. It may take several discussions with the patient or family members or both in order to obtain reliable information about the timing of psychotic and affective symptoms.

Concurrent or recent drug abuse constitutes another important aspect of the clinical presentation that complicates the diagnosis of schizophrenia. This judgment is often difficult because a person with schizophrenia is much more likely to have substance abuse or dependence disorder than a person without schizophrenia (see Mueser, Bellack, & Blanchard, 1992). Furthermore, there is evidence that stimulant abuse can lead to an earlier onset of schizophrenia in biologically vulnerable individuals as well as precipitate relapses in patients who already have the illness. Similarly, alcohol, cannabis, and hallucinogen abuse have also been linked to increased risk of relapse in schizophrenia. Thus, when diagnosing schizophrenia, the clinician is often faced with the assessment of patients with both psychotic symptoms and recent substance abuse and is therefore required to evaluate the role of substance abuse as a cause of the psychotic symptoms.

One "truism" that has been repeated often is that the presence of visual or tactile hallucinations or both is pathognomonic of substance abuse or withdrawal. The opposite has been purported to be true of auditory hallucinations, namely, that it is indicative of schizophrenia rather than drug abuse. However, surveys indicate that a wide range of different types of hallucinations are present in schizophrenia, with auditory hallucinations most common (72%), followed by visual (16%), tactile (17%), and olfactory/gustatory hallucinations (Mueser, Bellack, & Brady, 1990). Visual hallucinations are even more prevalent in samples of chronic schizophrenia patients, with some estimates exceeding 50% (Bracha, Wolkowitz, Lohr, Karson, & Bigelow, 1989). Thus, the diagnostician must use other evidence for ruling drug abuse in or out as an etiological factor in the presenting psychotic symptoms.

The differential diagnosis of schizophrenia or drug-induced psychosis is made primarily by examining the history and pattern of the drug abuse relative to the psychotic symptoms. In addition to the symptoms necessary for the diagnosis of schizophrenia, a deterioration in social and occupational functioning must be found to have occurred prior to the beginning of the suspected drug or alcohol abuse. It must be clearly established that the patient experienced psychotic symptoms in the absence of recent drug abuse.

We have found that patients readily admit their drug use when the interviewer carefully examines all classes of drugs. The interviewer places a list of drugs in front of the patient and asks him or her to identify the drugs that have been used (see Table 3). The Structured Clinical Interview for DSM-III-R utilizes this method, and it can be quite effective even when the patient initially denies drug use in superficial questioning.

Do's and Don't's

A well-conducted diagnostic interview has many essential components that have been discussed at length elsewhere. Instead of repeating information already available, we will discuss guidelines for interviewing schizophrenic patients in light of the special challenges they present. Psychotic patients are often interviewed at the height of an exacerbation after an involuntary admission to a psychiatric facility. The patient in this situation may be frightened due to hallucinations and delusions he or she is experiencing. Alternatively, he or she may be angry about the admission. Thus, it is possible that the interviewer will get little more than superficial cooperation from the patient. It is particularly important to develop empathy and rapport in order to maximize the usefulness of the interview. We will present a number of specific ways to achieve this. Interview procedures to avoid will also be presented.

Do's

Outline the information to be covered. It is important to help the patient be at ease by describing exactly what will happen in the interview. Even if the patient knows that there is information that he or she is not willing to reveal, it makes the interview more predictable and thus more comfortable for the patient (see the section entitled "Introducing the Interview" above).

Use both general and specific questions for difficult topics. When addressing an area about which the patient is upset, such as conflict with family members, it is useful to start with general questions and then gradually become more specific. This technique will help reduce the defensiveness that the patient may have about the topic. This approach is illustrated below.

TABLE 3.   Drugs Commonly Abused by Schizophrenia Patients[a]

Sedatives, hypnotics, anxiolytics ("downers"): Quaalude ("ludes"), Seconal ("reds"), Valium, Xanax, Librium, barbiturates, Miltown, Ativan, Dalmane, Halcion
Cannabis: marijuana, hashish ("hash"), THC, "pot," "grass," "weed," "reefer"
Stimulants ("uppers"): amphetamine, "speed," crystal meth, dexadrine, Ritalin, diet pills, "crank"
Opioids: heroin, morphine, opium, methadone, Darvon, codeine, Percodan, Demerol, Dilaudid
Cocaine: snorting, IV, freebase, "crack," "speedball"
Hallucinogens ("psychedelics"): LSD ("acid"), mescaline, peyote, psilocybin, STP, mushrooms
PCP: "angel dust," "peace pill"
Other: steroids, "glue," ethyl chloride, nitrous oxide ("laughing gas"), amyl or butyl nitrate ("poppers"), Extasy, Special K, MDA, MDM, nonprescription sleep or diet pills

---

[a]Adapted from Spitzer et al. (1990).

I: I understand that things were not going well between you and some of your family members before you came to the hospital. Could you tell me a little about that?

P: There ain't nothing to tell. It's all my sister's fault. If she wasn't so mean I wouldn't be here.

I: It sounds like you think she may not be on your side.

P: She just is sneaky and doesn't want me at home anymore. I didn't do anything to her. I don't know why she wants me gone.

I: Are there some things that you believe she does to you when you aren't watching.

P: I'm not sure, but I think it's with the food.

I: What do you think she is doing to your food?

P: Rat poison, what else? I really got her for it too. Zapped her right on the forehead. She won't forget that lesson for a while.

Use follow-up questions. The dialogue above also illustrates the importance of follow-up questions. By remaining on the topic and asking follow-up questions, the interviewer gradually acquires more information about a particular area. Follow-up is especially crucial for the assessment of delusions. If the patient is somewhat disorganized or exhibiting loosened associations, follow-up questions may be necessary to redirect the patient back to the topic. The clinician can say, for example: "You mentioned a moment ago that you felt your sister was doing something to hurt you, perhaps even poisoning you. Can you say more about why she would do this?" At other times, the interviewer can simply follow-up by asking: "Could you tell me a little more about that?"

Adjust language to the individual patient. To help the patient feel as comfortable as possible and understand the questions put to him or her, the interviewer should use the patient's language for describing symptoms or events. For example, if the patient describes the initial psychotic break or subsequent exacerbation of schizo-phrenia as "having a nervous breakdown," the clinician can ask: "You mentioned that you had a 'nervous breakdown' last year. Did you hear voices at that time?" The clinician should also recognize that a difference in education often exists between him or her and the patient and accordingly limit technical jargon and use plain language instead.

Gently pressure the patient only when necessary. Novice diagnostic interviewers often use pressure when faced with inconsistencies or with apparent attempts to conceal important information. It can be frustrating to interview a patient who is uncooperative or evasive when this information is sought. The interviewer needs to bear in mind that most people with schizophrenia have experienced negative social consequences when discussing their symptoms with others, such as being told they are "crazy" when talking about delusions or that auditory hallucinations are "just in their imagination." These unpleasant social reactions have the understand-able effect of making many patients reticent to discuss their private perceptions and thoughts. Pressure or confrontation should not be a routine interviewing technique, because it usually increases the patient's defensiveness. When inconsis-tencies appear in the patient's account of his difficulties, the interviewer can request more information about the topic without pointing out the contradiction. This may be done, for example, by asking a patient who had denied hallucinations prior to admission: "We were talking a minute ago about hearing voices. I noticed that you seemed distracted or bothered by something a moment ago. Can you tell me what you were seeing or hearing?"

Don't's

Don't apologize for questions. It is unnecessary for a clinician to apologize for the questions asked in a diagnostic interview, even if the interviewee reacts incredulously to queries about delusions or hallucinations. Some patients might initially deny these symptoms, and to apologize for asking may legitimize the denial.

Don't use leading questions. Leading questions imply to the patient what the correct answer is. An example of this type of question is: *"Weren't* you hearing voices when you first came to the hospital?" The preferable way of asking this question is: *"Were* you hearing voices when you first came to the hospital?" Likewise, the interviewer should be cautioned against asking leading questions that suggest that a particular symptom was *not* present, for example: *"You weren't* feeling sad or blue when you first started hearing the voices, *were you?"*

Don't repeat questions. When an interviewer believes that a symptom is present, despite the patient's denial of the symptom, do not simply keep repeating the same question in the hope that the patient will relent and say "Yes." For example, some clinicians might ask: "Did you feel that your family was trying to hurt you?" followed by "So you didn't feel your family was trying to do something to hurt you?" As an alternative, the interviewer might ask for more detailed information about the situation by saying: "I'd like you to describe a little bit about how you have been getting along with your family. Every family has disagreements, so I'd like you to tell me about some things that have bothered you about them or that they have complained about to you over the last month."

Don't try to correct the patient's delusional ideas. If the patient becomes upset when discussing symptoms, the interviewer should empathize with his or her feelings without colluding with the patient by implying that the psychotic beliefs are true [e.g., "It must be very upsetting for you to hear these voices putting you down all the time" (Shea, 1988)]. Attempts to convince schizophrenic patients that their delusions are false invariably fail, and often paradoxically increase the patient's degree of conviction about the belief. In rare instances, the patient may directly inquire whether the interviewer believes his or her delusion. In such cases, the interviewer may either refocus the patient back to discussing his or her experiences (e.g., "I would like to concentrate here on what *you* believe, rather than what *I* believe") or state frankly that they have a difference of opinion (e.g., "I don't think that you are being pursued by the FBI and the Mafia, but it's okay for you and I to have different opinions about this").

Don't redirect the interview unless necessary. Patients should be given as much time as possible to talk about their difficulties so that they feel free to give their version of events. Even in structured interviews, the patient should be given time to describe incidents, problems, or interpretations without frequent interruption so that he or she feels comfortable. Of course, patients who are more disorganized, tangential, or circumstantial will need more redirection and structure. Redirection can be accomplished in some such fashion as this: "Let's back up to where we were talking about when you left your residential home because I want to understand more about what that was like for you. Were you getting the feeling that the people there were going out of their way to give you a hard time or trying to hurt you?"

Summary

Schizophrenia is one of the most difficult psychiatric disorders to diagnose, both because its characteristic symptoms overlap with those of many other disorders and because patients are often reticent to discuss their symptoms. Until recently, the diagnosis of schizophrenia was considered by many to be a waste-basket diagnosis for patients with severe, psychotic symptoms that were not easily classified into other diagnostic categories. The development of operationalized diagnostic criteria and standardized interview instruments over the past 15 years has enabled schizophrenia to be reliably diagnosed.

Special care is required to conduct a diagnostic interview with a patient suspected of having schizophrenia. Efforts must be made to ensure that the patient is as comfortable as possible with the interview situation, to provide the patient with an opportunity to tell his or her story without excessive interruptions or challenges, and to follow up hints of delusions or hallucinations that may be critical to establishing the correct diagnosis. Additionally, other sources of information about the patient usually need to be tapped, such as medical records and reports of significant others. Despite the prominence of thought disorder in many schizo-phrenics, the vast majority of patients are cooperative during the diagnostic interview and are responsive to a warm, empathic, frank interpersonal style on the interviewer's part. Strong interviewing skills are necessary to confirm or rule out the diagnosis of schizophrenia, which subsequently has important pharmacologi-cal and psychotherapeutic treatment implications. Recent advances in pharmaco-logical interventions (Kane, Honigfeld, Singer, & Meltzer, 1988) and psychosocial treatments for schizophrenia (Mueser & Liberman, 1991) underscore the impor-tance of establishing an accurate diagnosis, in order to link these patients with the treatment services most likely to improve the prognosis of this chronic psychiatric illness.

References

American Psychiatric Association (1980). *Diagnostic and statistical manual of mental disorders*, 3rd ed. Washington, DC: Author.

American Psychiatric Association (1987). *Diagnostic and statistical manual of mental disorders*, 3rd ed., revised. Washington, DC: Author.

American Psychiatric Association (1993). *Diagnostic and statistical manual of mental disorders*, 4th ed., draft criteria. Washington, DC: Author.

Bleuler, E. (1950). *Dementia praecox or the group of schizophrenias*. Translated by J. Zinken (1911). New York: International Universities Press.

Bracha, H. S., Wolkowitz, O. M., Lohr, J. B., Karson, C. N., & Bigelow, L. B. (1989). High prevalence of visual hallucinations in research subjects with chronic schizophrenia. *American Journal of Psychiatry, 146,* 526–528.

Bruce, M. L., Takeuchi, D. T., & Leaf, P. J. (1991). Poverty and psychiatric status. *Archives of General Psychiatry, 48,* 470–474.

Buchsbaum, M. S. (1990). The frontal lobes, basal ganglia, and temporal lobes as sites for schizophrenia. *Schizophrenia Bulletin, 16,* 379–389.

Cornblatt, B. A., Lenzenweger, M. F., Dworkin, R. H., 7 Erlenmeyer-Kimling, L. (1992). Childhood attentional dysfunctions predict social deficits in unaffected adults at risk for schizophrenia. *British Journal of Psychiatry, 161 (Suppl. 18),* 59–64.

Crow, T. J. (1990). Meaning of structural changes in the brain in schizophrenia. In A. Kales, C. N. Stefanis, & J. Talbott (Eds.), *Recent advances in schizophrenia* (pp. 81–94). New York: Springer-Verlag.

Endicott, J., & Spitzer, R. L. (1978). A diagnostic interview: The Schedule for Affective Disorders and Schizophrenia. *Archives of General Psychiatry, 35,* 837–844.

Flaum, M., Arndt, S., & Andreasen, N. (1991). The reliability of "bizarre" delusions. *Comprehensive Psychiatry, 32,* 59–65.

Fox, J. W. (1990). Social class, mental illness, and social mobility: The social selection–drift hypothesis for serious mental illness. *Journal of Health and Social Behavior, 31,* 344–353.

Goldstein, J. M. (1988). Gender differences in the course of schizophrenia. *Journal of Psychiatry, 145,* 684–689.

Harding, C. M., Brooks, G. W., Ashikaga, T., Strauss, J. S., & Breier, A. (1987). The Vermont longitudinal study of persons with severe mental illness. I. Methodology, study sample, and overall status 32 years later. *American Journal of Psychiatry, 144,* 718–726.

Jablensky, A., & Sartorius, N. (1975). Culture and schizophrenia. In H. M. VanPraag (Ed.), *On the origin of schizophrenia psychoses* (pp. 99–124). Amsterdam: De Erven Bohn.

Kane, J., Honigfeld, G., Singer, J., & Meltzer, H. (1988). Clozapine for the treatment-resistant schizophrenic: A double-blind comparison with chlorpromazine. *Archives of General Psychiatry, 45,* 789–796.

Kay, S. R., & Sevy, S. (1990). Pyramidical model of schizophrenia. *Schizophrenia Bulletin, 16,* 537–545.

Kraepelin, E. (1919). *Dementia praecox and paraphrenia.* Edinburgh: Livingston.

Kramer, M. S., Vogel, W. H., DiJohnson, C., Dewey, D. A., Sheves, P., Cavicchia, S., Litle, P., Schmidt, R., & Kimes, I. (1989). Antidepressants in "depressed" schizophrenic inpatients. *Archives of General Psychiatry, 46,* 922–928.

Kuriansky, J. B., Deming, W. E., & Gurland, B. J. (1974). On trends in the diagnosis of schizophrenia. *American Journal of Psychiatry, 131,* 402–408.

Levinson, D. F., & Levitt, M. M. (1987). Schizoaffective mania reconsidered. *American Journal of Psychiatry, 144,* 415–425.

Lewine, R. R. J. (1990). A discriminant validity study of negative symptoms with a special focus on depression and antipsychotic medication. *American Journal of Psychiatry, 147,* 1463–1466.

Liberman, R. P., DeRisi, W. J., & Mueser, K. T. (1989). *Social skills training for psychiatric patients.* New York: Pergamon Press.

Matarazzo, J. D. (1983). The reliability of psychiatric and psychological diagnosis. *Clinical Psychology Review, 3,* 103–145.

Mattes, J. A., & Nayak, D. (1984). Lithium vs. fluphenazine for prophylaxis in mainly schizophrenic schizo-affectives. *Biological Psychiatry, 19,* 445–449.

Mellor, C. S. (1970). First rank symptoms of schizophrenia. *British Journal of Psychiatry, 117,* 15–23.

Morrison, R. L. (1988). Structured interviews and rating scales. In A. S. Bellack & M. Hersen (Eds.), *Behavioral assessment: A practical handbook,* (3rd ed., pp. 252–278). New York: Pergamon Press.

Mueser, K. T., Bellack, A. S., & Blanchard, J. J. (1992). Comorbidity of schizophrenia and substance abuse: Implications for treatment. *Journal of Consulting and Clinical Psychology, 60,* 845–856.

Mueser, K. T. Bellack, A. S., Brady, E. U. (1990). Hallucinations in schizophrenia. *Acta Psychiatrica Scandinavica, 82,* 26–29.

Mueser, K. T., Bellack, A. S., Morrison, R. L., & Wade, J. H. (1990). Gender social competence, and symptomatology in schizophrenia: A longitudinal analysis. *Journal of Abnormal Psychology, 99,* 138–147.

Mueser, K. T., Douglas, M. S., Bellack, A. S., & Morrison, R. L. (1991). Assessment of enduring deficit and negative symptom subtypes in schizophrenia. *Schizophrenia Bulletin, 17,* 565–582.

Mueser, K. T., & Glynn, S. M. (1990). Behavioral family therapy for schizophrenia. In M. Hersen, R. M. Eisler, & P. M. Miller (Eds.), *Progress in behavior modification* (Vol. 26, pp. 122–147). Newbury Park: Sage Publications.

Mueser, K. T., & Liberman, R. P. (1991). Schizophrenia, psychosocial treatment. *Encyclopedia of Human Biology, 6,* 755–767.

Robins, L. N., Helzer, J. E., Croughan, J., & Ratcliff, K. S. (1981). National Institute of Mental Health Diagnostic Interview Schedule: Its history, characteristics, and validity. *Archives of General Psychiatry, 38,* 381–389.

Robins, L. N., Helzer, J. E., Ratcliff, K. S., & Seyfried, W. (1982). Validity of the Diagnostic Interview Schedule, version II: DSM-III diagnoses. *Psychological Medicine, 12,* 855–870.

Roy, A. (1986). Suicide in schizophrenia. In A. Roy (Ed.), *Suicide* (pp. 97–112). Baltimore: Williams & Wilkins.

Shea, S. C. (1988). *Psychiatric interviewing: The art of understanding.* Philadelphia: W. B. Saunders.

Spitzer, R. L., Williams, J. B. W., Gibbon, M., & First, M. B. (1990). *Structured Clinical Interview for DSM-III-R—Patient Edition (SCID-P), Version 1.0.* Washington, DC: American Psychiatric Press.

Walker, E., & Lewine, R. J. (1990). Prediction of adult-onset schizophrenia from childhood home movies of the patients. *American Journal of Psychiatry, 147,* 1052–1056.

Walker, E., Downey, G., & Caspi, A. (1991). Twin studies of psychopathology: Why do the concordance rates vary? *Schizophrenia Research, 5,* 211–221.

Wing, J. K. (1970). A standard form of psychiatric Present-State Examination and a method for standardizing the classification of symptoms. In E. H. Hare & J. K. Wing (Eds.), *Psychiatric epidemiology: An international symposium* (pp. 93–108). London: Oxford University Press.

Zigler, E., & Glick, M. (1986). *A developmental approach to adult psychopathology.* New York: John Wiley.

6

Personality Disorders

PAUL H. SOLOFF

DESCRIPTION OF THE DISORDERS

Definitions

Personality is the sum total of an individual's enduring patterns of perception, cognition, and action in the interpersonal world. It is a habitual and predictable style of thinking, feeling, and acting, arising from the integration of constitutional endowment, early life experience, developmental achievement, and interpersonal, social, and cultural influences. By convention, the term *personality* has come to represent the whole person, the totality of the person's habitual psychological functioning. The term *character* has been reserved for those personal qualities that reflect the person's attitudes and adherence to moral and social values and the term *temperament* for the person's biological potential (Millon, 1981). We know our personality only in interaction with others and our limitations only when circumstances prove our patterned responses inadequate.

A personality *disorder* is defined as a chronically maladaptive pattern of interpersonal functioning, i.e., a pattern of thought, feeling, and action that repeatedly results in significant social impairment and personal distress. The diagnosis of personality disorder is fundamentally a social commentary on behavior deemed disturbing, eccentric, or excessive by the standards of a given social milieu.

Dimensional versus Categorical Models

Personality may be conceptualized as a synthesis of related behavioral dimensions or as a cohesive category organized around a defining etiology. The dimensional approach is favored by empiricists and the categorical by clinicians. Empirical psychologists, utilizing advanced statistical analyses, have produced a

PAUL H. SOLOFF • Western Psychiatric Institute and Clinic, University of Pittsburgh School of Medicine, Pittsburgh, Pennsylvania 15213.

Diagnostic Interviewing (Second Edition), edited by Michel Hersen and Samuel M. Turner. Plenum Press, New York, 1994.

bewildering array of two-dimensional models of interpersonal behavior. Patients are rated for severity on opposing dimensions such as dominance vs. submission, control vs. affection, active vs. passive, introversion vs. extroversion. With increasing complexity and statistical sophistication, multiple arrays of two-dimensional factors can be arranged in a circle (like the spokes of a wheel) around orthogonal axes (usually dominance or power vs. affiliation) to yield a circumplex model (Wiggins, 1982). As the complexity of the model increases, related dimensions fuse into crude approximations of clinical typologies.

For the clinician, the categorical model holds the greatest appeal and utility. Personality dimensions are related to a hypothetical etiology or central organizing principle, which then becomes a focus for treatment. Efforts to classify behavior according to prototypical patterns date back (at least) to the four personality types of Hippocrates and the four defining humors. The modern concept of personality disorder derives from 19th century efforts to classify patterns of eccentric, asocial, and deviant behavior as forms of "moral insanity" and relate them to hypothetical hereditary defects. Although the organizational principles around which prototypes are classified vary greatly (from the "psychopathic degeneration" of Cesare Lombroso to Freud's instinct theory), each prototype defines an easily recognizable clinical entity.

Our most recent classification of personality disorders, the *Diagnostic and Statistical Manual of Mental Disorders*, 4th edition (DSM-IV), is an amalgam of dimensional and categorical approaches. Ten prototypical disorders are defined, but *without reference to any etiological principles* (American Psychiatric Association, 1994). Instead, in an effort to enhance reliability of diagnosis, specific trait criteria are defined for each category—representing dimensional factors most often associated with the prototype. A quantitative structure is imposed to assure that sufficient dimensional traits are present to warrant a categorical diagnosis. In accommodating the obvious overlap of traits among real people (not ideal types), multiple personality diagnoses are allowed. DSM-IV also defines a category for a personality disorder ("not otherwise specified") in which traits of more than one specific personality disorder may be present but fail to meet full diagnostic criteria for any one disorder (APA, 1994). This quasi-empirical classification enhances the *reliability* of diagnoses based on observable data at the expense of a commonsense understanding of the unity of personality. Nonetheless, the empirical definitions lend themselves well to development of structured interview methods of assessment.

STRUCTURED INTERVIEW METHODS

In recent years, research in the field of personality disorders has focused attention on structured clinical interviews as a method to standardize the interview process and provide for testing of reliability, sensitivity, and specificity of diagnoses. In these interviews, diagnostic criteria derived from the DSM are systematically sought through predetermined questions. The strength of the structured interview method lies in the systematic evaluation of all criteria, control of interrater variability, and quantitative expression of the results. The weakness of the method is an excessive reliance on the patient's response, with an unrealistic assumption of insight, candor, and truthfulness on the patient's part.

The structured interview offers a standardized way to phrase questions about critical diagnostic dimensions of personality and a controlled context in which to make clinical observations of interpersonal style, i.e., the process of the interview. For these reasons, the student of diagnostic interviewing should become familiar with the use of structured interviews in personality assessment. Two of the most widely studied research interviews for personality disorders are the Structured Interview for DSM-III-R Personality (Pfohl, Stangl & Zimmerman, 1983) and the Personality Disorder Examination (Loranger, Susman, Oldham, & Russakoff, 1985). Both demonstrate sufficient sensitivity and specificity for clinical use. These structured interview methods usefully supplement diagnostic data gleaned from the content and process of the interpersonal assessment.

INTERPERSONAL ASSESSMENT

The essence of personality is its predictability, i.e., a habitual pattern of response in affect, thought, and action to the stimuli of the interpersonal world. The diagnostic task begins with a search for this pattern as it is manifested in the patient's developmental, social, and vocational history. The therapist is very much a detective, uncovering his patient's modus operandi (i.e., his track record) in an interpersonal assessment. The data for this interpersonal assessment are to be found in the *content* of the patient's history, past and present, and in the *process* of the clinical interaction itself. The patient's recall of his own history is subject to the distortions of his current mental state, his adult perspective, and his immediate needs within the interview. The interaction with the clinician, the process of the interview, represents a characteristic interpersonal exchange available for study. Both the process and the content of the interview provide clues to discovering dimensions of personality that define the patient's predictability.

This task begins with a historical reconstruction of early life experiences, more specifically the history of interpersonal relationships through childhood, adolescence, and adulthood. To add order to the investigation, the clinician may utilize one of many theoretical schemata to conceptualize milestones or critical phases in interpersonal development. The developmental models of Erickson, Sullivan, and Freud are particularly useful in that they provide specific anchor points in a life history for evaluation of mastery of that particular psychosocial phase. At each phase, dominant personality traits may be identified until a pattern emerges through life.

By definition, personality disorder is a *maladaptive* pattern of functioning. This pattern is represented in the history by a track record of interpersonal *failures*. The personality-disordered patient wears his maladaptive attitudes, defenses, and coping styles like a suit of armor (Reich, 1945). His rigid and stereotyped responses to interpersonal relationships are apparent throughout adult life and are manifest in the relationship with the clinician. We recognize the limits of this character armor through the patient's inability to respond to a wide variety of interpersonal demands with flexible adaptation. In reviewing the history, the examiner looks for a pattern of maladaptive stereotyped responses to the normal developmental stressors of life, among which are separations and loss, sexuality and intimacy, social and vocational identity, and parenting. Prominent personality traits may be differentiated from personality disorder by the degree to which the traits are clearly and repetitively maladaptive or lead to interpersonal and social impairment. Also important is the degree to which the traits are rigidly related, with a specific presentation of affect, highly selective cognitive mode, defenses, attitudes, and response patterns. The diagnostic process is a careful examination of how the patient experiences his inner and outer worlds.

THE TEN PERSONALITY DISORDERS

The ten DSM-IV personality prototypes are conceptually grouped into three thematic clusters: a dramatic group, an anxious–fearful group, and an odd–eccentric group (Table 1). Within each group, one may define specific cognitive modes, i.e., characteristic styles of experiencing and thinking about the world and related affective styles and interpersonal response patterns (Shapiro, 1965).

DRAMATIC GROUP

Histrionic Personality Disorder

Interpersonal Assessment

The best studied of the dramatic group are the histrionic personalities—flamboyant, theatrical individuals who experience the world as a series of intense emotional stimuli. Their perception is highly distractible and easily captivated by emotionally laden stimuli. Their cognition is marked by a defect in sustained intellectual concentration and an impressionistic mode of thinking (Shapiro, 1965). The patient does not examine or analyze the content of perception, but reacts emotionally to an initial impression as though it were final reality. The result is a superficial experience of the real world in which details are lost in an overly romanticized, exaggerated affective picture. The patient experiences the sense of

TABLE 1.   DSM-IV Personality Disorders[a]

Dramatic group	Anxious–fearful group	Odd/eccentric group
Histrionic	Compulsive	Paranoid
Antisocial	Avoidant	Schizoid
Narcissistic	Dependent	Schizotypal
Borderline		

[a]From APA (1993). DSM-IV also codes a "Personality Disorder, Not Otherwise Specified."

self in a similar manner as an exaggerated, untempered impression of a romantic or tragic figure. The impressionistic intake of the world has its parallel in the uncontrolled spontaneity of the patient's emotional output. Feelings are expressed (or reported) with exaggerated intensity, but are usually of short duration and more superficial than profound. In response to stress, the impressionistic cognitive style leads to disorganization of thinking, increased intensity of affect, and often a loss of behavioral controls (colloquially referred to as "hysterics").

In the diagnostic interview, one is struck by the degree to which the patient attempts to control or manipulate the clinician through affect and behavior. If allowed to by an inexperienced interviewer, the patient creates an illusion of instant rapport and emotional contact, sets a highly emotional tone to each session, and leads the interview by dramatic, angry, sad, or sexualized cues. The histrionic patient presents with a theatrical quality that, if unchecked by the interviewer, dominates and controls the flow of the interview, manipulating the clinician's attention, conveying an impression of great distress with little substantive detail. Because the patient experiences the world impressionistically, the historical narrative is more a collage of affects than facts. The examiner is drawn away from the details of history into a coquettish social banter of "pseudointimacy" as stimulating as it is deceiving. A loud, angry, but poorly focused tirade may serve the same defensive purpose. A lability of mood and explosiveness of affect betray the pressure of underlying issues that the patient makes every effort to avoid through manipulation of the interview. As in theatrical dialogue, the patient may utilize an "aside" or a "stage direction" to assure the examiner that things are not quite as bad as they appear, that he or she is fully aware of the performance quality of the presentation. The end result of such a misdirected interview is a broad display of affect, but little intellectual understanding of the patient's concerns.

Example

This is the third interview with Mrs. A, an attractive, socially prominent woman who entered therapy following the termination of an affair.

Mrs. A walks in and begins talking immediately, even before she sits down. She speaks with intensity and angry gestures.

MRS. A: I just got on the elevator and a girl got in, six feet tall, blonde and thin. She stood as close to me as she could to show me how pretty she is, the little bitch . . . [Pause] Well? Aren't you going to ask me anything, or should I begin?

DR.: How are you this week?

MRS. A: [Loudly] I've been starving myself, haven't eaten for days—food is absolute poison. Sugar makes me depressed and preservatives are the worst! You're going to laugh, aren't you? Why doesn't someone write these things down?

DR.: Why are you so worried about food?

MRS. A: Look, I'm 43. It's hard enough when you're 30, but 43! You've got to look as good undressed as you do outside. Don't you know there are nine women for every man? Don't you ever read anything? And they're all cheats, all of them.

DR.: Even John [the ex-lover]?

MRS. A: He was big and beautiful and male. He was my size. And he's such a liar and cheat and every woman wants him. He's the worst. He has women everywhere and he fell for that big dumb secretary—she's only 24 and thought he was so great—she's big, dumb and tall.

The overall effect is dramatic and stimulating. The therapist is captivated by the patient's anger and theatrical flair. She controls the interview with her loud, rapid speech and angry tone. Without limits, she will wander from topic to topic venting her affect without discussing the facts of the matter at hand. Her style entertains, intimidates, and manipulates the clinician away from the key dynamic issues—in Mrs. A's case, the lost relationship.

The challenge in interviewing the histrionic patient comes in resisting the seductiveness of the patient's affective style and keeping to the task of obtaining the facts. A stubborn and sustained insistence on the historical details behind the affect offers a measure of cognitive structure—and limits—to the patient's impulsive affective excess. With the hysteric, the clinician must play detective and get the facts, though this task can be exasperating.

The clinician may set limits by focusing on the facts of history or interpreting the process of the interview—for example: "You're angry that John left you for another woman. Tell me what happened between you." At a more process level: "You wander from topic to topic with a lot of angry feelings but don't talk about what brought you here. Why won't you talk about your loss?" The Boston analyst Elvin Semrad taught that hysterics suffer from a "separation of head and heart." The clinician repairs this breach.

The factual history—when finally obtained—will reveal characteristic disturbances in interpersonal relationships reflecting the same style. Histrionic patients typically view their partners as uncaring, unreliable, rejecting, or emotionally unresponsive. They, in turn, are described (by the partner) and experienced (by the clinician) as demanding, manipulative, and dependent.

Antisocial Personality Disorder

The impulsive dimensions of personality that characterize the dramatic group appear to be transmitted across generations and expressed through a cultural pattern of sex typing into female histrionic and male sociopathic personality styles. While the relative roles of nature and nurture have yet to be clearly defined in this transmission, the increased prevalence of male sociopathy and female hysteria within the same families suggests a close diagnostic relationship.

Interpersonal Assessment

The antisocial patient experiences his perception, thinking, and action as dominated by irresistible internal impulse or commanded by external stimulus. His cognitive style is passive and reactive, easily attracted by opportunity for immediate gratification of prevailing needs, without reflection on consequences. As a result, the patient often complains that he has no control over his actions. Impulse is immediately translated into action without delay or reflection on prior experience, values, or morality. The sociopathic patient rarely has any long-term interests and acts to gratify short-term needs according to current mood and opportunities. Because the patient lacks a background of sustained or continuous interests, his behavior lacks a sense of purpose in relation to any long-term goals. The inability to reflect, delay gratification, or inhibit impulse is expressed socially as a lack of conscience, morality, or values. The patient presents himself with a casual insincerity that betrays a lack of critical reflection on his behavior. As with the histrionic patient, the sociopath views the diagnostic interview as an opportunity to impress the clinician with his own point of view. He is often less interested in what he says than in how he says it (Shapiro, 1965).

The "performance" quality of the patient's interview poses a unique challenge to the clinician. Both patient and doctor understand society's condemnation of the antisocial behaviors that characterize the sociopathic patient. How does one obtain factual history from a patient who is more intent on making a favorable impression than on talking straight? Furthermore, when the history is a catalogue of socially offensive behaviors (some of which may still carry legal consequences), the interview itself becomes a threat to the patient.

Fortunately, most sociopathic patients are less defensive about the past than about the present. The impulsive pattern of the adult has a long track record extending back into adolescence. Major manifestations of the disorder are clearly evident before the age of 15 and are found in histories of truancy, fighting, running away, and juvenile delinquency. To obtain this history, the interviewer must not only adopt a nonjudgmental attitude but also actively encourage a complete rendition by implying that childhood behavior no longer counts. The patient is encouraged to talk freely about his wild times, his pranks, appealing to his sense of bravado, supporting his self-esteem. He is assured that no stigma is attached to his childhood hell raising—indeed, that the interviewer understands and is empathic with his account. The interview takes on a casual atmosphere, the doctor "giving permission" for admission of deviant behavior, asking such questions as: "Lots of kids play hooky from school—did you?" "Ever play pranks on animals?" "How about fights? Ever have to put somebody in his place—stand up for yourself in school?" "How about making it with the girls? Ever get in trouble?" *The purpose is diagnostic—not therapeutic; the method is manipulative.* One risk is that the patient may actually embellish his account to please the clinician. Nonetheless, the traditional interviewer's position of neutrality will fail with the antisocial patient, who interprets the examiner's impassiveness as judgmental.

All dramatic cluster patients actively manipulate a response from the clinician. Interviewing the sociopathic patient is one of the few clinical situations in which these roles may be reversed. Having confirmed the diagnosis through a nonjudgmental review of childhood, one may then return to adult behavior to identify the interpersonal consequences of sociopathy. The patient lacks an ability to sustain interpersonal relationships, parental responsibilities, or vocational stability. The inability to reflect on a stable system of values or morality is manifest in an absence of empathy for others, a lack of loyalties, and disregard of social norms. At the extreme, the sociopath is criminal; in milder form, a chronically irresponsible, inadequate individual. The patient's inadequacy is most glaring in interpersonal relationships.

Example

A 24-year-old single man was referred for psychiatric evaluation in preparation for a legal defense on felony charges of aggravated assault, involuntary deviate sexual intercourse, and unlawful restraint. The patient was accused of picking up a teenage girl in his car, forcing her to commit sexual acts, then attempting to choke her with a belt while stabbing her superficially in the stomach. This was a first arrest for this man, who, prior to arrest, was well thought of in the community and worked as a police dispatcher, a volunteer fireman, and a volunteer rescue paramedic. He was casually dressed, polite, and cooperative for the interview. While he denied the allegations against him, the patient created a distinct impression concerning his relationships with women. This was the only topic of his history presented with strong feeling and language.

T: When did you begin dating?

P: Around 17.

T: Was that early or late for your crowd?

P: It was pretty late I guess. I was pretty shy.

T: When did you begin your sexual life with women?

P: I knocked up my first piece of ass in high school. She got pregnant right away.

T: You didn't take any precautions?

P: Well, she didn't seem to care, so I didn't either.

T: What happened to the pregnancy?

P: She was opposed to abortion so we got married.

T: How long did that last?

P: Oh, about 9 months. She would always call the cops on me and her father would come over and beat me up.

T: Why?

P: She didn't like my going out drinking with the boys, wanted me to stay at home all the time . . .

The patient goes on to describe a second relationship of 2 years' duration that ended for similar reasons. He views himself as being used and overly controlled in a long-term relationship.

T: Have you seen anyone recently?

P: No, I'm tired of getting fucked, so now I'm out just to get a piece of ass.

T: Did you know Jamie [the alleged victim]?

P: Yeah, she was a young punk dope smoker, hung around with the low-life crowd. A hard-looking chick.

T: Were you ever interested in her?

P: We all knew better, she's only 16, jail bait . . .

T: Have you ever been involved sexually with guys?

P: No, doc, I'm strictly straight. Everything's just average, nothing kinky or unusual.

T: Have you ever been worried about being attacked sexually?

P: Well, me being smaller, the smaller guys are the ones who always get shit on.

T: Has that always been true for you?

P: Yeah.

T: How about now?

P: Well, I'm scared to death of jail, you know, being meat.

In dealing with the sociopathic patient, the clinician must attend not only to what is said—but also to how it is said. The patient is trying to convey an impression through language, tone, and gesture. An independent perspective, obtained through corollary history from family or friends, is imperative to understand the full meaning of the patient's presentation. In this case, family provided a critical perspective. By history, he was the youngest and least successful of four children born to a middle-class family. As a child, he participated in minor delinquent activities such as setting fires and teasing animals, but had avoided any arrest. He was sensitive to the fact that he was physically smaller than average and took great pride in his masculine appearance and activity. In addition to working with the police, fire, and rescue squads of his local community, the patient also participated actively in karate and rifle club activities. The coarseness of his language was in striking contrast to his mild and pleasant social manner, his presentation of himself as a bright, middle-class young man. In light of his history, his presentation suggested an exaggerated defense of his masculinity, a defense motivated both by unconscious factors and by the wish to impress on the examiner his straight masculine orientation as well as his rebuttal of the implication of sexual inadequacy in the charges against him. His sociopathic style of relationship is clearly manifest in a lack of empathy and sexual exploitation of his partners as well as the overt manipulation of the interviewer.

The criteria for diagnosis of antisocial personality disorder are largely historical, adding to the statistical reliability of the diagnosis. Getting a valid history of conduct disorder before age 15 and antisocial behavior after age 15 requires considerable patience and use of multiple data sources. The diagnostic criteria are behavioral manifestations of a core construct of psychopathy, defined by a lack of concern for others, disregard of social norms, incapacity to maintain relationships, low frustration tolerance, high degree of impulsivity and aggressivity, absence of remorse, and failure to profit from punishment.

Narcissistic Personality Disorder

Interpersonal Assessment

The narcissistic personality shares with the antisocial person a disregard for the needs and expectations of others. These patients are specialists in looking to themselves for support and reward. Unlike antisocial patients, the narcissistic patients' motivations are not dominated by active pursuit of gratification, but by a pervasive overvaluation of the self that assures them that they are *entitled* to have their needs met and need not pursue reinforcement actively (Millon, 1981). It is the hallmark of this egotistical pattern that these patients flatter and reward themselves, that perception, cognition, and action serve the purpose of supporting their inflated self-images. Such patients present with a pretentious, pompous disdain for others that borders on arrogance. They selectively interpret others' behavior toward them as supporting their self-importance and discount or deny experience to the contrary.

The egotistical pattern is often seen as a defensive posture, reactive to a vulnerable self-esteem and to feelings of worthlessness or inadequacy barely beyond awareness. Confronted with reversals in reality, these patients make even louder demands on others to acknowledge and support their overinflated presentation of self. When all else fails and reality seems unavoidable, the narcissistic patient resorts to fantasy and the restitutional healing of the daydream. With continued intolerable stress, depression and transient psychotic symptoms may appear.

The attitude of the patient in the following interview reflects this general style. He is self-assured and pretentious, unwilling to adopt even the rudimentary cultural deference customary to the patient role. While referral to a psychiatrist generally results from a failure of the patient's egotistical defense, there is little acknowledgment of fault. Humility and self-searching criticism are not part of the narcissist's psychological makeup. The patient behaves as though he is indifferent to the clinician's perspective. Eventually, the grandiose exaggeration of self, attitude of entitlement, and devaluation of the clinician evoke anger in the interviewer, offering valuable insight into the difficulties the patient experiences in the interpersonal world.

Example

Mr. D was a 39-year-old schoolteacher who was referred by his psychiatrist for hospital admission for excessive drug and alcohol abuse following separation from his wife. The precipitating event leading to admission was his learning that his wife had moved in with another man shortly after their separation, resulting in depression and suicidal ideation. The patient's presenting complaint was couched in a long, angry tirade about his wife's infidelity. There was no spontaneous concern about his resort to drug or alcohol abuse or any apparent sincerity in his suicidal statements. We were most impressed, however, by his accent—a distinct South African accent in a man born and raised in West Virginia! Inquiry revealed that Mr. D had worked in South Africa for 3 months many years earlier and had adopted the accent, which appeared only at times of stress. In his initial interview, the patient asked (with a straight face) if we had any medical explanation for the episodic slurred speech, staggering gait, and loss of coordination that alarmed his colleagues at school. He seemed surprised to hear of his drug problem.

When he finally admitted the problem (with little emotion), he berated the clinician for the "primitiveness" of the treatment offered. Each approach was rejected as inadequate to his level of sophistication. For example, group therapy was rejected because "Other patients have nothing to teach me" and "The staff is poorly read"; behavioral approaches to relaxation were "for amateurs," the patient noting that "I studied meditation with a yoga master." Mr. D left the hospital against advice after 10 days, indignant at the ignorance of the university hospital but no longer concerned about his wife. The South African accent had also disappeared.

Borderline Personality Disorder

Interpersonal Assessment

The borderline patient is the most extreme, and thereby the most impaired, of the dramatic group. Defined by pathological vulnerability in the areas of impulse, affect, and cognition, the borderline disorder represents a conceptual border with more severe psychiatric syndromes, including those of psychotic proportion.

Given structure and support in the interpersonal sphere, borderline patients function at the level of their intellectual capacity, with apparent control of cognition, impulse, and affect. Under stress, especially perceived loss or rejection, the patient manifests his or her inherent instability in brief but extreme reactions such as transient psychotic thoughts, self-destructive behavior, or impulsive aggression toward others. The borderline patient's history is a pattern of "stable instability," with crisis and calm alternating in response to the stress of the patient's interpersonal relationships.

When first seen, the borderline patient will most likely be in such a crisis. His or her affect is generally angry or depressed, with marked lability. A recent history of dramatic, impulsive behavior is usually evident. These behaviors are self-destructive and include drug overdose, wrist cuts, self-mutilation, or loud suicidal threats. Impulsive aggression against others presents as real or threatened assault, temper tantrums, or destruction of property. More subtle but equivalent impulsive behaviors include binges of alcohol or drug use, sexual promiscuity, or compulsive eating. This behavior appears both self-punitive and manipulative, typically following a perceived loss or rejection and arising out of a pattern of chaotic interpersonal relationships. The relationships of the borderline patient may be overly dependent and masochistic or hostile and sadistic, but all betray manipulation of the partner in a characteristic manner. The patient uses others to gratify needs with little regard for their individual and separate needs. In the crisis setting, the patient may be angry and demanding or depressed and withdrawn, both being presentations meant to coerce care from the clinician.

As with the hysteric, the borderline patient's more dramatic demands must be countered with direct limit-setting; e.g., shouting, screaming, and throwing things are unacceptable if the interview is to proceed. Similarly, self-abuse (in front of the clinician) is not tolerated. Once the ground rules for the interview are made verbally explicit, the clinician focuses on details of history, limiting affective demonstrations by structured questioning. If the patient is unable to discuss the current crisis (presumably a perceived rejection) without loss of affective and behavioral controls, the clinician should focus on the past track record for details, reserving the most painful exploration for a more controlled time or setting. Common sense should prevail in how far to push for details of the current stressor, taking into account the patient's vulnerability, the setting, and the purpose of the interview (e.g., current history may not be as necessary in making the characterological diagnosis as in judging whether the patient needs medication or hospital care).

While the episodic impulsive–destructive reactions and chaotic interpersonal relationships are the most discriminating diagnostic criteria, the borderline patient reveals many enduring traits during periods of relative calm. Borderline patients complain of not having a good sense of self, of identity, values, and goals. As with other patients having severe dependent needs, a sense of separateness is often sacrificed in the wish to be part of someone else. The exquisite rejection sensitivity of the borderline patient is based on chronically low self-esteem, heightened by the patient's wish for dependent nurturance. The patient complains of an inner sense of emptiness, an internal void experienced primitively as a true physical sensation, prompting often frantic efforts to "fill" the void. (These efforts may include excessive alcohol and drug use, binge eating, or sexual promiscuity.) The patient describes a hunger for companionship, an intolerance of being alone. Borderline patients tend to identify with those less fortunate in life and go out of their way to involve themselves with the sick and needy. By identifying with the object of their care (projective identification), they meet some of their own needs for nurturance in a socially acceptable pattern. Stray dogs and cats may also become the beneficiaries of this dynamic.

In relationships with others, the borderline patient tends to present only one aspect of personality, typically keeping separate the hostile or competitive traits from the tender and submissive ones. This defensive process, termed *splitting*, results in the creation of dyadic relationships that are grossly inconsistent but, taken together, represent the totality of the patient's needs. The borderline patient is a very different person to each significant other. In the hospital setting, as in the patient's friendship circle, this splitting process can produce conflict among the dyadic partners, an internal conflict that is acted out outside the patient. In interview, the splitting is problematic, since the therapist sees only one perspective of the patient without "outside" help.

The borderline patient uses primitive defenses such as projective identification and splitting as part of his or her characteristic style. Under duress, cognition may become further disrupted and truly psychotic defenses appear, resulting in distortions of perception (derealization, depersonalization), referential thinking, and paranoid ideation.

Example

The patient was a 22-year-old single woman referred by her family for long-term psychotherapy following multiple hospitalizations for suicidal behavior and self-inflicted injuries. She was unable to hold a job or remain in school for more than a few months at a time and appeared without direction in life. Repeated psychiatric hospitalizations of brief duration and aggressive pharmacotherapy had failed to stabilize her highly reactive moods and her sensitivity to rejection (both real and fantasized).

Historical review disclosed that the patient had been adopted in infancy and was temperamentally very different from her emotionally reserved parents. She was raised in a middle-class home as an only child. Her parents were college-educated, industrious people who worked in white-collar occupations and expected their daughter to do the same. Instead, she had become progressively disruptive in the home through her dramatic mood swings and demandingness. By age 13, she was responding to limits and perceived rejection with temper outbursts and self-abuse, primarily wrist-cutting. She was a rebellious adolescent, who identified with a drug-using, promiscuous, punk peer group. Her outrageous behavior and dress resulted in her being expelled from eight schools in the four years of high school. (She shaved the sides of her head and spiked her hair in punk fashion, dyed her hair black, and wore black lipstick, nail polish, and clothes.) After a long period of sexual promiscuity, using her body to command attention and "caring" from men, she settled on a lesbian life style, reserving heterosexual contact for sadomasochistic prostitution.

It was in the context of her first committed relationship, at age 18, that her pattern of rejection sensitivity and self-abuse became life-threatening. She would provoke her lover into physical fights in which she was beaten and (temporarily) abandoned, precipitating a pattern of wild "street" behavior that ended in overdose, wrist cuts, and hospitalization. This cycle was repeated many times in the 3-year relationship. In her own words: "If she didn't hit me, she didn't love me. Without her, I hibernated, did S&M, whored, and did crack, obliviated myself because she wasn't there."

The formal diagnosis of borderline personality disorder is made from a history of emotional instability, rejection sensitivity, repeated suicide attempts, and identity confusion. A history of unstable interpersonal relationships often reflects the patient's low self-esteem and intense dependency needs. In our example, angry rebellion masked the patient's impaired self-esteem during adolescence and was later seen more clearly in her dependence on her partners and dramatic attention-seeking behaviors. Her identity confusion was apparent in the choice of sexual partners (first heterosexual, then homosexual) and sexual behaviors (promiscuity, sadomasochistic prostitution as a dominatrix), but ultimately in her inability to define a life-style or life goals based on a stable set of values.

ANXIOUS–FEARFUL GROUP

Obsessive–Compulsive Personality Disorder

Interpersonal Assessment

While dramatic personalities make loud demands on others and manipulate the environment through affect and behavior, the anxious–fearful group are defined by excessive inhibition and self-control. The best studied of the group are the obsessive–compulsive personalities, whose efforts at self-control produce a rigidity of thought, a formality of affect, and deliberateness of action unequaled by others. The obsessive–compulsive person views the world with a degree of intellectual effort and deliberateness that controls all spontaneous affect. This style is manifest by a rigid control over perception and attention, an intense preoccupation with details, and an analytical mode of cognition. Impulse and affect are the enemy of the obsessive–compulsive and are contained by a set of rigid moral directives or rules for action that tend to be overbearing and inflexible. The obsessive–compulsive patient develops an internal bureaucracy of conscience, with rules and regulations governing thought, affect, and action. Authoritarian dogma in the cognitive realm is matched by a lack of spontaneity in the affective sphere. Without rules, the patient becomes paralyzed by choices, an ambivalence that makes free choice intolerable. The patient avoids novel situations in which creative solutions are required. Rigidity of thinking prevents creativity. At the extreme, the obsessive–compulsive patient is a caricature of control, a technocrat obsessed with details, unresponsive to the affective value of a situation, unable to appreciate spontaneous impulse or creative choice (Shapiro, 1965).

The interview style of the obsessive–compulsive patient is marked by intellectual monotony. The patient recounts his history in lengthy detail, somehow missing the point. There is often a glaring incongruity between the content of conversation and the patient's affective tone. Highly emotional issues and conflicts may be presented with characteristic intellectual calm, while seemingly trivial events produce an outpouring of righteous indignation. The affect associated with personally hot issues is typically isolated away, the issue intellectualized, until the affect can be displaced onto another (impersonal) target. The patient defends against experiencing emotion in the interview by focusing on details, by intellectualizing or rationalizing events or—when all else fails—by obsessing. Under real interpersonal pressure, the patient may fall silent and count books on the clinician's shelf, solve a mind puzzle, contemplate world events—all far removed from the emotional situation at hand. The obsessive–compulsive patient shares with the histrionic patient a "separation of head and heart." In contrast to the hysteric, who is dominated by affect and blind to reason, the obsessive–compulsive is dominated by thought. The more painful the emotion, the more rigid, dogmatic, and intellectual the obsessive defense.

Example

A 40-year-old engineer recently learned that his wife has been unfaithful to him. The therapist tries to elicit some emotional response.

T: What did she tell you?

P: Everything, the whole thing. You know, now I understand why she's been so nervous lately. I thought she was a little crazy or something.

T: How do you feel about it?

P: Well it sure helped me see a lot that I missed before, you know, put the pieces together. Now they all fit—like a puzzle.

T: What was it like for you?

P: At first I tried to figure out why she did it. If she was unhappy, why didn't she say something? Then I figured she must have met him at the convention. Maybe she was lonely or something. She's not a drinker. Maybe she had too much to drink.

T: She said that to you?

P: No, but there's got to be a reason. She never said anything. It's not like we've been fighting or anything.

T: Must have been a surprise.

P: I try to see things from her point of view. Maybe she just wanted a change, things are too dull.

T: [Insistent] So your wife tells you she has an affair—so how is it for you?

P: That's what I've been saying. I understand more of what's been happening at home. It's like that book up there [refers to a textbook on the shelf] *Hazards of Medication*—hazards is right.

T: What? I don't understand.

P: Well, that's what happened to her—all the nerves at home—from the affair—a hazard.

T: [Laughs] I'm trying to get you to talk and you're reading my books! Look, how would you tell this to a really close friend. I mean, what would you say?

P: What kind of friend? I have all kinds—friends at work, neighbors, at the train club. Talking to a psychiatrist is not exactly easy. Not like talking to a friend, you know.

T: So how would you tell it?

P: Well I'd find out what went wrong. The way I understand it, I'm responsible for a kind of fault too, ah, a kind of social infidelity and she's responsible for a sexual one. I admit it. I've been a lump for a number of years. So I asked myself what was meant by love. I figure there are three parts—understanding, companionship, and passion. So I've decided to unlump myself, exercise regularly, lose some weight, go out more. I told her we would take the week off from work and just spend all the time together. We'll talk it over and figure out what went wrong. We need a second honeymoon. I figure we can go out to dinner every night—like a real honeymoon and straighten this out.

T: Are you angry? Hurt?

P: I suppose. It was quite a surprise but it really explained everything.

T: You *suppose*! You don't *know*?

The session ends without any real expression of feeling, despite the therapist's obvious exasperation. The following day, the patient phoned to ask the therapist to clarify what he meant by "talking to a friend" ("I wanted you to know that I do have friends, but talking to a psychiatrist is different").

This example illustrates the defensive use of intellectualization and rationalization as the patient avoids his painful feelings. Because of deep-seated conflicts concerning powerlessness and dependency, interpretation of the patient's responsibility for his problems will be viewed as critical judgments by a powerful authority. Even the therapist's attempt to be disarming with humor and mild sarcasm (to evoke an affective response) is met by a rigid, stubborn insistence on an alternative intellectual solution. In this example, the patient has a new "understanding" of his wife's nervous behavior—rather than a gut reaction to her infidelity. He works out a plan to deal with the problem rather than responding emotionally. The irrelevance of his rambling rationalization is obvious from his preoccupation with the therapist's meaning in asking about his friends.

The obsessive–compulsive patient will often wander far away from the emotional business at hand in a long-winded litany of endless and meaningless detail. In the extreme case, the patient may actually confront the therapist with a written agenda, notes in hand, in an effort to control the interchange and defend against spontaneous feeling.

To work with an obsessive–compulsive personality requires an active, intrusive process. The clinician must follow the affect and encourage its expression. A quiet, reflective position merely complements the patient's defenses. The interview deteriorates into an academic, intellectual exercise in which the patient's motivation is defined and explained but not changed. The role of patient is inherently uncomfortable for the patient, whose concerns with dependence and power require keeping the therapist at a distance. The clinician should avoid being drawn into meaningless intellectual arguments, power struggles in which the patient views the therapist as a hostile, critical opponent. On the other hand, the clinician must actively cut through rambling discourse to expose the affective issues. A light-handed, uncritical sense of humor and emotional spontaneity are strong assets for those who would deal with the obsessive–compulsive patient.

Avoidant, Dependent, and Passive–Aggressive Personality Disorders

Although less well established, the remaining three disorders of the anxious–fearful group are defined by conflicts involving a desire for social approval and fears of rejection, the dimension of intimacy vs. distance in interpersonal relations. These personality disorders are each organized around a single behavioral dimension, raising the theoretical issue of whether they should more properly be considered trait disturbances. With the understanding that overlapping patterns exist, the authors of DSM-IV have represented each separately.

Avoidant Personality Disorder

Interpersonal Assessment

Avoidant individuals suffer from social anxieties, fears of rejection, humiliation, and criticism. While desiring to be accepted, they actively withhold themselves from the social setting, creating sufficient distance to feel safe. They suffer from a lack of self-confidence, expressed in a passive, unassertive, fearful lifestyle, avoiding competition and aggression. At the core of the personality is low self-esteem.

In the interview setting, the patient presents as shy, fearful, awkward. Rejection sensitivity is apparent from the patient's scanning observational style and painful self-consciousness. Affect and physical movement are overly controlled in a consciously deliberate manner. The patient is hesitant, awkward in speech and unspontaneous. He or she appears sensitive, mistrustful, vulnerable.

Example

A 24-year-old single graduate student was referred to the university counseling center by his academic advisor for difficulty completing his course requirements for graduation. Although he clearly possessed adequate knowledge and had demonstrated ability on exams, he was chronically late with his assignments and missed critical deadlines for papers. A review of his academic career revealed a pattern of procrastination around decisions that would produce changes in his life. His associations to graduation focused on the theme of leaving the sheltered life of the university, a life that was highly structured, though, as history revealed, intensely lonely. The patient had few friends, was painfully shy, and had never dated. The companionship of classmates and the socialization of the school setting had not led to close friendships, but had filled a social need that he felt incapable of meeting on his own, that is, in the real world outside the university.

His interview presentation revealed him to be introverted and emotionally guarded, sharing little affect. He was very self-conscious and fearful of attracting attention, lest people ridicule or reject him, yet he desperately wanted to be part of the crowd. His fantasy life reflected both an intense desire for acceptance by peers (especially women) and rage over his interpersonal failures. He was often preoccupied with violent fantasies of revenge for presumed rejections. His extracurricular life centered around solitary activities, bike riding and weight lifting, with little apparent effort to join others. His "academic problem" proved, in fact, to be a defense against anxiety over being "forced" out of a marginal social life into a friendless world.

Dependent Personality Disorder

Interpersonal Assessment

The dependent person has a similar need for approval and dread of rejection. His solution is total submission to the wishes of his benefactor. He is the master of the "inferior role" (Millon, 1981). Motivated by a fear of rejection, disapproval, and abandonment, he inhibits his own assertiveness and initiative in the service of maintaining the dependent bond. At the extreme, the dependent individual presents as self-effacing, ingratiating, and helpless. At best, the patient earns his position by complementing his partner's needs for dominance, power, or benevolence, masking his own degree of dependence by loyal service.

In the interview, the dependent person is deferential to excess, overly cooperative, and eager to please the therapist. Angry feelings or resentful thoughts are suppressed, even when justified (e.g., when the clinician is late or cancels or changes appointment times on short notice). The absence of initiative is apparent in the context of the interview. The clinician feels pressed to lead the patient, to keep the flow of the interview moving. Without explicit direction, the patient waits. Once the clinician's interests are apparent, the dependent patient will elaborate this topic despite absence of relevance in his life. The interview may deteriorate into a repetitious account of behavior that the patient feels the clinician wishes to hear. The passivity and submissiveness of the dependent patient must themselves become the focus of work.

Example

A 45-year-old man presented to the clinic requesting help for anger and depression precipitated by the remarriage of his mother after 13 years of widowhood and the sale of the family home. He was the oldest of four children born to a poor family and raised on a farm. The patient's father had been a chronic alcoholic and grossly negligent in caring for the patient and his three younger siblings. As a result, from an early age, the patient felt he had become a surrogate husband to his mother and father to his brothers. Raised in a small rural community and isolated on the farm, he made few friends outside his immediate family. He stated that he always had difficulty relating to people and felt uncomfortable in social settings. Although he had completed a college degree in accounting at a local college, he had not succeeded in finding work as an accountant. He had one brief dating relationship (at age 28), but no relationships with women since then. With the exception of two brief attempts to live on his own, he had remained with his mother in the parental home, assuming more responsibility following the father's death and supporting the household by driving a cab. His mother's decision to remarry and sell the family home left him feeling "used," "abandoned," and "incapable of functioning in society on my own."

A pervasive pattern of dependent and submissive behavior defines the dependent personality disorder in DSM-IV. These patients have an excessive need to be taken care of, lack confidence in their ability to care for themselves, and go to excessive lengths to seek support from others.

Passive–Aggressive Personality Disorder

In DSM-IV, the passive–aggressive personality is no longer considered a full disorder, but is treated as a trait disturbance under "personality disorder, not otherwise specified." The passive–aggressive trait fits easily into the anxious–fearful group.

Interpersonal Assessment

The passive–aggressive individual desires the approval of others, but is covertly resentful of the degree of compliance needed to guarantee results. He is torn between being passive or assertive, dependent or autonomous, to meet his needs. It is the intensity of these conflicting dynamics that makes the pattern pathological. As a result, his behavior is erratic and vacillates between sullen acquiescence and contradictory, often covert, opposition. Demands by others are met with a negative, resistant attitude as though all are unreasonable. The patient makes a great show of his efforts to please others or engender guilt at his apparent suffering on their account. The martyr role invariably masks a manipulative, often malicious intent. Despite the overt display, the passive–aggressive patient typically manifests his resentment through studied inefficiency and intentional ineptness. The patient may be pessimistic, discontented, complaining, or sullen, but rarely risks the overt display of anger that threatens dependent ties.

Example

A 28-year-old dental hygienist was admitted to hospital for depression associated with a fight with her roommate of long standing. The roommate was soon to be married and wanted the patient to move out of their apartment in favor of the couple. The patient responded to loss of the interpersonal tie by fighting over the apartment. She describes her method:

P: I'll kill her with kindness. I'll be so sickeningly sweet. She hates that. Anyhow, she can't throw me out when I'm in the hospital.

T: Why don't you ask her to move in with Don?

P: She would see that as a rejection. After all, she is supposed to be my best friend.

T: But she *is* getting married.

P: She doesn't have to be so nasty about it.

In the interview setting, the passive–aggressive patient complains about the degree to which he or she serves the needs of others, the little he or she receives in turn, and how little he or she is appreciated. These attitudes extend to the clinician. The patient complains that he or she is given too little direction, but when suggestions are made, each is found to be unacceptable. He or she is simultaneously demanding, yet rejecting of help.

The passive–aggressive patient shrinks from responsibility, preferring the security of a dependent position—reserving the right to complain. If the clinician suggests a specific course of action (e.g., psychological or vocational testing), the patient may grudgingly comply, but accepts no responsibility for the decision. If the project fails—perhaps due to lack of real effort on the patient's part—he accepts no blame. Low self-esteem is apparent in the patient's depressive, pessimistic outlook on life, but serves the purpose of luring the clinician into further efforts to be directive and helpful. The patient is envious of others—including the clinician—and complains that others are withholding and can give more. As with all dependent individuals, the complaining stops short of actual anger, the aggression is passive and masked. A spilled ashtray or cup of coffee in the doctor's office conveys the message of discontent despite profuse and abject apologies from the patient.

The key criterion for diagnosis of the passive–aggressive personality disorder in DSM-IV is a pervasive pattern of passive resistance and general obstructiveness in response to the expectations of others.

ODD/ECCENTRIC GROUP

Interpersonal Assessment

The paranoid, schizoid, and schizotypal personalities comprise the odd or eccentric group. Characterized by social and emotional distance and peculiarities of thought, patients in this group bear a distinct but superficial resemblance to those with psychotic disorders (e.g., paranoid and schizophrenic disorders). All share profound deficits in their ability to relate warmly in personal relationships or form enduring, trusting ties to others. Their oddness and isolation derive primarily from peculiarities of perception and thought, rather than social anxiety or shyness.

Among the eccentrics, the paranoid is the most striking and the most functional. His perception and interpretation of the interpersonal world are organized around a basic mistrust and a suspicious attitude. Suspiciousness is a style of thinking brought to bear on all interpersonal events and is served by a vigilant, hypersensitive, searching mode of attention. The paranoid scans the world, seeking out potential sources of external threat, discounting the face value of events in favor of an interpretation of hidden motives allied to the patient's suspicions. He approaches novel situations with controlled affect and movement, ready for action, as though each interaction posed a threat to self-esteem, autonomy, or control. Much of the patient's thought is occupied with a fear of being dominated or controlled by others. Warm, spontaneous emotions are suppressed as indicators of vulnerability (to external control), while fearful affects are projected, leading to the perception of threat from others. The patient's inner experience of emotion is restricted, the outward expression of feeling controlled (Shapiro, 1965).

While the paranoid's mistrust may lead to aggressive defenses and confrontational tactics, the schizoid individual withdraws from emotional interactions, appearing to function with little or no affective spontaneity. Described by Bleuler as "people who are comfortably dull, at the same time sensitive," schizoids perceive any affective arousal as distressing, avoiding interpersonal ties that demand or stimulate emotion (Siever, 1981). The schizoid patient may elaborate an inner fantasy world, an autistic environment to which he retreats for comfort from the threatening emotional world of interpersonal reality.

The schizotypal individual is one step closer to autistic functioning and experiences true distortions of reality in response to affective arousal. Such individuals not only experience the world as threatening but also defend themselves from it with near psychotic dissociation (derealization, depersonalization), referential thinking, and mild paranoid ideation. The world is perceived through a cognitive style subject to autistic distortion under stress.

An interview with a paranoid, schizoid, or schizotypal patient is marked on the patient's part by the absence of emotional rapport or even superficial trust that characterizes most doctor–patient exchanges. The clinician feels the suspicion of the paranoid, the emotional distance of the schizoid, and the bizarreness of the schizotypal patient. The scanning hypervigilance of the patient makes the clinician uncomfortably aware that his gestures and words are being examined for hidden meaning or signs of threat. Success in interviewing the paranoid patient hinges on one's ability to be open and candid in the face of suspicion and mistrust. While the patient seeks hidden meanings to validate his beliefs, the clinician must respond with detailed and explicit discussion of all areas under suspicion, however trivial they may seem.

The patient's initial testing of the relationship may begin with the mechanics of arranging the first interview. The operation of the office (or clinic), the hours available, the clinician's expectations and fee may provide an early focus for suspicion. The negotiation of the first visit may represent a first test of power dynamics. With a little forewarning, the clinician anticipates these concerns, explains the format as openly as possible, and gives the patient as much choice as possible—wherever possible (e.g., office hours).

The paranoid patient's need to maintain distance and resist the dependency inherent in the patient role may lead to confrontations, argument, or challenging of the clinician's authority, knowledge—and even credentials. Reasonable inquiry should be answered directly, before asking why the question was asked. (It is wise to delay the investigation of the patient's motivation until it is clear that he will remain a patient!) A lighthearted sense of humor, uncritical and benign, helps with the more blatant confrontations. The paranoid patient is fearful of being controlled and humiliated in the relationship with any authority. A mild, soft-spoken manner and physically unassuming presence are reassuring to the patient. It is important for the clinician to be emotionally visible and responsive. The blank screen of analytic lore only provokes projection by the paranoid patient. The therapist's silence will be interpreted as hostility. The patient wishes to know where you are emotionally and physically. To form a therapeutic alliance, one must let him know.

To this point, our discussion assumes the patient is cooperative and not severely impaired, that the interview has been scheduled with some opportunity for preparation. In the emergency setting, or in crisis intervention, the patient may be functioning with less control of reality testing. The more impaired the patient, the more explicit the clinician must be about the realities of the interview situation. In the extreme case, one in which the patient is using psychotic projection and distortion to deal with stress, the clinician must actually help the patient test the reality of his fears and set limits on the use of the psychotic defenses. Ideas of reference and persecutory fears can be tested directly, by asking such questions as: "Who is talking about you?" "How do they know you?" "Why you?" If the patient is anxious or agitated, offer to change the routine to meet his needs (within reason). For example, a patient fearing attack may be interviewed in an open area, a waiting room, or an office with the door open. If the patient is fearful that the room is bugged, he should be encouraged to look until satisfied that there are no bugs. This paradoxical method forces the patient to confront his own delusional perception with direct challenge by the clinician. The paranoid patient should be able to test the reality of his distortions given the cognitive structure imposed by the interviewer and a nonthreatening, supportive atmosphere. If the patient is unable to test the reality of his perceptions, the diagnosis warrants revision.

Example

A 41-year-old married woman was referred for treatment in an outpatient therapy clinic with an accompanying warning from the intake team that she had been very uncooperative in giving information, had been secretive and vague about facts in her life, and had angered her psychiatrist intake interviewer by challenging his motives and credentials. She was an articulate, college-educated mother of two who quickly listed many grievances about how she was treated by others. Specifically, she complained about the coldness and distance in her marriage to a man whom she chose for his financial stability and self-reliance. She complained that she often felt rejected by others, that other people were "out to get her" and caused problems for her at work and through her children. As a result, she had significant difficulty holding a job and frequent conflicts with her children's teachers. Previous attempts to get help ended when she became suspicious of the motives of the clinic staff and detected "conspiracies" between the agency, the school, and her employers. At times of personal stress, she responded with a marked increase in these accusations, in angry confrontations with authority figures, including husband, boss, school, and therapists. This was the state in which she had presented to the intake team.

To engage this patient in treatment, it was necessary to provide an open, nonconfrontational setting in which she could vent her grievances, keep her secrets, and test the trustworthiness of the therapist. She was not confronted with demands for information, but was allowed to control as much as possible the content of the sessions and the time and duration of visits. (Getting her to come and stay was itself an accomplishment.) It was apparent early on that she had the ability to test the reality of her beliefs, that she recognized that her fears worsened during time of personal stress. This was critical in distinguishing between a delusional process and a chronic interpersonal style of paranoid perception and projection. In time, she conformed to a more traditional therapy format and would accept interpretation of her paranoid defenses without defensive anger. She even accepted the occasional prescription of low-dose neuroleptic medication when the paranoid defenses became too disruptive.

The critical dimension of the paranoid patient is a *pervasive distrust* and *suspiciousness of others*. This is the belief that leads to unwarranted fears of harm or exploitation by others, to perception of attacks on one's character (when none is apparent), to reluctance to confide in others, and to the tendency to bear grudges persistently.

Schizoid Personality Disorder

Interpersonal Assessment

While the paranoid patient establishes distance and control in the interview through a suspicious and argumentative style, the schizoid shrinks from any affective arousal, appearing insensitive and indifferent to interpersonal relationships. The patient does not respond with the casual social graces that are taken for granted by others. Social pleasantries, greetings, jokes, small talk in the office that precede or follow a session fail to bring the customary responses. The clinician is faced with an unresponsive, bland patient whose emotional tone seems reduced to a bare minimum. An eerie feeling of being out of contact, not on the same wavelength, characterizes this interview.

The schizoid patient's withdrawal and isolation provide a focus for investigation in the interview. If the clinician assumes this to be a motivated defensive adaptation, the work of the interview lies in uncovering the painful origins of this life-style. Engaging the patient in this process takes considerable enthusiasm and activity on the clinician's part. A spontaneous, emotionally active approach is needed to stimulate, manipulate, and even provoke the schizoid patient into recalling painful events. Whenever possible, the clinician labels and encourages the patient's expression of emotion: "You look sad. That must have been painful for you. It's okay to cry." The patient may be given permission to express feeling: "That would have made anyone angry—how did you feel about it?" When a socially expected response is inhibited, the clinician can get his point across with a well-timed exaggeration: "You weren't angry? Not at all? Not even a little bit?" This would be followed by the more tactful inquiry: "If you weren't—why weren't you?" One pokes and prods the schizoid patient, cajoling and coercing until the historical origins of the social withdrawal are clarified and the associated affect is appropriately acknowledged and felt.

Example

Tom was a 32-year-old single man referred to the clinic by his mother. His chief complaint and self description defined the problem: "I don't fit in. I don't belong. I'm not wanted. I feel numb, empty, and unhappy." Tom described a childhood in which he had few friends, "drifted" between social groups without any well-defined sense of belonging. Although a high school graduate, he had no sense of motivation, of personal or vocational goals. He had 15 jobs in a 7-year period, and was unable to develop any enthusiasm for a vocation. He appeared content to support himself in a marginal life-style, on and off welfare. His longest employment was a 4-year enlistment in the Navy, which ended in a rejection of his request to reenlist. Relationships with women were sporadic and characterized by him as "brief infatuations." He had abruptly ended his last effort at psychotherapy when he became infatuated with his female therapist. He was surprisingly eloquent in describing his poor self-concept ("a vagabond"), his aversion to responsibility or commitment, personally and vocationally: "The world is a dark, senseless place. I have little inclination to participate in its hypocrisy." On interpersonal relationships: "I look for security, not love." Security meant being supported until emotional demands were made on him, at which point he would "drift on out of boredom."

Tom was generally disheveled, unkempt, and malodorous, though he was employed at the time of his clinic visits. He showed little concern for the social impression he made on others despite complaining about frequent rejection. He avoided eye contact and spoke in monologue as though his therapist were not present. His voice and affect did not express the emotional content of his words. He was, in sum, odd in appearance, flat of affect, and tedious to sit with.

The key diagnostic criterion for the schizoid patient in DSM-IV is a pervasive pattern of detachment from social relationships and restricted range of expression of emotions in interpersonal settings.

Schizotypal Personality Disorder

Interpersonal Assessment

The schizotypal patient differs from the schizoid in the presence of overt manifestations of mild thought disorder. While research has uncovered no clear empirical evidence for a biological link between the schizoid personality and schizophrenia, the schizotype appears to be in a genetic spectrum shared by the more severe forms of thought disorder. Schizotypal patients share the paranoid's mistrust and the schizoid's emotional isolation, but demonstrate true cognitive slippage under emotional duress. The patient appears to suspend reality testing transiently under stress, only to correct the distortions in a conflict-free time or place. In the realm of perception, the schizotype experiences dissociative episodes (derealization, depersonalization), illusions, and even non-Schneiderian (e.g., nonschizophrenic) hallucinosis under duress.

The schizotypal personality experiences cognitive and perceptual distortions such as ideas of references, magical thinking, and illusions. While the patient cannot report on the oddness of his thought and speech, a mild thought disorder in both form and content is often apparent to the examiner. An example of "primary process" thinking is illustrated in the following letter received by a therapist from his patient in the course of a long- term psychodynamic psychotherapy. The patient, a college-educated, professionally trained woman, tries to explain her frequent lapses into silence during therapy. This is being explored by the therapist as a resistance to sharing painful experiences.

Example

If I speak words I'll feel, I won't be. I have too many thoughts to speak just one. Feelings expose and magnetize me to others but I want to live. I live in my head. How can I tell you anything if I won't get myself back? I will be connected to you and then I won't be me. I'll be all gone. For example, if I speak sex I'll be sex-bound. I'll want you and I don't want you. I want my feelings and thoughts to go with my husband and his feelings and thoughts. I'll feel violated if I trust. Sharing words will turn into sexual feelings and that would be messy and oh so connected.

The mild looseness of association and idiosyncratic usage of words illustrate defects in the form of thought, while the content describes a loss of ego boundaries and a primitive fusion fantasy more common in psychotic patients.

Writers who view the schizotype as one step removed from schizophrenia point to the patient's cognitive distortions and autistic thinking as a primary process, while the more dramatic quasi-delusional symptoms appear only in response to stress. The schizotype's difficulties in achieving satisfaction (anhedonia) or resolving conflicting desires (ambivalence) may be indicators of a general distortion of the personality in the direction of schizophrenia.

Psychotic Symptoms and Personality Disorder

With the odd/eccentric personality group, the patient's symptoms resemble milder forms of more severe paranoid and schizophrenic phenomena. While the DSM restricts the use of the term *psychotic* to "gross impairment in reality testing" as manifested by the presence of either delusions or hallucinations, it is clear that the psychological function of reality testing appears particularly vulnerable in some patients with "nonpsychotic" personality disorders, especially the odd/eccentric groups and the dramatic cluster. In particular, paranoid and schizotypal patients appear to have frequent cognitive distortions reflecting a tenuous hold on reality, while the borderline, histrionic, and narcissistic types require significant interpersonal stressors to reveal transient loss of reality testing. Psychoanalytic writers make a distinction between the absolute loss of reality testing in the true psychotic and a diminished *sense* of reality (or the "suspension" of reality testing) in the stress-vulnerable personalities. The distinction is important diagnostically and is testable in the clinical interview. With the structure of the interview, the stress-vulnerable personality will reorganize and "test" irrational "micropsychotic" experience. The truly psychotic individual generally cannot do so.

Do's and Don't's

Diagnostic interviewing is not therapy. Although the effect may be therapeutic, the intent of the diagnostic interview is to gather data from the content and process of the interview to make an accurate assessment. Because time is often limited, the methods of diagnostic interviewing may be more active, intrusive, or even manipulative compared to those of long-term psychotherapy. Unlike the therapist, the diagnostician has a structured format for his thinking (e.g., predetermined categories used to sort developmental history, symptom presentation, and interview observations). He actively includes or rules out diagnostic categories as the patient presents his problem. An initial impression leads to formulation of a differential diagnosis and a list of related disorders to be considered. Resolution of the differential diagnosis requires active investigation for historical or symptomatic criteria needed to make specific diagnoses.

The clinical approach to the patient must be adapted to the patient's dominant defensive style. Patients from the dramatic group must have a more structured interview to elicit factual history and contain lability of affect and flights of fantasy. The diagnostic interview uses the cognitive limits of structured questioning to help patients organize the thoughts behind their experiences in a coherent manner. In contrast, anxious–fearful patients suffer from cognitive overcontrol and must be pressed for affective responses in painful areas to complete the diagnostic process. Odd/eccentric patients will need an open, accepting, and uncritical clinician to develop trust enough to relate history. With each interview, the diagnostician reviews his checklist of criteria until satisfied by the fit between data and diagnosis.

Personality disorder is not episodic. One must examine the patient's life experience—a longitudinal perspective—to make an accurate diagnosis. The cross-sectional perspective obtained during a hospital admission or crisis interview is rarely sufficient due to distortion by anxieties, depressions, or stress responses superimposed on the personality style. In DSM terminology, Axis I disorders often obscure and confound the diagnosis of comorbid Axis II personality disorders. One is occasionally embarrassed by the "disappearance" of an Axis II personality disorder along with remission of Axis I depression. On the other hand, one must not "biologize" behavior, i.e., force the affective and cognitive reactions of the personality into artificial biological constructs. Not every depressed mood is a major affective disorder or every cognitive slip an underlying schizophrenia.

Accuracy of diagnosis is proportional to the number of perspectives. The patient does not exist in a vacuum, but is defined (insofar as personality is concerned) by his interactions with others. Additional perspectives should be sought from family and friends to test the clinician's experience. The patient presents his own history in a self-conscious and self-interested fashion. A biased presentation may be unconscious and unintentional, or consciously manipulative, depending on the patient's motivation. The clinician should not hesitate to test his own perceptions against the experience of others.

The general task of the diagnostic interviewer is best likened to that of a detective, whose job is to get the facts. It is useful to view the patient's symptoms and defensive maneuvers as forms of self-deception, an avoidance of a painful inner reality. As the diagnostic process unfolds, the clinician helps the patient acknowledge some of these realities, express and bear the associated feelings, and place them in perspective. Success in this process will lead to an accurate diagnosis, psychodynamic formulation, and assessment of potential for therapeutic change.

Finally, personality disorder is more than a matrix for episodic mental illness. It is a disabling disorder in its own right, more devastating for its subtlety and chronicity and all the more deserving of therapeutic effort. To dismiss the symptoms of disordered personality as "problems of living," unworthy of the most serious attention, is to deny the poet's admonition that "character is destiny."

SUMMARY

Recent advances in the study of personality disorders have resulted in the development of criteria-based diagnoses and structured interview methods to enhance reliability. For the practicing clinician, these tools offer a framework for clinical interviewing and a guide for understanding the psychopathology of the patient with personality disorders. Modern diagnostic practice is an amalgam of dimensional and categorical perspectives on personality, defining characteristic and habitual styles of perceiving, thinking, feeling, and acting for ten prototypical personality disorders. These disorders must be interpreted within an interpersonal, social and cultural context.

This chapter discusses the ten prototypical personality disorders of DSM-IV from the perspective of the clinical interviewer. The personality disorders are conceptually organized into three dimensional clusters, the dramatic, anxious–fearful, and odd/eccentric personality types, each with its own interactional style. An understanding of how each patient perceives the interpersonal world and operates within a specific cognitive and affective structure helps the clinician modify the interview process to achieve a collaborative and accurate result.

REFERENCES

American Psychiatric Association (1994). *Diagnostic and statistical manual of mental disorders*, 4th ed. Washington, DC: Author.

Bleuler, E. (1924). Textbook of Psychiatry (A. A. Brill, Trans.). London: Allen and Unwin.

Loranger, A. W., Susman, V. L., Oldham, J. M., & Russakoff, L. M. (1985). *Personality Disorder Examination (PDE): A structured interview for DSM-III-R Personality Disorders*. Unpublished manuscript, New York Hospital–Cornell Medical Center, Westchester Division, White Plains.

Millon, T. (1981). *Disorders of personality: DSM-III Axis II*. New York: John Wiley.

Pfohl, B., Stangl, D., & Zimmerman, M. (1983). *Structured interview for DSM-III personality disorders. SIDP* (2nd ed.). Unpublished manuscript, University of Iowa College of Medicine, Iowa City.

Reich, W. (1945). *Character analysis*, 3rd ed. (1980). Translated by Vincent R. Carfagno. New York: Farrar, Strauss & Giroux.

Shapiro, D. (1965). *Neurotic styles*. New York: Basic Books.

Siever, L. J. (1981). Schizoid and schizotypal personality disorders. In J. R. Lion (Ed.), *Personality disorders: Diagnosis and management*, 2nd ed. Baltimore: Williams & Wilkins.

Wiggins, J. S. (1982). Circumplex models of interpersonal behavior in clinical psychology. In P. C. Kendall & J. N. Butcher (Eds.), *Handbook of research methods in clinical psychology* (pp. 183–221). New York: John Wiley.

7

Alcohol Problems

Linda C. Sobell, Tony Toneatto, Mark B. Sobell,
and Jennifer-Ann Shillingford

Description of the Disorder

Many people experience problems related to their use of alcohol. These problems can be quite diverse, including, for example, accidents, family conflicts, impaired work performance, and cirrhosis of the liver. Whatever their nature, alcohol problems impose a heavy burden on society. It has been estimated that the cost of alcohol problems in the United States in 1990 was $136.3 billion (National Institute on Alcohol Abuse and Alcoholism, 1990). The costs occur in a wide range of domains, such as excessive morbidity and mortality, lost productivity at work, and disrupted families.

This chapter provides an overview of critical areas that need to be addressed in assessing and diagnosing individuals with alcohol problems. The clinical utility of various interviewing strategies and diagnostic instruments is reviewed, and case examples are presented to demonstrate the value of selected assessment instruments.

Alcohol problems have in common that individuals suffer adverse consequences related to their drinking. This being the case, there can be no modal description of this disorder. In its minimal form, for example, a person may simply become mildly intoxicated on occasion, provoking marital disputes. At the extreme, a person's life can revolve around obtaining and consuming alcohol even though the person knows that further consumption may be life-threatening.

Although research shows that alcohol problems are best conceptualized as

The views expressed in this chapter are those of the authors and do not necessarily reflect those of the Addiction Research Foundation.

Linda C. Sobell and Mark B. Sobell • Addiction Research Foundation, Toronto, Ontario, Canada M5S 2S1; Department of Psychology, University of Toronto, Toronto, Ontario, Canada M5S 1A1; and Department of Behavioural Science, University of Toronto, Toronto, Ontario, Canada M5S 1A8. Tony Toneatto • Addiction Research Foundation, Toronto, Ontario, Canada M5S 2S1; and Department of Behavioural Science, University of Toronto, Toronto, Ontario, Canada M5S 1A8. Jennifer-Ann Shillingford • Toronto General Hospital, Toronto, Ontario, Canada M5G 2C4.

Diagnostic Interviewing (Second Edition), edited by Michel Hersen and Samuel M. Turner. Plenum Press, New York, 1994.

lying on a continuum—from none to mild to moderate to severe—historically, the population of major concern to workers in the alcohol field has been persons who are severely dependent on alcohol. Many years ago, this focus was expected because severely dependent individuals were those most likely to go to the few available alcohol treatment facilities. Today, while many more treatment programs exist, the emphasis is still on severe cases. This situation is unfortunate, as the field has neglected individuals whose alcohol problems are not severe. As can be seen in Figure 1, the population of persons with identifiable alcohol problems but no severe signs of dependence is many times greater than the population that exhibits severe dependence. The conservative and liberal estimates shown in Fig. 1 reflect the fact that different studies have used different criteria and population samples (see M. B. Sobell & L. C. Sobell, 1993b). Regardless of how one slices the pie, not only do problem drinkers vastly outnumber severely dependent cases, but also the cost of alcohol problems goes far beyond those attributable to severely dependent cases (for a review, see M. B. Sobell & L. C. Sobell, 1993b).

Problem drinkers, individuals who are not severely dependent on alcohol, are characteristically different from severely dependent alcohol abusers (Edwards, 1986; Hill, 1985; M. B. Sobell & L. C. Sobell, 1993b). In particular, problem drinkers do not have a history of physical dependence, especially major withdrawal symptoms, and usually have a shorter history of drinking problems and greater social and economic stability than severely dependent individuals. They also often respond well to nonintensive outpatient interventions (M. B. Sobell & L. C. Sobell,

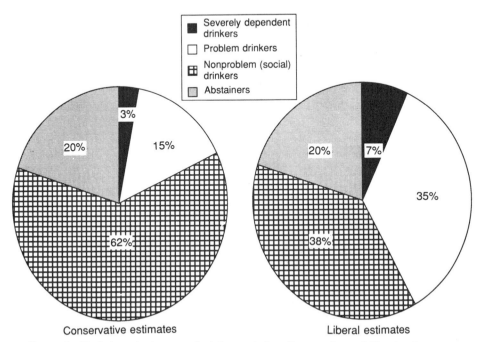

FIGURE 1. Alcohol use in the general adult population: Conservative and liberal estimates.

1993b). The next section of this chapter reviews several instruments that can distinguish problem drinkers from more severely dependent alcohol abusers.

In most health care fields, when interventions occur as early as possible, not only are success rates higher, but also the costs of intervening are lower. In this regard, a "treatment-tiering" approach, as used in other health fields, could be very cost-effective for the alcohol field (see M. B. Sobell & L. C. Sobell, 1993b). For example, in the medical field, if a person is diagnosed with mild hypertension, then the first intervention would probably be a dietary change and increased exercise, with more intensive interventions (e.g., medication) considered only if other strategies fail. Although the same approach has applicability in the alcohol field, too often the most intensive treatment is recommended for all cases (Hansen & Emrick, 1983). A more reasonable approach would be keyed to the needs of each client, based on the assessment and diagnosis, which determine the types of treatment needed.

Epidemiology

In Western societies, alcohol is a widely used psychoactive drug. Most studies indicate that at least 75% of adults surveyed report some drinking. However, knowing how many people drink and knowing how many have drinking problems are two very different issues. In fact, determining the incidence of alcohol problems in the general population is difficult because of a lack of consensus about how to define and measure such problems. It has been shown that the method of measuring alcohol problems affects the estimates derived (see Hilton, 1989). For example, requiring "Yes" responses to at least four items on the Short Michigan Alcoholism Screening Test (SMAST) (Selzer, Vinokur, & van Rooijen, 1975) produced estimates of 3.7 million male and 1.5 million female alcohol abusers, whereas requiring "Yes" responses to at least two SMAST items produced drinking problem estimates of 8.8 million men and 4.2 million women (Hilton, 1989).

Progressivity

One reason problem severity has been a neglected issue in the alcohol field may relate to conventional views of alcoholism that consider the disorder to be progressive—the condition will worsen unless the individual stops drinking. Despite conventional wisdom, however, several well-designed scientific studies have failed to support the progressivity concept (e.g., Cahalan, 1970; Fillmore, 1988; Hasin, Grant, & Endicott, 1990). These longitudinal studies show that symptom severity increases over time for only a minority of cases (25–30% by most estimates). For most individuals, the natural history of the disorder can best be described as vacillating between periods of drinking problems of varying severity and periods of abstinence or of nonproblem drinking. Thus, if a person is experiencing alcohol problems at one time, it is not possible to predict what the individual's circumstances will be at a later time (Mandell, 1983). For example, Hasin et al. (1990) found that some individuals who were diagnosed at one point as alcohol-dependent were diagnosed at a later time as alcohol abusers (i.e., less

severe symptoms). Conclusions from the progressivity studies have serious implications (see Fillmore, 1988; M. B. Sobell & L. C. Sobell, 1986/1987). Because
individuals who are not severely dependent (i.e., problem drinkers) have been
considered to be in the "early stages" of the progressive development of the disease
of alcoholism, they have been viewed as needing the same treatment as severe
cases. The evidence against progressivity suggests that less severe cases might
require alternative treatments.

Mortality and Morbidity

Suffice it to say that there are multiple causes of alcohol-related deaths. Death
rates are considerably higher for alcohol abusers than for nonproblem drinkers.
Likewise, suicide rates among alcohol abusers also are higher than for the general
population (National Institute on Alcohol Abuse and Alcoholism, 1990).

Depending on the amount consumed and the pattern of drinking, excessive
drinking can cause a variety of medical problems. These problems will not be
reviewed in this chapter, as several other detailed reviews address medical complications and consequences (Babor, Kranzler, & Lauerman, 1987; Gallant, 1987;
Wartenberg & Liepman, 1987). It should be noted, however, that while most people
drink in moderation, a small percentage of drinkers—those who drink excessively—
are responsible for the high incidence of alcohol-related mortality and morbidity
as well as social consequences.

PROCEDURES FOR GATHERING INFORMATION

Assessment, the cornerstone of treatment (Mash & Terdal, 1976; Sobell, Sobell,
& Nirenberg, 1988), can be viewed as a continuous and interactive process that
occurs before, during, and following treatment. Clinical assessments are critical for
two reasons: (1) They delineate the nature of the problems being treated and
(2) they form a basis for evaluating response to treatment.

As discussed in other reviews, the last 20 years has seen the development of a
number of behavioral assessment techniques in the alcohol field (L. C. Sobell &
M. B. Sobell, 1983; Sobell, Sobell, & Nirenberg, 1988; Vuchinich, Tucker, & Harllee,
1988). Most of these reviews, however, have critiqued the assessment literature from
a research perspective. Rarely have reviews evaluated the clinical utility of assessment techniques and instruments. For purposes of this chapter, procedures for
gathering information will be reviewed from a clinical perspective—the various
techniques will be discussed in relation to their clinical utility and limitations.

The assessment of an alcohol abuse disorder is a complex task, as it involves
considerably more than the mere measurement of alcohol use. For example, events
that trigger the use of alcohol, as well as short-term and long-term consequences of
alcohol use, need to be identified for each client. Such events and consequences are
critical for understanding the functions that alcohol serves in a client's life. Also, a
detailed evaluation of these functions is critical to the development of a treatment
plan and related strategies.

Although direct observation is one way of assessing an individual's alcohol problem, it is seldom possible to observe clients while they are intoxicated. Moreover, even if observation were possible, it would need to occur in a broad range of situations and circumstances in order to identify the array of factors related to an individual's drinking. Consequently, in the alcohol field, most behaviors in which clinicians and researchers are interested cannot be observed, but must be obtained through retrospective self-reports (Babor, Brown, & Del Boca, 1990; L. C. Sobell & M. B. Sobell, 1990).

Can Alcohol Abusers' Self-Reports Be Trusted?

From a practical standpoint, self-reports are a valuable, inexpensive, and reasonable source of information. Despite the folklore, several reviews of this literature have concluded that alcohol abusers' self-reports are generally veridical if interviews are conducted in a clinical or research setting, when clients are alcohol-free, and when they are given assurances of confidentiality (Babor et al., 1990; Babor, Stephens, & Marlatt, 1987; O'Farrell & Maisto, 1987; L. C. Sobell & M. B. Sobell, 1990). There is one condition, however, when alcohol abusers' self-reports are often invalid and underestimated—when they have a positive blood alcohol level when interviewed. Thus, it is very important to ensure that clients are alcohol-free at the time they are interviewed.

Basic Areas of Assessment

Diagnostic interviews and assessments will vary from client to client. However, at a general level, they can be conceptualized as structured interviews that are guided by a series of questions in the form of a decision tree. These structured interviews are intended to help clinicians develop a meaningful treatment plan for clients. An example of a decision tree that can be used to assess a client with a possible alcohol problem is illustrated in Figure 2.

In an earlier review (Sobell, Sobell, & Nirenberg, 1988), key assessment areas and issues that need to be considered in treatment planning for substance abusers were outlined. This chapter updates and expands those areas with respect to recent developments. Following this discussion, techniques and instruments that can be used to assess these various areas are reviewed. At a basic minimum, the following key areas should be included in the assessment of individuals who have alcohol problems.

Specific Quantities and Frequency of Alcohol Use

First and foremost, the extent and pattern of alcohol use and abuse should be carefully assessed. It is important to obtain *specific* drinking information. Estimates of average drinking patterns are sometimes misleading, since instances of atypical but clinically important levels of alcohol consumption (i.e., sporadic days of heavy drinking) are often not identified by averaging (i.e., quantity–frequency) methods (Room, 1990; L. C. Sobell & M. B. Sobell, 1992). Knowledge of high-risk drinking

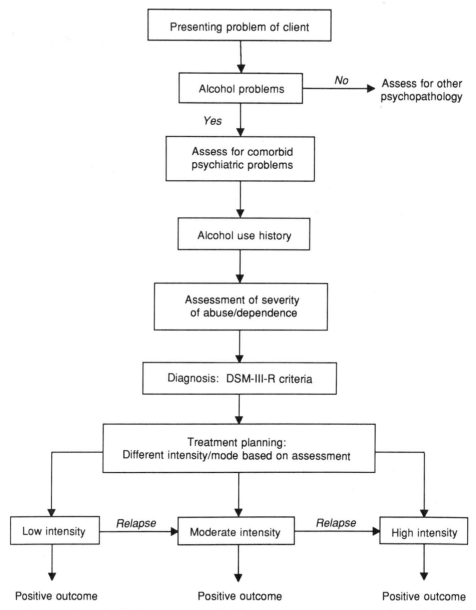

FIGURE 2. Example of a decision tree used in diagnostic interviews to assess alcohol abuse.

days obviously is extremely important when assessing potential health risks associated with alcohol consumption.

Positive and Negative Mood States

While it has been commonly accepted that alcohol abusers drink during negative emotional states (i.e., when depressed or anxious), recent evidence suggests that some problem drinkers drink when they are feeling good (i.e., positive emotional states) (Berg & Skuttle, 1986; M. B. Sobell & L. C. Sobell, 1993a). Knowledge of mood states associated with alcohol use, therefore, may help identify high-risk situations.

Medical Problems

Medical problems associated with or exacerbated by alcohol use should be evaluated. For example, ulcers, hypertension, and insomnia are just some of the problems that should be considered. For more information, readers are referred to publications that address the medical consequences of alcohol use (American Medical Association, 1977; Wartenberg & Liepman, 1987).

Comorbid Psychiatric Problems

Psychiatric problems experienced by substance abusers should also be identified. Clinicians treating alcohol abusers who have another psychiatric disorder, whether primary or secondary, should be aware that the literature shows that such clients have poorer outcomes compared to clients with only an alcohol abuse problem (see the section entitled "Diagnosis of Alcohol Problems").

History of Past Alcohol Withdrawal Symptoms

Characteristic alcohol withdrawal symptoms are defining features for a diagnosis of alcohol dependence using the DSM-IV criteria (APA, 1993). Further, a history of past withdrawal symptoms as well as reports of recent heavy ethanol consumption should alert clinicians that possible withdrawal symptoms are likely to occur on cessation of drinking. Also, in many cases, although not all (reviewed in M. B. Sobell & L. C. Sobell, 1986/1987), a relationship between severe dependence and abstinence (vs. moderation) outcomes has been reported. Thus, if an alcohol abuser has a history of severe dependence on alcohol, a goal of moderation would probably not be indicated.

Frequent Thoughts of Drinking or Urges to Drink

Reports of frequent thoughts of drinking or urges to drink can be assessed and monitored through self-monitoring logs. Such information can be used to identify events and mood states that have triggered or could trigger further drinking (Sobell, Bogardis, Schuller, Leo, & Sobell, 1989).

Multiple Drug Use

In the past several years, there has been a trend for abuse of other drugs to accompany alcohol abuse (Craddock, Bray, & Hubbard, 1985; Hubbard, Marsden, Rachal, Cavanaugh, & Ginzburg, 1989; Sobell, Sobell, & Nirenberg, 1988; Wilkinson, Leigh, Cordingley, Martin, & Lei, 1987). In addition to use of illicit drugs, use of tobacco and caffeine has been shown to correlate strongly with alcohol consumption (Istvan & Matarazzo, 1984). For example, 80–90% of alcohol and drug abusers smoke cigarettes, in contrast to a 30% prevalence rate in the general population (reviewed in Sobell, Sobell, Koslowski, & Toneatto, 1990). The combined use of alcohol and other drugs is a serious problem. Some drugs are synergistic with alcohol, resulting in a multiplicative rather than an additive effect when used concurrently. Also, for individuals who want to simultaneously stop using alcohol and other drugs, consideration should be given to what problems might be encountered by simultaneously giving up more than one psychoactive substance at a time.

Prior History of Alcohol Treatment and Control over Other Appetitive Behaviors

A review of prior successes and failures in treatment can prove useful in formulating treatment plans. Clearly, a clinician does not want to reinsert a client into a treatment situation that has failed previously. On the other hand, knowledge of prior success experiences with other appetitive behaviors (e.g., eating disorders, smoking, gambling) could be helpful, as social learning theory predicts that previous mastery experiences should provide for increased self-efficacy in dealing with the current behavior.

Consideration of a Nonabstinent Treatment Goal

In the case of alcohol abusers for whom a nonabstinent treatment drinking goal might be considered, the risks associated with such a goal must be evaluated. Currently, evidence suggests that those individuals more likely to be successful at moderation are less severely dependent on alcohol, younger, and socially stable (Heather & Robertson, 1983; M. B. Sobell & L. C. Sobell, 1987). In assessing the feasibility of a nonabstinent treatment goal, a key factor is whether there are existing medical problems that could be exacerbated by drinking and whether aiming for such a goal might jeopardize other aspects of a client's life (e.g., a client's spouse would leave if any drinking occurred).

ASSESSMENT/DIAGNOSTIC INSTRUMENTS

The preceding section outlined a minimum set of areas that should be evaluated when assessing individuals who have alcohol problems. In this section, we examine the clinical utility of different assessment techniques and instruments.

The alcohol field has no shortage of assessment instruments, as illustrated by a large compendium of such instruments published several years ago (Lettieri,

Nelson, & Sayers, 1985). When selecting particular instruments, clinicians and researchers should consider two things: First, the psychometric characteristics (reliability and validity) of the instrument are important because they determine the confidence one can have in data gathered by that instrument. Such information can be found in the original source publication describing the instrument. Second, the instruments selected should be clinically useful and user-friendly. The clinical utility of an instrument will depend on what clinicians or researchers want to know about their clients. For example, if it is known that a client has a very serious alcohol problem, then administering a screening test such as the Michigan Alcoholism Screening Test (Selzer, 1971) would provide redundant information. In terms of user friendliness, an important characteristic is how labor-intensive or demanding it is to complete or interpret an instrument. While assessment instruments will not replace the clinical interview, they can be useful adjuncts.

Drinking Assessment Instruments

Drinking is the key variable of interest for clinicians and researchers assessing alcohol use disorders. Before choosing a drinking assessment instrument, one must decide what kind of information is desired [i.e., level of precision and time frame (e.g., past 30 days, 12-month pretreatment, lifetime)] (L. C. Sobell & M. B. Sobell, 1992; Sobell, Sobell, & Nirenberg, 1988). This section provides guidance about when to use four popular assessment methods: (1) Lifetime Drinking History (Skinner & Sheu, 1982; Sobell, Sobell, Leo, & Cancilla, 1988), (2) Quantity–Frequency Methods (e.g., see Cahalan & Room, 1974; Polich, Armor, & Braiker, 1981; Straus & Bacon, 1953), (3) Timeline Follow-back (Sobell, Maisto, Sobell, & Cooper, 1979; L. C. Sobell & M. C. Sobell, 1992), and (4) Self-Monitoring (Nelson & Hayes, 1981; L. C. Sobell & M. B. Sobell, 1973; Sobell et al., 1989). Since two previous reviews have discussed in detail the advantages and disadvantages of these drinking assessment procedures, only their key features will be reviewed here (L. C. Sobell & M. B. Sobell, 1992; Sobell, Sobell, & Nirenberg, 1988).

Since alcoholic beverages vary in their alcohol concentration and in drink size, it is important for interviewers and clients to agree on what constitutes a "drink." One way to deal with this problem is to have clients report their drinking using a standard drink conversion (e.g., 1 standard drink = 12 ounces of 5% beer = 1½ ounces of 80-proof spirits = 5 ounces of 12% wine; each drink contains about 13.6 g absolute ethanol). Standard drink conversions have been used with several populations of alcohol abusers (e.g., Maisto, Sobell, Cooper, & Sobell, 1979; O'Farrell, Cutter, Bayog, Dentch, & Fortgang, 1984; L. C. Sobell & M. B. Sobell, 1992; Stockwell, Blaze-Temple, & Walker, 1991). Reporting of standard drinks also facilitates the description of occasions on which more than one type of alcoholic beverage is consumed (e.g., 3 beers and 5 ounces of spirits).

Lifetime Drinking History

The Lifetime Drinking History (LDH) was developed to assess a person's entire drinking behavior history. It takes about 20–30 minutes to complete and requires recalling drinking behavior in discrete phases reflecting major changes in a person's average drinking patterns. The LDH would be recommended if a picture of a person's lifetime drinking is needed (e.g., from adolescence to adulthood) or when the period to be recalled occurred in the distant past (Sobell, Sobell, & Toneatto, 1992). While the LDH has reasonably high reliability for an aggregate index of drinking (Skinner & Sheu, 1982), it lacks precision for the most recent drinking period (i.e., the last year). Thus, if information about recent drinking is needed, the LDH would not be an appropriate assessment method.

Quantity–Frequency Methods

Quantity–frequency (QF) methods were among the earliest to be used to assess drinking behavior (reviewed in Room, 1990). While several QF methods exist, all require respondents to report their "average" consumption pattern [e.g., "How many days (in a specified time interval) *on average* did you drink beer, and when you drank beer, *on average* how many beers did you drink?"]. The procedure typically ignores occasional days of heavy and light drinking as well as days when more than one type of alcoholic beverage was consumed. While QF methods provide some reliable information about overall consumption and frequency of drinking (reviewed in L. C. Sobell & M. B. Sobell, 1992), they fail to identify atypical heavy drinking days—days that are often associated with alcohol-related problems—and they cannot provide a picture of unpatterned drinking. QF methods should therefore be used only when time is at a premium and, when information about atypical drinking is not required.

Timeline Follow-Back

The Timeline Follow-Back (TLFB) is a drinking estimation method developed for the retrospective collection of daily drinking data. As reviewed extensively elsewhere, several memory aids (e.g., calendar, dates of personal significance, standard drink reporting format) can be used to enhance recall (L. C. Sobell & M. B. Sobell, 1992). The TLFB uses a calendar and asks subjects to provide retrospective estimates of their daily drinking over a specified time period ranging up to 12 months. For clinical populations, 25–30 minutes are required to gather 12 months of data and approximately 10 minutes to gather 90 days of data. The method can be interviewer-administered or self-administered and has been shown to have good psychometric characteristics with a variety of drinker groups (reviewed in L. C. Sobell & M. B. Sobell, 1992). If one wants to evaluate specific changes in drinking (e.g., before and after treatment) or one needs a fairly accurate picture of heavy and light drinking days and drinking patterns, then the TLFB method is recommended. Excerpts from three clients' TLFB calendars are presented and discussed later in the "Case Examples" section.

Self-Monitoring

Unlike the preceding methods, Self-Monitoring (SM) is a prospective method in which clients routinely record various aspects of their drinking (e.g., amount, frequency, mood, time, urges, consequences). SM is a popular behavioral technique that can take a variety of forms such as logs or diaries (see Nirenberg, Sobell, Ersner-Hershfield, & Cellucci, 1983; Sobell, Sobell, & Nirenberg, 1988; Sobell et al., 1989). As a prospective assessment method, SM is subject to fewer memory problems than retrospective procedures when used appropriately (i.e., filled out at the time the behavior occurs). However, SM has two major drawbacks: First, not all clients comply with instructions (Sanchez-Craig & Annis, 1982). Second, because it is prospective, it cannot provide a retrospective assessment of drinking. Finally, although SM has been shown to provide slightly more accurate information than the TLFB, the added information does not appear to significantly change the evaluation of the severity of a person's drinking problem (Samo, Tucker, & Vuchinich, 1989; Sobell et al., 1989). SM does have clinical utility, however, in that (1) it provides feedback about treatment effectiveness, (2) it can identify situations that pose a high risk of relapse, and (3) it gives clients an opportunity to discuss their drinking behavior between treatment sessions.

Assessing Drug Use

Instruments for assessing multiple psychoactive drug use are scarce (Sobell, Sobell, & Nirenberg, 1988). Measurement of drug use is also complicated by several factors (Wilkinson, Leigh, Cordingley, Martin, & Lei, 1987). First, it is often difficult to determine how much of an active ingredient was consumed or, in some cases, even what type of drug was consumed. Second, because there is no logical equivalency across drug types, use of one type of drug cannot be seen as equivalent to the use of another drug. Third, the route of administration (e.g., nasal vs. injection) can affect both the speed of onset and drug potency. While there is no commonly accepted manner of combining data on drug use into a single drug use measure, it is generally accepted that use of several drug types can be assessed separately using a drug use history (see Hubbard et al., 1989; Wilkinson et al., 1987). Drug use within each drug class can be assessed along a number of dimensions: (1) frequency of use (e.g., number of days per month), (2) route of administration, (3) number of years used, (4) year last used, (5) year of heaviest use, and (6) frequency of use per day. Although little has been published on the psychometric characteristics of these instruments, the available literature suggests that such data can be reliably gathered (Harrell, 1985; Maisto, McKay, & Connors, 1990).

Nicotine Dependence

Since the majority of alcohol and drug abusers also smoke cigarettes, clinicians and researchers may wish to assess nicotine dependence. While the Fagerström Tolerance Questionnaire, a short 13-item scale that assesses the severity of nicotine dependence (Fagerström, 1978), has come under criticism for not assessing dependence adequately (Pomerleau, Pomerleau, Majchrzak, Kloska, & Malakuti, 1990), a revised 6-item scale (Fagerström Test for Nicotine Dependence) is now recommended (Heatherton, Kozlowski, Frecker, & Fagerström, 1991). It has been suggested that one question on this scale may be particularly telling: "How many minutes upon waking until the first cigarette is smoked?" This question is strongly correlated with dependence (discussed in Pomerleau et al., 1990). For example, a response of smoking within 30 minutes upon waking is predictive of nicotine dependence (Kozlowski, Director, & Harford, 1981).

Consequences of Alcohol Use

Using the DSM-IV, a diagnosis of alcohol dependence is defined by specific adverse consequences experienced as a result of ethanol consumption. Two types of consequences are commonly experienced—psychosocial consequences and dependence symptoms usually manifested as withdrawal symptoms on cessation of drinking. Several short self-administered scales have been developed to assess psychosocial consequences and dependence symptoms related to alcohol abuse. Unfortunately, none of the scales is ideal. Paramount among the problems is a lack of agreement on what constitutes the core dependence symptoms (for an excellent discussion of these problems, the reader is referred to an article by Davidson, 1987). Three of the more common scales developed to assess elements of the alcohol dependence syndrome will be reviewed: (1) the Severity of Alcohol Dependence Questionnaire (SADQ) (Stockwell, Murphy, & Hodgson, 1983), (2) the Alcohol Dependence Scale (ADS) (Skinner & Allen, 1982), and (3) the Short Alcohol Dependence Data Questionnaire (SADD) (Raistrick, Dunbar, & Davidson, 1983).

The SADQ, a 20-item scale that can be used with chronic populations, is not as sensitive as the other two scales for evaluating low-dependence alcohol abusers. The ADS, a 25-item scale that is generally applicable to adult alcohol abusers, has been used with a variety of problem drinking populations. The ADS appears to have satisfactory test–retest reliability and correlates highly with measures of similar constructs (Kivlahan, Sher, & Donovan, 1989; Ross, Gavin, & Skinner, 1990; Skinner & Allen, 1982; L. C. Sobell & M. B. Sobell, 1992). It is particularly helpful for distinguishing low dependence (i.e., problem drinkers) from moderate and more severely dependent alcohol abusers. It also can be used to help screen clients for appropriateness of a reduced-drinking goal (Skinner & Horn, 1984). The third measure, the SADD, is a 15-item scale aimed at the general alcohol problem population with a focus on those who are mildly to moderately dependent on alcohol. Although assessments of this instrument's psychometric characteristics are sparse, it has been shown to have adequate content validity (Davidson & Raistrick, 1986).

This section would not be complete without mentioning the 24-item Michigan Alcoholism Screening Test (MAST) (Hedlund & Vieweg, 1984; Selzer, 1971). This instrument, which takes about 5 minutes to administer, has been used for several years as a scaled measure of alcohol-problem severity. A shorter 13-item version has also been found to be reliable (SMAST) (Selzer et al., 1975). A problem with the MAST and with other similar consequence scales is that they have face validity (i.e., people can easily prevent an invalid profile). Consequently, such scales are not useful for identifying alcohol problems in persons who do not wish to be identified as having problems.

Considering all the work that has gone into developing scales to identify alcohol problems, it is interesting to note that two studies (Cyr & Wartman, 1988; Woodruff, Clayton, Cloninger, & Guze, 1976) conducted a decade apart showed that the most sensitive question "was the straightforward yet less traditional question 'Have you ever had a drinking problem?'" (Cyr & Wartman, 1988, p. 54). Thus, in a physician's office or a health care practice where time is at a premium and the object is to identify persons who have a drinking problem, incorporating this one question into a routine medical history would be recommended.

Assessing Risk Situations and Self-Efficacy

Since relapse rates among treated alcohol abusers are extremely high, assessment of high-risk drinking situations is extremely important (Allsop & Saunders, 1989; Marlatt & Gordon, 1985). Two instruments, developed by Annis and her colleagues, both with adequate psychometric characteristics, yield profiles of high-risk situations: (1) Inventory of Drinking Situations (IDS) (Annis, 1986; Annis & Davis, 1988, 1989) and (2) Situational Confidence Questionnaire (SCQ) (Annis & Davis, 1988, 1989; Solomon & Annis, 1989, 1990).

The IDS requires clients to evaluate 100 different situations and to indicate on a 4-point scale the frequency with which they drank heavily in each situation in the past year. Sample questions are noted in the "Case Examples" section later in this chapter, where three client IDS profiles are discussed in some detail. The SCQ contains items parallel to the IDS but assesses situational self-efficacy, a client's perceived ability to resist drinking heavily in particular situations. Clients are asked to imagine themselves in each situation and to indicate on a 6-point scale how confident they are that they will be able to resist urges to drink heavily in that situation.

The items comprising the IDS and SCQ constitute eight subscales, based on research by Marlatt and Gordon (1985). The subscales are: unpleasant emotions, physical discomfort, pleasant emotions, testing control over alcohol, urges and temptations to drink, conflict with others, social pressure from others to drink, and pleasant times with others. For research studies, a short version of each scale has been developed: a 42-item IDS (Annis & Davis, 1989) and a 39-item SCQ (Annis & Graham, 1988).

The IDS can provide a picture of the person's high-risk drinking situations in the past year (M. B. Sobell & L. C. Sobell, 1993a), whereas the SCQ can show areas in which the client currently lacks confidence for resisting drinking. While both scales can be used clinically to enhance the treatment plan, the scales identify only generic situations or general problem areas. To explore idiosyncratic high-risk situations or areas in which the client lacks self-confidence for resisting drinking, clinicians can explore specific situations with clients. For example, clients could be asked to describe their three highest-risk situations in the last year. Such an exercise can look for differences and similarities between the general risk areas on the IDS and the client's personal high-risk situations. When such comparisons were made, considerable convergence was found between the IDS and personal risk situations (M. B. Sobell & L. C. Sobell, 1993a). This adds confidence to the information obtained on the IDS as well as the clinical interview.

Assessing Recent Ethanol Use

Earlier, it was noted that alcohol abusers' self-reports are generally valid when obtained under specific conditions. However, when clients have any alcohol in their systems, their self-reports are often invalid (M. B. Sobell & L. C. Sobell, 1975). This same study found that clinician's judgments of clients' states of intoxication were no more accurate than the clients' self-reports (M. B. Sobell & L. C. Sobell, 1975), probably because of the phenomenon of tolerance and because alcohol abusers have learned to "mask" many of the typical signs of intoxication (e.g., slurred speech, gait). Fortunately, recent use of ethanol can be detected through tests of different bodily fluids such as urine, sweat, breath, and blood. Some methods (e.g., blood, urine assays) require laboratory assessment and therefore cannot provide immediate feedback. However, several portable testers, differing in cost and level of precision, are now commercially available and can provide a reasonably accurate estimate of a client's level of intoxication (e.g., M. B. Sobell & L. C. Sobell, 1975). It should be noted that many of the portable testers are not specific for ethanol; thus, on rare occasions, false-positives may occur.

The alcohol dipstick, a relatively new technique for determining ethanol concentration in urine, saliva, or blood, can be used in a variety of clinical settings (e.g., doctors' offices, emergency rooms). The dipstick reacts with the carrier fluid and provides quantifiable differences in color intensity associated with different ethanol levels. It has been shown to have fair reliability and validity (Kapur & Israel, 1983, 1984; Tu, Kapur, & Israel, 1992). The advantage of alcohol dipsticks and portable breath alcohol testers is that they provide clinicians and researchers in a variety of settings with a reliable and quick objective indicator (i.e., yes or no) of ethanol consumption.

Alcohol Use over Extended Periods

Besides self-reports, one of the most common ways to assess alcohol use over extended time periods is liver function tests. Several studies have found that elevations in some biochemical tests (e.g., GGTP, HDL) correlate with recent heavy drinking (Holt, Skinner, & Israel, 1981; Leigh & Skinner, 1988; Levine, 1990; Morgan, 1980). These tests, however, have several problems (see Levine, 1990; O'Farrell & Maisto, 1987). For example, there is considerable intersubject variability (Morgan, 1980), some tests are more affected by certain drinking patterns (Devenyi, Robinson, Kapur, & Roncari, 1981; Skinner, Holt, Schuller, Roy, & Israel, 1984), and some tests are affected by medical conditions (e.g., heart failure, diabetes, other psychoactive drug use) (Morgan, Colman, & Sherlock, 1981; Shaw, Korts, & Stimmel, 1982/1983). Finally, while it is often asserted that abnormal liver function tests will return to normal within 3–4 weeks of abstinence, they do not always do so (see Leigh & Skinner, 1988). In summary, the major clinical utility of liver function tests is as probable, rather than definite, indicators of recent heavy ethanol consumption. Although several studies have suggested that diagnostic accuracy can be increased by using several tests in combination (reviewed in Bernadt, Mumford, Taylor, Smith, & Murray, 1982; Leigh & Skinner, 1988; Levine, 1990), it has also been found that questionnaires were often superior to liver function tests in identifying alcohol consumption in alcoholics (also see Petersson, Trell, & Kristensson, 1983).

Because no data source, including official records, is error-free, it has been recommended that the best strategy for obtaining valid information is to gather data from multiple sources and cross-check the sources (e.g., collaterals, records, objective tests) (O'Farrell & Maisto, 1987; L. C. Sobell & M. B. Sobell, 1990). This approach has been referred to as *convergent validity* (L. C. Sobell & M. B. Sobell, 1980).

CASE EXAMPLES

The following case examples are from actual cases and are intended to illustrate the clinical utility and value of the Inventory of Drinking Situations (IDS) and the Timeline Follow-Back (TLFB) for treatment planning. As explained earlier, the IDS provides a "user friendly" summary of high-risk drinking situations for the client over the preceding year. A few general points about using IDS profiles should be mentioned before the actual cases are described.

First, situations identified by the IDS have been only *associated with* heavy drinking. Therefore, while one may conjecture about a causal link between the types of situations and drinking, it is always possible that a third variable may explain the association (e.g., a person may have poor social skills that make him or her likely to experience interpersonal conflict and that also lead the person to barroom drinking as a way of gaining social acceptance).

Second, as scaled data that form a profile, IDS findings may be viewed from at least three perspectives: (1) *magnitude of responses* (how high the person's scale scores are in general as compared to others in the sample—people who drink more heavily and more frequently would be expected to have higher-magnitude scores), (2) *scatter of the scale scores* (the extent to which the profile is differentiated or undifferentiated—are some scores high and others low or are most of the scores at about the same level), and (3) *pattern of the scale scores* (if some scores are high and others low, which particular scales are involved and do other persons show a similar profile?). Each of these perspectives can convey useful information. In the case examples, we focus on contrasting patterns in the profiles, as the profiles are most clinically useful when a person's profile is differentiated (some high, some low), whereas the magnitude of scores usually relates to how frequently heavy drinking has occurred.

A few general points about using the TLFB are also relevant. Timeline data, because they are continuous variables with a data point for each day, are very valuable for quantitative description and for scientific purposes such as group outcome comparisons (reviewed in L. C. Sobell & M. B. Sobell, 1992). In clinical situations, it is usually not necessary to statistically summarize the Timeline data;

rather, it is more helpful to simply study the completed Timeline calendar and to see whether clients have indicated on the Timeline the occurrence of specific events associated with their drinking (e.g., drinking on Thursdays, during sporting events). Timeline entries should be interpreted as reflecting a person's best *estimate* of what his or her drinking was like, and it should be expected that there will be some amount of error (reviewed in L. C. Sobell & M. B. Sobell, 1992). In most cases, however, these errors will not affect the clinical utility of the Timeline, for the magnitude and frequency of drinking will still be relatively accurate (i.e., clinically, it makes little difference whether a heavy drinking day involved 17 drinks or 20 drinks). Finally, the results from the TLFB and the IDS should be discussed with the client.

As with the IDS, the Timeline has its greatest clinical utility when the pattern is differentiated, including days of nondrinking and days of drinking at various levels. As the person's pattern gets closer to one of daily heavy drinking, there will be little variance in the data. The three case descriptions that follow have been selected for their utility, and thus it should not be assumed that all cases will be as easily interpreted as those presented here. All the clients participated in a brief outpatient treatment program (M. B. Sobell & L. C. Sobell, 1993a).

Case 1

The patient was a 35-year-old married male with a college education who was employed full time at an office job. He reported that his drinking had been a problem for 5 years, although the only consequences he identified were hangovers and a strong felt need for alcohol. When he entered treatment, he reported being stressed as a result of his having been relocated by his employer from a small city to a very large city.

His IDS profile, shown in Figure 3, indicates a clear relationship between negative affective states and heavy drinking. The client had strongly endorsed items such as "I drank heavily when I felt empty inside" and "I drank heavily when pressure would build up at work because of the demands of my supervisor." His Timeline, an excerpt from which also appears in Figure 3, shows daily drinking that varied between days of limited consumption (≤ 3 standard drinks) and days of heavier consumption, typically ranging between 7 and 10 drinks. His Alcohol Dependence Scale score of 10 placed him within the first quartile (i.e., low dependence on alcohol) compared to the norms for clinical samples.

His goal was to reduce his drinking to an average of 1 drink per day on about 4 days per week, occasionally allowing himself a day of consumption of up to 4 drinks. When asked about his most serious problem drinking situations, he identified "Having a bad day at the office—I'm alone at home and there is a supply of liquor"; "Personality conflicts at home [related to] too many demands . . . can't relax and do things the way I planned or wanted"; and "Business meetings or trips . . . need to feel at ease with others." His IDS profile and his self-reports of high-risk situations were similar. Treatment planning for this client focused on becoming skilled in using alternative coping responses.

Case 2

The patient was a 49-year-old male employed full time at a white-collar job. He had 14 years of education and was separated from his wife. Although his Alcohol Dependence Scale score

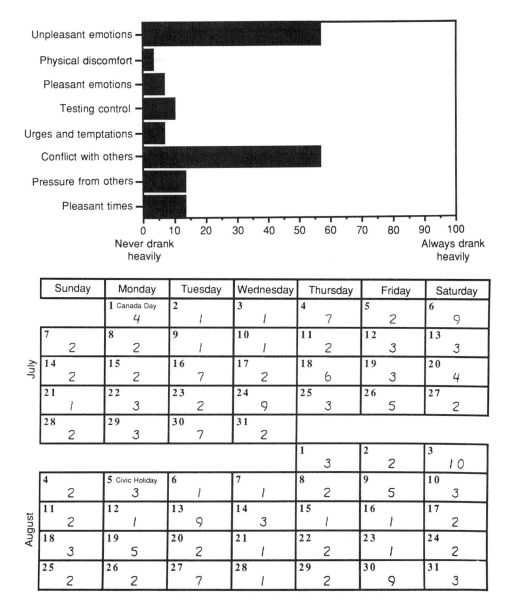

FIGURE 3. Case 1:   IDS profile and Timeline Follow-back calendar excerpt.

was only 8, lower than that of Case 1, he reported more consequences and consequences of greater severity than Case 1 (i.e., serious interpersonal difficulties, minor financial problems, effects on his work performance). He also reported having been advised by his physician to cut down or stop his drinking, and he had one prior alcohol-related arrest. This case shows that it is important to ask about specific consequences, as the consequences suggested a slightly more serious problem than reflected in the Alcohol Dependence Scale. In contrast to Case 1, this client's IDS, shown in Figure 4, indicated what might be referred to as a "good times/social pressure" drinking pattern. His highest-risk circumstances were when he was feeling good, and he would drink to feel even better. On the IDS, he strongly endorsed items like the following: "I drank heavily when I felt confident and relaxed" and "I drank heavily when I would be at a party and other people would be drinking."

His Timeline, an excerpt from which also appears in Figure 4, reveals an apparent weekend and holiday heavy drinking pattern. His drinking was also lighter at the beginning of the 1-year pretreatment interval than toward the time he entered treatment. His goal was to reduce his drinking to no more than 3 drinks per day on no more than 5 days per week. His self-reported most serious problem drinking situations were when "At home in the evening alone . . . [from which he would] feel indulged and self satisfied"; "Long parties with friends I am comfortable with . . . I just never refuse the next drink," and "Sailing in the summer months . . . it is a very happy time and is part of sailing and the club atmosphere."

His treatment focused on practical ways of limiting his drinking (e.g., interspersing nonalcoholic drinks, drinking nonalcoholic beverages before going to a party, drinking beer because of its lower alcohol concentration), engaging in activities incompatible with heavy drinking (e.g., initiating more activities with his children, more physical recreation), and restructuring his social life so as to spend less time in the company of heavy-drinking single males.

Case 3

The patient was a 50-year-old female with some college education, married, and employed full time in a library. This case is included as a contrast to Case 2. As can be seen in Figure 5, the IDS profile for this case can also be described as indicating "good times/social pressure" situations as high risk for heavy drinking. However, this profile is much lower in magnitude than that for Case 2. This client had an Alcohol Dependence Scale score of 9, and reported consequences of cognitive impairment, interpersonal difficulties, becoming verbally abusive, effects on work performance, and blackouts. She considered herself to have had a drinking problem for 10 years, and described herself as a weekend drinker. She stated that her husband drank more than she did, a factor that threatened to complicate treatment. She did not answer any IDS item as "Almost always," but she did respond "Frequently" to a few items, such as "I drank heavily when I would be in a situation in which I was in the habit of having a drink" and "I drank heavily when I would want to celebrate special occasions like Christmas or birthdays."

Her Timeline, excerpted in Figure 5, shows that most of her heavier drinking was confined to Fridays, although the absolute level of the "heavy" drinking was only about 5 or 6 drinks per day. The types of situations she self-reported as high-risk, however, also had an element of negative affect that was not readily apparent from the IDS profile. She indicated as high-risk "Drinking at home after a troubling situation at work . . . hoping to fill some emotional void;" "Drinking at a bar after work with friends, needing to get high so I could talk to people around me . . . extreme feeling of shyness"; and "Drinking at a party, social gathering, to get over the shyness of meeting people (usually men)." She described low-risk

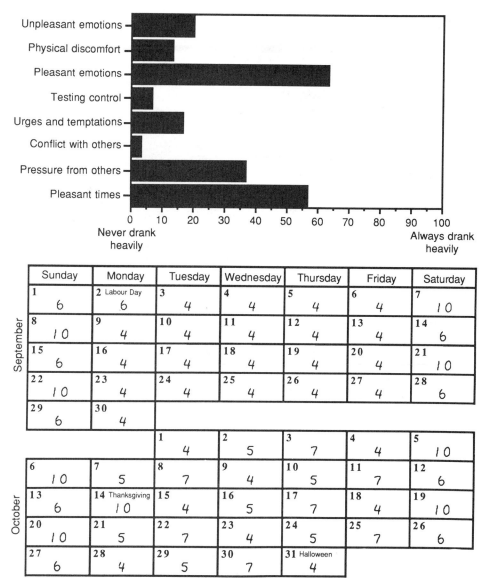

FIGURE 4. Case 2:   IDS profile and Timeline Follow-back calendar excerpt.

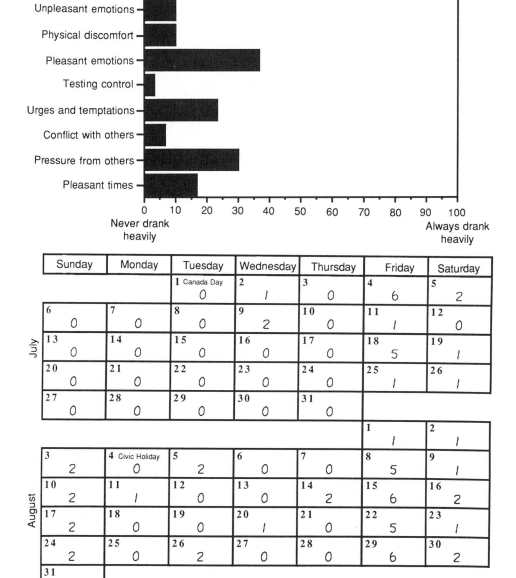

Figure 5. Case 3:   IDS profile and Timeline Follow-back calendar excerpt.

situations as involving "Coming home after work after a good day or when I feel strong, or meeting friends for lunch on a Saturday afternoon."

This case illustrates that while the IDS is helpful, it should not replace clinical interviewing. The treatment in this case was targeted largely at practical ways of limiting drinking.

DIAGNOSIS OF ALCOHOL PROBLEMS

The classification of alcohol problems has evolved considerably over the last two decades, reflecting both the state of knowledge and changing attitudes. Continuing revisions to the diagnostic nomenclature of the American Psychiatric Association [i.e., the *Diagnostic and Statistical Manual of Mental Disorders* (DSM)] reflect this ongoing process. For instance, the DSM-III (APA, 1980) diagnoses for alcohol disorders consisted of two types: "1) abuse, requiring a pattern of pathological use and social or occupational impairment, and 2) dependence, requiring either physiological tolerance or withdrawal and in addition to pathological use and/or social or occupational impairment" (Rounsaville, Kosten, Williams, & Spitzer, 1987, p. 351). The revised edition of DSM-III, DSM-III-R (APA, 1987), however, had alcohol dependence as its major category, with alcohol abuse retained primarily as a residual diagnosis for individuals who had only recently begun to abuse alcohol or who had used alcohol in a manner damaging to their biopsychosocial functioning (e.g., drunk driving arrest) but failed to meet the criteria for dependence. In DSM-III-R, the diagnostic criteria also formed a diagnostic index so that alcohol dependence is no longer defined by any particular symptom. That is, not all the core symptoms comprising the dependence syndrome need always be present, or present with the same magnitude on any given occasion, for dependence to be diagnosed. Furthermore, the criteria for a dependence diagnosis were broadened to incorporate behavioral, physiological, and cognitive symptoms of alcohol abuse. DSM-III-R also viewed alcohol dependence as a graded phenomenon, ranging from mild (one or more psychosocial consequences, but no major withdrawal symptoms, e.g., problem drinkers) to severe (major withdrawal symptoms and pervasive drug seeking, e.g., chronic alcohol abusers who have experienced delirium tremens).

One critical advance of DSM-IV over previous versions is in trying to empirically define as many characteristics as possible (Nathan, 1991). With respect to substance use and abuse, there are three major differences between DSM-III-R and DSM-IV: (1) DSM-IV includes "two options regarding tolerance and withdrawal: one requiring either symptom for a dependence diagnosis, the other subtyping and dependence diagnosis according to the presence or absence of these physical indicators" (p. 338) (Rounsaville, Bryant, Babor, Kranzler, & Kadden, 1993); (2) besides the nine DSM-III-R items, two new items are considered in DSM-IV (items 8 and 10 in the next paragraph); and (3) "the DSM-IV abuse diagnosis includes a broader range of criteria referring to substance-related consequences or substance use that produces risk of these consequences" (p. 338) (Rounsaville et al., 1993).

As noted in a recent paper comparing DSM-III-R and DSM-IV, the following 11 items constitute DSM-IV criteria for Substance Use Disorders including alcohol, of which at least three need to be present for a dependence diagnosis to be made: (1) tolerance; (2) the characteristic withdrawal syndrome for the substance; (3) the same substance is often taken to relieve or avoid withdrawal symptoms; (4) the substance is often taken in larger amounts or over a longer period than intended; (5) any unsuccessful effort or persistent desire to cut down or control substance use; (6) a great deal of time is spent in activities necessary to obtain the substance, take the substance, or recover from its effects; (7) recurrent substance use resulting in inability to fulfill major role obligations at work, school, or home; (8) recurrent substance use in situations in which it is physically hazardous; (9) important social, occupational, or recreational activities given up or reduced because of substance use; (10) recurrent substance-related legal or interpersonal problems; and (11) continued substance use despite knowledge of a persistent or recurrent problem(s) caused or exacerbated by the use of the substance.

Psychiatric Comorbidity

The comorbidity of other psychiatric disorders among alcohol abusers has been well demonstrated in recent years in treatment studies (Cox, Norton, Swinson, & Endler, 1990; Regier, 1990; Ross, Glaser, & Germanson, 1988; Wilson, 1988). The prevalence of psychiatric comorbidity in alcohol abusers varies, with reported rates ranging from 7% to 75% (see Mezzich, Arria, Tarter, Moss, & Van Thiel, 1991).

Although mood and anxiety disorders comprise the two most common Axis I disorders associated with alcohol problems, an Axis II diagnosis of antisocial personality disorder also occurs with some frequency (e.g., Ross et al., 1990; Schuckit, 1985). The lifetime prevalence of antisocial personality disorder among alcohol abusers has ranged between 40% and 50% when DSM-III criteria have been used (Hesselbrock, Meyer, & Keener, 1985; Ross et al., 1988). The prevalence of major affective disorder also varies among studies: Lifetime rates range from 18% to 25% (Hesselbrock et al., 1985; Powell, Read, & Penick, 1987; Weissman & Meyers, 1980), with current rates for treated alcohol abusers ranging from 9% to 38% (Dorus, Kennedy, Gibbons, & Ravi, 1987; Keeler, Taylor, & Miller, 1979). Anxiety disorders are also prevalent with alcohol abusers, with current rates ranging from 6% to 69% (reviewed in Kushner, Sher, & Beitman, 1990).

Finally, rates for an additional diagnosis of antisocial personality among alcohol abusers appear to vary considerably (Ross et al., 1990; Schuckit, 1985). The diagnosis of concurrent psychopathology has recently been viewed as having important treatment implications (Kessler, 1991). Studies show very different patterns of outcome depending on the presence or absence of comorbid diagnoses (see Rounsaville, Dolinsky, Babor, & Meyer, 1987). While a comprehensive diagnostic assessment must include the possibility that additional psychiatric disorders may be present, a uniform approach to the treatment of alcohol abusers with psychiatric disorders is not recommended because of the marked individual differences in dysfunction (Kushner et al., 1990). Rather, it would seem important to individualize treatment for such clients (Nace, David, & Gaspari, 1991).

Primary versus Secondary Alcohol Dependence

A diagnosis of alcohol dependence must distinguish between a disorder that is secondary to other psychiatric disorders and a primary disorder that can produce other psychiatric disorders. When ethanol is ingested chronically or in high doses, its pharmacological effects can give rise to syndromes closely resembling mood, anxiety, or psychotic disorders. For example, psychotic symptoms in an individual who abuses alcohol may be diagnosed as primary alcohol dependence with secondary psychosis or as an acute psychotic disorder with secondary alcohol dependence. The former diagnosis implies that the psychotic symptoms will disappear once the drinking remits, while the latter diagnosis suggests that the psychotic symptoms require direct treatment. A thorough history of a person's drinking and psychiatric functioning is necessary to disentangle the primary disorder.

Multiple Drug Use/Abuse

As with a diagnosis of comorbidity, a diagnosis of polydrug abuse also has important treatment implications. For example, treatment for multiple substance abuse may not parallel that for individuals who abuse only one drug (Battjes, 1988; Burling & Ziff, 1988; Kaufman, 1982). However, very few empirically based guidelines exist regarding how to treat such individuals. A major question concern simultaneous vs. sequential cessation of the abused substances. This issue is most clearly exemplified in concurrent abuse of tobacco and alcohol (Bobo, 1989; Burling & Ziff, 1988; Kozlowski, Jelinek, & Pope, 1986; Sobell et al., 1990). While simultaneous cessation of use has been hypothesized to increase the risk of relapse, conditioning theory might suggest the opposite. At this time, decisions as to whether to treat multiple drug problems concurrently or sequentially should be made on a case-by-case basis (Sobell et al., 1990).

Structured and Semistructured Interviews

Several structured and semistructured schedules exist that yield DSM-III-R diagnoses. Among the most frequently used are the Structured Clinical Interview for DSM-III-R (SCID) (Spitzer, Williams, Gibbon, & First, 1988), the Diagnostic Interview Schedule (DIS) (reviewed in Jacobson, 1989; Robins, Helzer, Croughan, & Ratcliff, 1981), and the Composite International Diagnostic Interview (CIDI) (World Health Organization, 1987). The SCID has been found to yield highly reliable DSM-III-R diagnoses, especially for psychoactive substance use disorders, and has been recommended for studies that assess comorbid psychiatric disorders (Riskind, Beck, Berchick, Brown, & Steer, 1987; Skre, Onstad, Torgersen, & Kringlen, 1991). The CIDI is frequently used in epidemiological investigations and can be administered by nonclinicians.

Utility of Diagnostic Formulations

An accurate diagnosis is essential to the assessment process because it permits classification of the problem behavior in a manner that can be easily communicated to other clinicians and researchers. The diagnostic formulation, in concert with other assessments, will provide an initial understanding of the problem behavior as well as a solid beginning for effective treatment planning.

Assessing Feasibility of the Treatment Goal

Assessment of drinking goals for alcohol abusers is very important. Traditionally, most alcohol abuse treatment programs have required an abstinence goal for all clients (see Riley, Sobell, Leo, Sobell, & Klajner, 1987; M. B. Sobell & L. C. Sobell, 1986/1987); this goal is usually based on the rationale of irreversibility. For example, in this reformulation of the disease concept of alcoholism, Kissin (1983) hypothesized that physically dependent alcohol abusers are biologically incapable of achieving nonabstinence drinking goals. This conceptualization not only has a tenuous empirical foundation, but also excludes the large number of individuals with alcohol problems who do not exhibit significant physical dependence (i.e., problem drinkers), and therefore are not presumed incapable of achieving moderation outcomes.

There are multiple rationales for alternative goals to abstinence: (1) Alcohol is legally available and its use in moderation is socially sanctioned; (2) when used in moderation, it does not produce marked impairment or dysfunction; (3) abstinence has not succeeded as an enduring outcome for most alcohol abusers (M. B. Sobell & L. C. Sobell, 1986/1987); (4) for some individuals, especially young males, a rigid adherence to abstinence may be unacceptable; (5) a key feature of successful interventions with problem drinkers is that they frequently invoke a moderation rather than abstinence outcome (Heather & Robertson, 1983; Hester & Miller, 1990; M. B. Sobell & L. C. Sobell, 1986/1987); and (6) as discussed earlier, several studies have shown that many persons evaluated as having significant alcohol problems at a given time may be drinking in moderation and without problems at a later time (even with abstinence-oriented treatments). Permitting some clients, especially low-dependence problem drinkers, to choose their own drinking goals (unless contraindicated) has become an increasingly common feature of many behavioral treatment programs. Such a goal-choice procedure is thought to increase motivation for change and to contribute to treatment success (reviewed in Miller, 1986/87; M. B. Sobell & L. C. Sobell, 1986/1987; Sobell, Sobell, Bogardis, Leo, & Skinner, 1992).

INTERVIEWING STRATEGIES

Interviewing Style

A critical factor in gathering information on alcohol use is *interviewing style*. It has been noted that therapist style, often ignored in outcome research, can be a major factor related to treatment success (Cartwright, 1981). For example, a client's responses can be affected by the way the interviewer asks questions (Mandell, 1983; Miller & Rollinick, 1991). While certain strategies and techniques (e.g., memory aids, calendars, probing) can aid the interview process (e.g., L. C. Sobell & M. B. Sobell, 1992; Sobell, Sobell, & Riley, 1988), others can significantly hinder it. This section discusses several important issues in interviewing.

Open-Ended versus Closed Questions

A detailed probing of reported events not only allows for individualized explanation, but also helps to minimize errors (Brown & Harris, 1978; Gorman, 1990; Katschnig, 1986). Previous research with alcohol abusers (L. C. Sobell & M. B. Sobell, 1992) and other populations (Miller & Salter, 1984; Sobell, Toneatto, Sobell, Schuller, & Maxwell, 1990) has shown that on probing, some initially reported events are revised with regard to whether or when they occurred. Also, free-flowing interviews are felt to elicit fuller contextual information about situations (Bradburn & Sudman, 1979; Katschnig, 1986; Miller & Salter, 1984; Miller & Rollinick, 1991).

Careful History Taking: What's in a Word?

Diagnostic, clinical, and research interviews are all dependent on clients' self-reports. An important part of the interviewing process is the terms that are used. The following examples illustrate some of the problems that might be encountered when interviewing alcohol abusers.

When asking about *blackouts*, it is important to determine that clients understand that this refers to time-bound amnesic episodes while drinking or taking drugs and not to loss of consciousness or to unclear memories about events (Goodwin, Crane, & Guze, 1969). The latter are known as *grayouts* and are not amnesic episodes. Another critical term that often causes clients some confusion is delirium tremens or *DT's*. This term, frequently confused with minor withdrawal symptoms such as psychomotor agitation, must include actual delirium.

A similarly important term that needs clarification is *morning drinking*, which is meant to identify drinking engaged in shortly after waking specifically *to escape or avoid withdrawal symptoms*. Such relief drinking is associated with heavy prolonged drinking engaged in by severely dependent alcohol abusers. However, when this question is asked as "Have you ever drunk in the morning or before noon?," affirmative responses may confuse true relief drinking with champagne breakfasts, drinking before noon on holidays, or drinking that occurs in the morning, but several hours after waking.

Other unprofitable ways of interviewing alcohol abusers include asking them "how often they get drunk or high." Similarly, reports of being "sober" or "not drunk" are not useful. Because of tolerance, it is not unusual for alcohol abusers to report being sober or not high when they have consumed large amounts of alcohol. It is better to ask about specific amounts of alcohol consumed than to rely on subjective descriptions of intoxication.

One final term that deserves mention is *cirrhosis*. Our experience has shown this term to be a source of confusion for clients and physicians. Cirrhosis can be diagnosed only by liver biopsy—not by a blood test (e.g., Galambos, 1975). However, over the years, we have encountered a number of clients who have reported being told by their physicians that they had cirrhosis. On probing, however, we found that they were only given a blood test that assessed acute hepatic dysfunction. Acute hepatic dysfunction will often dissipate shortly after cessation of drinking (e.g., Chick, Kreitman, & Plant, 1981; Leigh & Skinner, 1988).

Empathy

Research has indicated that being empathic is related to decreased client resistance and to increased long-term behavior change (Miller & Sovereign, 1989; Miller, Taylor, & West, 1980; Valle, 1981). A key element of empathy is *reflective listening*. According to Miller and Rollinick (1991), "The reflective listener forms a reasonable guess as to what the original meaning was, and gives voice to this guess in the form of a statement" (p. 74) that is "less likely to evoke resistance" than a question. Empathy also helps the interviewer gain the acceptance and trust of clients. Success in doing so can be gauged by the amount of spontaneous taking in which a client engages. Spontaneous talking can be encouraged by asking open-ended questions such as "Tell me more about your drinking habits," rather than a question leading to only a "Yes" or "No" answer such as "Do you get into problems because of your drinking?" Asking open-ended questions does not mean that everyone will readily divulge information, but it offers clients the opportunity to do so in an accepting manner.

Periodic Summary

Miller and Rollinick (1991) recommended the use of periodic summarizing throughout the interview process. Doing so allows the interviewer to synthesize the information gathered and allows the client to give the interviewer feedback about his or her understanding of the information.

Flexibility

One of the more important factors relating to interview style, especially with resistant clients, is *flexibility*. Sometimes the interview may get into an area that the client finds threatening or is reluctant to discuss. When this occurs, the interviewer should display flexibility or, in the words of Miller and Rollinick (1991), "roll with resistance." One strategy is to respond with nonresistance and reflective listening. Another is to emphasize that it is the client's personal choice whether the matter will be discussed or not. Perceived loss of control often brings about resistance.

Confrontation

Confrontation and argumentation should be avoided when possible (Miller & Rollinick, 1991). Research has indicated that confrontational strategies can be potentially damaging (Annis & Chan, 1983; Lieberman, Yalom, & Miles, 1973). For example, it was found that problem drinkers randomly assigned to confrontational counseling had higher levels of resistance (Miller & Sovereign, 1989).

Labeling

Clients are generally reluctant to be labeled as "alcoholic," and researchers have recommended that *labeling* be deemphasized, as it has *no clinical advantages*. In fact, labels may hinder recognition of an alcohol problem (see Sobell, Sobell, & Toneatto, 1992). Roman and Trice (1968) have suggested that individuals who fear the sanctions of being labeled "alcoholic" may be reluctant to divulge information about their alcohol use. In fact, several studies have found that alcohol abusers reported they either delayed (e.g., Thom, 1986) or avoided (Sobell et al., 1992) entry into treatment because of concerns about being labeled an alcoholic.

Beginning Treatment: Assessing Commitment to Change

A final assessment issue but a critical one is the need to evaluate the client's motivation for and commitment to change. According to Miller and Rollinick (1991), "Motivation is a *state* of readiness or eagerness to change, which may fluctuate from one time or situation to another. This state is one that can be influenced" (p. 14). Thus, rather than a "trait," motivation is conceived as a "state" that is subject to the influence of several variables. One way to assess a client's level of motivation is to use a decisional-balance exercise wherein the costs and the benefits of the client's use of alcohol are evaluated (Appel, 1986; Janis & Mann, 1977; Miller & Rollinick, 1991). It is important to keep in mind that it is the client's subjective perceptions of costs and benefits that are important. Differences between the client's perceptions and those from a more objective perspective may constitute important topics to be considered in treatment. Other methods of assessment include asking clients about their readiness to change.

Once an assessment of the client's readiness to change has been accomplished, the next step is to strengthen the client's motivation. Several motivational approaches have been suggested by Miller and Rollinick (1991): (1) The interviewer should identify the problem, stress the importance of change, and get the client to develop a specific course of action; (2) obstacles to treatment should be identified and addressed; (3) clear and realistic goals should be set by the client; and (4) personal choice should be encouraged.

SUMMARY

A thorough and in-depth assessment has become an increasingly important element of the treatment process for individuals with alcohol problems. The need for accurate diagnosis of alcohol and other concurrent disorders is integral to the assessment process, and the assessment is critical to the development of meaningful treatment plans. As this chapter has shown and as illustrated by the case studies, alcohol abusers are a very heterogeneous population; the interviewing procedure must therefore be sufficiently flexible to be able to provide clinicians with a valid profile of the alcohol problem. The assessment instruments described in this chapter can be used to obtain information relevant to the assessment process. Furthermore, the implications of assessment data for treatment issues, such as drinking goals and treatment intensity, show how the clinical interview can significantly impact on treatment. Finally, several clinically useful strategies can be incorporated into the assessment process to enhance the validity of the information obtained from clients and to enhance clients' motivation for behavior change.

ACKNOWLEDGMENTS.   The authors with to thank Ms. Joanne Jackson for her patience and diligence in typing repeated drafts of this manuscript and Ms. Gloria Leo for the preparation of the figures.

REFERENCES

Allsop, S., & Saunders, B. (1989). Relapse and alcohol problems. In M. Gossop (Ed.), *Relapse and addictive behaviour* (pp. 11–40). New York: Tavistock/Routledge.

American Medical Association (1977). *Manual on alcoholism* (3rd ed.). Chicago: Author.

American Psychiatric Association (1980). *Diagnostic and statistical manual of mental disorders*, 3rd ed. Washington, DC: Author.

American Psychiatric Association (1987). *Diagnostic and statistical manual of mental disorders*, 3rd ed., revised. Washington, DC: Author.

American Psychiatric Association (1993). *Diagnostic and statistical manual of mental disorders*, 4th ed., draft criteria. Washington, DC: Author.

Annis, H. M. (1986). A relapse prevention model for the treatment of alcoholics. In W. R. Miller & N. Heather (Eds.), *Treating addictive behaviors: Processes of change* (pp. 407–435). New York: Pergamon Press.

Annis, H. M., & Chan, D. (1983). The differential treatment model: Empirical evidence from a personality typology of adult offenders. *Criminal Justice and Behavior, 10*, 159–173.

Annis, H. M., & Davis, C. S. (1988). Assessment of expectancies. In D. M. Donovan & G. A. Marlatt (Eds.), *Assessment of addictive behaviors* (pp. 84–111). New York: Guilford Press.

Annis, H. M., & Davis, C. S. (1989). Relapse prevention. In R. K. Hester & W. R. Miller (Eds.), *Handbook of alcoholism treatment approaches: Alternative approaches* (pp. 170–182). New York: Pergamon Press.

Annis, H. M., & Graham, J. M. (1988). *Situational Confidence Questionnaire (SCQ 39): User's guide*. Toronto: Addiction Research Foundation.

Appel, C. P. (1986). From contemplation to determination: Contributions from cognitive psychology. In W. R. Miller & N. Heather (Eds.), *Treating addictive behaviors: Processes of change* (pp. 59–90). New York: Plenum Press.

Babor, T. F., Brown, J., & Del Boca, F. K. (1990). Validity of self-reports in applied research on addictive behaviors: Fact or fiction? *Addictive Behaviors, 12*, 5–32.

Babor, T. F., Kranzler, H. R., & Lauerman, R. J. (1987). Social drinking as a health and psychosocial risk factor: Anstie's limit revisited. In M. Galanter (Ed.), *Recent developments in alcoholism*, Vol. 5 (pp. 373–402). New York: Plenum Press.

Babor, T. F., Stephens, R. S., & Marlatt, G. A. (1987). Verbal report methods in clinical research on alcoholism: Response bias and its minimization. *Journal of Studies on Alcohol, 48*, 410–424.

Battjes, R. J. (1988). Smoking as an issue in alcohol and drug abuse treatment. *Addictive Behaviors, 13*, 225–230.

Berg, G., & Skuttle, A. (1986). Early intervention with problem drinkers. In W. R. Miller & N. Heather (Eds.), *Treating addictive behaviors: Processes of change* (pp. 205–221). New York: Plenum Press.

Bernadt, M. R., Mumford, J., Taylor, C., Smith, B., & Murray, R. M. (1982). Comparison of questionnaire and laboratory tests in the detection of excessive drinking and alcoholism. *Lancet, 1*, 325–328.

Bobo, J. K. (1989). Nicotine dependence and alcoholism epidemiology and treatment. *Journal of Psychoactive Drugs, 21,* 323–329.

Bradburn, N. M., & Sudman, S. (1979). *Improving interview method and questionnaire design.* San Francisco: Jossey-Bass.

Brown, G. W., & Harris, T. (1978). *Social origins of depression: A study of psychiatric disorder in women.* London: Tavistock.

Burling, T. A., & Ziff, D. C. (1988). Tobacco smoking: A comparison between alcohol and drug inpatients. *Addictive Behaviors, 13,* 185–190.

Cahalan, D. (1970). *Problem drinkers: A national survey.* San Francisco: Jossey-Bass.

Cahalan, D., & Room, R. (1974). *Problem drinking among American men.* New Brunswick, NJ: Rutgers Center of Alcohol Studies.

Cartwright, A. K. J. (1981). Are different therapeutic perspectives important in the treatment of alcoholism? *British Journal of Addiction, 76,* 347–361.

Chick, J., Kreitman, N., & Plant, M. (1981). Mean cell volume and gamma-glutamyl-transpeptidase as markers of drinking in working men. *Lancet, 1,* 1249–1251.

Cox, B. M., Norton, R. G., Swinson, R. P., & Endler, N. S. (1990). Substance abuse and panic-related anxiety: A critical review. *Behaviour Research and Therapy, 28,* 385–393.

Craddock, S. G., Bray, R. M., & Hubbard, R. L. (1985). *Drug use before and during drug abuse treatment: 1979–1981 TOPS admission cohorts* (DHHS Publication No. ADM 85-1387). Rockville, MD: National Institute on Drug Abuse.

Cyr, M. G., & Wartman, S. A. (1988). The effectiveness of routine screening questions in the detection of alcoholism. *Journal of the American Medical Association, 259,* 51–54.

Davidson, R. (1987). Assessment of the alcohol dependence syndrome: A review of self-report screening questionnaires. *British Psychological Society, 26,* 243–255.

Davidson, R., & Raistrick, D. (1986). The validity of the Short Alcohol Dependence Data (SADD) questionnaire: A short self-report questionnaire for the assessment of alcohol dependence. *British Journal of Addiction, 81,* 217–222.

Devenyi, P., Robinson, G. M., Kapur, B. M., & Roncari, D. A. K. (1981). High-density lipoprotein cholesterol in male alcoholics with and without severe liver disease. *American Journal of Medicine, 71,* 589–594.

Dorus, W., Kennedy, J., Gibbons, R. D., & Ravi, S. D. (1987). Symptoms and diagnosis of depression in alcoholics. *Alcoholism: Clinical and Experimental Research, 11,* 150–154.

Edwards, G. (1986). The alcohol dependence syndrome: A concept as stimulus to enquiry. *British Journal of Addiction, 81,* 171–184.

Fagerström, K. O. (1978). Measuring degree of physical dependence on tobacco smoking with reference to individualization of treatment. *Addictive Behaviors, 3,* 235–241.

Fillmore, K. M. (1988). *Alcohol use across the life course: A critical review of 70 years of international longitudinal research.* Toronto: Addiction Research Foundation.

Galambos, J. T. (1975). The course of alcoholic hepatitis. In J. M. Khanna, Y. Israel, & H. Kalant (Eds.), *Alcoholic liver pathology* (pp. 97–111). Toronto: Addiction Research Foundation.

Gallant, D. M. (1987). *Alcoholism: A guide to diagnosis, intervention, and treatment.* New York: Norton.

Goodwin, D. W., Crane, J. B., & Guze, S. B. (1969). Alcoholic "blackouts": A review and clinical study of 100 alcoholics. *American Journal of Psychiatry, 126,* 191–198.

Gorman, D. M. (1990). Data collection in studies of life events and the harmful use of alcohol. *Drug and Alcohol Review, 9,* 67–74.

Hansen, J., & Emrick, C. D. (1983). Whom are we calling "alcoholic"? *Society of Psychologists in Addictive Behaviors, 2,* 164–178.

Harrell, A. V. (1985). Validation of self-report: The research record. In B. A. Rouse, N. J. Kozel, & L. G. Richards (Eds.), *Self-report methods of estimating drug use: Meeting current challenges to validity* (NIDA Research Monograph No. 57, pp. 12–21). Rockville, MD: National Institute on Drug Abuse.

Hasin, D. S., Grant, B., & Endicott, J. (1990). The natural history of alcohol abuse: Implications for definitions of alcohol use disorders. *American Journal of Psychiatry, 147,* 1537–1541.

Heather, N., & Robertson, I. (1983). *Controlled drinking,* 2nd ed. New York: Methuen.

Heatherton, T. F., Kozlowski, L. T., Frecker, R. C., & Fagerström, K.-O. (1991). The Fagerström Test for Nicotine Dependence: A revision of the Fagerström Tolerance Questionnaire. *British Journal of Addiction, 86,* 119–1127.

Hedlund, J. L., & Vieweg, B. W. (1984). The Michigan Alcoholism Screening Test (MAST): A comprehensive review. *Journal of Operational Psychiatry*, *15*, 55–65.

Hesselbrock, M. N., Meyer, R. E., & Keener, J. J. (1985). Psychopathology in hospitalized alcoholics. *Archives of General Psychiatry*, *42*, 1050–1055.

Hester, R. K., & Miller, W. R. (1990). Self-control training. In R. K. Hester & W. R. Miller (Eds.), *Handbook of alcoholism treatment approaches: Effective alternatives* (pp. 141–149). New York: Pergamon Press.

Hill, S. Y. (1985). The disease concept of alcoholism: A review. *Drug and Alcohol Dependence*, *16*, 193–214.

Hilton, M. E. (1989). How many alcoholics are there in the United States? *British Journal of Addiction*, *84*, 459–460.

Holt, S., Skinner, H. A., & Israel, Y. (1981). Early identification of alcohol abuse. 2. Clinical and laboratory indicators. *Canadian Medical Association Journal*, *124*, 1279–1295.

Hubbard, R. L., Marsden, M. E., Rachal, J. V., Cavanaugh, E. R., & Ginzburg, H. M. (1989). *Drug abuse treatment: A national survey of effectiveness*. Chapel Hill: University of North Carolina Press.

Istvan, J., & Matarazzo, J. D. (1984). Tobacco, alcohol, and caffeine use: A review of their interrelationships. *Psychological Bulletin*, *95*, 301–326.

Jacobson, G. R. (1989). A comprehensive approach to pretreatment evaluation. 1. Detection, assessment, and diagnosis of alcoholism. In R. K. Hester & W. R. Miller (Eds.), *Handbook of alcoholism treatment approaches: Alternative approaches* (pp. 17–53). New York: Pergamon Press.

Janis, I. L., & Mann, L. (1977). *Decision-making: A psychological analysis of conflict, choice, and commitment*. New York: Free Press.

Kapur, B. M., & Israel, Y. (1983). A dipstick methodology for rapid determination of alcohol in body fluids. *Clinical Chemistry*, *29*, 1178.

Kapur, B. M., & Israel, Y. (1984). Alcohol dipstick for ethanol and methanol. *Clinical Biochemistry*, *17*, 201.

Katschnig, H. (1986). Measuring life stress—a comparison of the checklist and the panel technique. In H. Katschnig (Ed.), *Life events and psychiatric disorders: Controversial issues* (pp. 74–106). New York: Cambridge University.

Kaufman, E. (1982). The relationship of alcoholism and alcohol abuse to the abuse of other drugs. *American Journal of Drug and Alcohol Abuse*, *9*, 1–17.

Keeler, M. H., Taylor, I., & Miller, W. C. (1979). Are all recently detoxified alcoholics depressed? *American Journal of Psychiatry*, *136*, 586–588.

Kessler, R. G. (1991). Comorbidity of substance use disorders and other psychiatric disorders: An ADAMHA report of prevalence, etiology, implications for prevention, course of illness and research. Unpublished manuscript, University of Michigan.

Kissin, B. (1983). The disease concept of alcoholism. In R. G. Smart, F. B. Glaser, Y. Israel, H. Kalant, R. E. Popham, & W. Schmidt (Eds.), *Research advances in alcohol and drug problems: Volume 7* (pp. 93–126). New York: Plenum.

Kivlahan, D. R., Sher, K. J., & Donovan, D. M. (1989). The Alcohol Dependence Scale: A validation study among inpatient alcoholics. *Journal of Studies on Alcohol*, *50*, 170–175.

Kozlowski, L. T., Director, J., & Harford, M. A. (1981). Tobacco dependence, restraint and time to the first cigarette of the day. *Addictive Behaviors*, *6*, 307–312.

Kozlowski, L. T., Jelinek, L. C., & Pope, M. A. (1986). Cigarette smoking among alcohol abusers: Continuing and neglected problem. *Canadian Journal of Public Health*, *77*, 205–207.

Kushner, M. G., Sher, K. J., & Beitman, B. D. (1990). The relation between alcohol problems and the anxiety disorders. *American Journal of Psychiatry*, *147*, 685–695.

Leigh, G. L., & Skinner, H. A. (1988). Physiological assessment. In D. M. Donovan & G. A. Marlatt (Eds.), *Assessment of addictive behaviors* (pp. 112–136). New York: Guilford Press.

Lettieri, D. J., Nelson, J. E., & Sayers, M. A. (Eds.) (1985). *Alcoholism treatment assessment research instruments (NIAAA Treatment Research Series 2)*. Rockville, MD: National Institute on Alcohol Abuse and Alcoholism.

Levine, J. (1990). The relative value of consultation, questionnaires, and laboratory investigation in the identification of excessive alcohol consumption. *Alcohol and Alcoholism*, *25*, 539–553.

Lieberman, M. A., Yalom, I. D., & Miles, M. B. (1973). *Encounter groups: First facts*. New York: Basic Books.

Maisto, S. A., McKay, J. R., & Connors, G. J. (1990). Self-report issues in substance abuse: State of the art and future directions. *Behavioral Assessment*, *12*, 117–134.

Maisto, S. A., Sobell, M. B., Cooper, A. M., & Sobell, L. C. (1979). Test–retest reliability of retrospective self-reports in three populations of alcohol abusers. *Journal of Behavioral Assessment, 1*, 315–326.

Mandell, W. (1983). Types and phases of alcohol dependence. In M. Galanter (Ed.), *Recent developments in alcoholism*, Vol. 3 (pp. 415–448). New York: Plenum Press.

Marlatt, G. A., & Gordon, J. R. (Eds.) (1985). *Relapse prevention*. New York: Guilford Press.

Mash, E. J., & Terdal, L. (1976). Behavior-therapy assessment: Diagnosis, design, and evaluation. In E. J. Mash & L. G. Terdal (Eds.), *Behavior therapy assessment* (pp. 15–32). New York: Springer.

Mezzich, A. C., Arria, A. M., Tarter, R. E., Moss, H., & Van Thiel, D. H. (1991). Psychiatric comorbidity in alcoholism: Importance of ascertainment source. *Alcoholism: Clinical and Experimental Research, 15*, 893–898.

Miller, P. M., & Salter, D. P. (1984). Is there a short-cut? An investigation into the life event interview. *Acta Psychiatrica Scandinavica, 70*, 417–427.

Miller, W. R. (1986/87). Motivation and treatment goals. *Drugs & Society, 1*, 133–151.

Miller, W. R., & Rollinick, S. (1991). *Motivational interviewing: Preparing people to change addictive behavior*. New York: Guilford Press.

Miller, W. R., & Sovereign, R. G. (1989). The check-up: A model for early intervention in addictive behaviors. In T. Løberg, W. R. Miller, P. E. Nathan, & G. A. Marlatt (Eds.), *Addictive behaviors: Prevention and early intervention* (pp. 219–231). Amsterdam: Swets & Zeitlinger.

Miller, W. R., Taylor, C. A., & West, J. C. (1980). Focused versus broad-spectrum behavior therapy for problem drinkers. *Journal of Consulting and Clinical Psychology, 48*, 590–601.

Morgan, M. Y. (1980). Markers for detecting alcoholism, and monitoring for continued abuse. *Pharmacology, Biochemistry & Behavior, 13*, 1–8.

Morgan, M. Y., Colman, J. C., & Sherlock, S. (1981). The use of a combination of peripheral markers for diagnosing alcoholism and monitoring for continued abuse. *British Journal of Alcohol and Alcoholism, 16*, 167–177.

Nace, E. P., David, C. W., & Gaspari, J. P. (1991). Axis II comorbidity in substance abusers. *American Journal of Psychiatry, 148*, 118–120.

Nathan, P. E. (1991). Substance use disorders in DSM-IV. *Journal of Abnormal Psychology, 100*, 356–361.

National Institute on Alcohol Abuse and Alcoholism (1990). *Seventh Special Report to the U.S. Congress on Alcohol and Health* [U.S. Department of Health and Human Services Publication No. (ADM) 90-1656]. Washington, DC: U.S. Government Printing Office.

Nelson, R. O., & Hayes, S. C. (1981). Theoretical explanations for reactivity in self-monitoring. *Behavior Modification, 5*, 3–14.

Nirenberg, T. D., Sobell, L. C., Ersner-Hershfield, S., & Cellucci, A. J. (1983). Can disulfiram precipitate urges to drink alcohol? *Addictive Behaviors, 8*, 311–313.

O'Farrell, T. J., & Maisto, S. A. (1987). The utility of self-report and biological measures of alcohol consumption in alcoholism treatment outcome studies. *Advances in Behaviour Research and Therapy, 9*, 91–125.

O'Farrell, T. J., Cutter, H. S. G., Bayog, R. D., Dentch, G., & Fortgang, J. (1984). Correspondence between one-year retrospective reports of pretreatment drinking by alcoholics and their wives. *Behavioral Assessment, 6*, 263–274.

Petersson, B., Trell, E., & Kristensson, H. (1983). Comparison of γ-glutamyltransferase and questionnaire test as alcohol indicators in different risk groups. *Drug and Alcohol Dependence, 11*, 279–286.

Polich, J. M., Armor, D. J., & Braiker, H. B. (1981). *The course of alcoholism: Four years after treatment*. New York: Wiley.

Pomerleau, C. S., Pomerleau, O. F., Majchrzak, M. J., Kloska, D. D., & Malakuti, R. (1990). Relationship between nicotine tolerance questionnaire scores and plasma cotinine. *Addictive Behaviors, 15*, 73–80.

Powell, B. J., Read, M. R., & Penick, E. C. E. (1987). Primary and secondary depression in alcoholic men: An important distinction? *Journal of Clinical Psychiatry, 48*, 98–101.

Raistrick, D., Dunbar, G., & Davidson, R. (1983). Development of a questionnaire to measure alcohol dependence. *British Journal of Addiction, 78*, 89–95.

Regier, D. A., Farmer, M. D., Rae, D. S., Locke, B. Z., Keith, S. J., Judd, L. L., & Goodwin, F. K. (1990). Comorbidity of mental disorders with alcohol and other drug abuse. *Journal of the American Medical Association, 264*, 2511–2518.

Riley, D. M., Sobell, L. C., Leo, G. I., Sobell, M. B., & Klajner, F. (1987). Behavioral treatment of alcohol problems: A review and a comparison of behavioral and nonbehavioral studies. In W. M. Cox (Ed.), *Treatment and prevention of alcohol problems: A resource manual* (pp. 73–115). New York: Academic Press.

Riskind, J. H., Beck, A. T., Berchick, R. J., Brown, G., & Steer, R. A. (1987). Reliability of DSM-III diagnoses for major depression and generalized anxiety disorder using the Structured Clinical Interview for DSM-III. *Archives of General Psychiatry, 44,* 817–820.

Robins, L. N., Helzer, J. E., Croughan, J., & Ratcliff, K. S. (1981). National Institute of Mental Health Diagnostic Interview Schedule. *Archives of General Psychiatry, 38,* 381–389.

Roman, P. M., & Trice, H. M. (1968). The sick role, labelling theory and the deviant drinkers. *International Journal of Social Psychiatry, 14,* 245–251.

Room, R. (1990). Measuring alcohol consumption in the United States: Methods and rationales. In L. T. Kozlowski, H. M. Annis, H. D. Cappell, F. B. Glaser, M. S. Goodstadt, Y. Israel, H. Kalant, E. M. Sellers, & E. R. Vingilis (Eds.), *Research advances in alcohol and drug problems,* Vol. 10 (pp. 39–80). New York: Plenum Press.

Ross, H. E., Gavin, D. R., & Skinner, H. A. (1990). Diagnostic validity of the MAST and the Alcohol Dependence Scale in the assessment of DSM-III alcohol disorders. *Journal of Studies on Alcohol, 51,* 506–513.

Ross, H. E., Glaser, F. B., & Germanson, T. (1988). The prevalence of psychiatric disorders in patients with alcohol and other drug problems. *Archives of General Psychiatry, 45,* 1023–1031.

Rounsaville, B. J., Bryant, K., Babor, T., Kranzler, H., & Kadden, R. (1993). Cross system agreement for substance use disorders: DSM-III-R, DSM-IV and ICD-10. *Addiction, 88,* 337–348.

Rounsaville, B. J., Dolinsky, Z. S., Babor, T. F., & Meyer, R. E. (1987). Psychopathology as a predictor of treatment outcome in alcoholics. *Archives of General Psychiatry, 44,* 505–513.

Rounsaville, B. J., Kosten, T. R., Williams, J. B. W., & Spitzer, R. L. (1987). A field trial of DSM III-R psychoactive substance dependence disorders. *American Journal of Psychiatry, 144,* 351–355.

Samo, J. A., Tucker, J. A., & Vuchinich, R. E. (1989). Agreement between self-monitoring, recall, and collateral observation measures of alcohol consumption in older adults. *Behavioral Assessment, 11,* 391–409.

Sanchez-Craig, M., & Annis, H. M. (1982). "Self-monitoring" and "recall" measures of alcohol consumption: Convergent validity with biochemical indices of liver function. *British Journal of Alcohol and Alcoholism, 17,* 117–121.

Schuckit, M. A. (1985). The clinical implications of primary diagnostic groups among alcoholics. *Archives of General Psychiatry, 42,* 1043–1049.

Selzer, M. L. (1971). The Michigan Alcoholism Screening Test: The quest for a new diagnostics instrument. *American Journal of Psychiatry, 127,* 89–94.

Selzer, M. L., Vinokur, A., & van Rooijen, L. (1975). A self-administered Short Michigan Alcoholism Screening Test (SMAST). *Journal of Studies on Alcohol, 36,* 117–126.

Shaw, S., Korts, D., & Stimmel, B. (1982/1983). Abnormal liver function tests as biological markers for alcoholism in narcotic addicts. *American Journal of Drug and Alcohol Abuse, 9,* 345–354.

Skinner, H. A., & Allen, B. A. (1982). Alcohol dependence syndrome: Measurement and validation. *Journal of Abnormal Psychology, 91,* 199–209.

Skinner, H. A., & Horn, J. L. (1984). *Alcohol Dependence Scale (ADS) user's guide.* Toronto: Addiction Research Foundation.

Skinner, H. A., Holt, S., Schuller, R., Roy, J., & Israel, Y. (1984). Identification of alcohol abuse using laboratory tests and a history of trauma. *Annals of Internal Medicine, 101,* 847–851.

Skinner, H. A., & Sheu, W. J. (1982). Reliability of alcohol use indices: The lifetime drinking history and the MAST. *Journal of Studies on Alcohol, 43,* 1157–1170.

Skre I., Onstad, S., Torgersen, S., & Kringlen, E. (1991). High interrater reliability for the Structured Clinical Interview for DSM-III-R Axis I (SCID-I). *Acta Psychiatrica Scandinavica, 84,* 167–173.

Sobell, L. C., Maisto, S. A., Sobell, M. B., & Cooper, A. M. (1979). Reliability of alcohol abusers' self-reports of drinking behavior. *Behaviour Research and Therapy, 17,* 157–160.

Sobell, L. C., & Sobell, M. B. (1973). A self-feedback technique to monitor drinking behavior in alcoholics. *Behaviour Research and Therapy, 11,* 237–238.

Sobell, L. C., & Sobell, M. B. (1980). Convergent validity: An approach to increasing confidence in treatment outcome conclusions with alcohol and drug abusers. In L. C. Sobell, M. B. Sobell, & E.

Ward (Eds.), *Evaluating alcohol and drug abuse treatment effectiveness: Recent advances* (pp. 177–185). New York: Pergamon Press.

Sobell, L. C., & Sobell, M. B. (1983). Behavioral research and therapy: Its impact on the alcohol field. In K. D. Craig & R. J. McMahon (Eds.), *Advances in clinical behavior therapy* (pp. 175–193). New York: Brunner/Mazel.

Sobell, L. C., & Sobell, M. B. (1990). Self-report issues in alcohol abuse: State of the art and future directions. *Behavioral Assessment, 12*, 91–106.

Sobell, L. C., & Sobell, M. B. (1992). Timeline Follow-Back: A technique for assessing self-reported ethanol consumption. In J. Allen & R. Z. Litten (Eds.), *Measuring alcohol consumption: Psychosocial and biological methods* (pp. 41–72). New Jersey: Humana Press.

Sobell, L. C., Sobell, M. B., Kozlowski, L. T, & Toneatto, T. (1990). Alcohol or tobacco research versus alcohol and tobacco research. *British Journal of Addiction, 85*, 263–269.

Sobell, L. C., Sobell, M. B., Leo, G. I., & Cancilla, A. (1988). Reliability of a timeline method: Assessing normal drinkers' reports of recent drinking and a comparative evaluation across several populations. *British Journal of Addiction, 83*, 393–402.

Sobell, L. C., Sobell, M. B., & Nirenberg, T. D. (1988). Behavioral assessment and treatment planning with alcohol and drug abusers: A review with an emphasis on clinical application. *Clinical Psychology Review, 8*, 19–54.

Sobell, L. C., Sobell, M. B., Riley, D. M., Schuller, R., Pavan, D. S., Cancilla, A., Klajner, F., & Leo, G. I. (1988). The reliability of alcohol abusers' self-reports of drinking and life events that occurred in the distant past. *Journal of Studies on Alcohol, 49*, 225–232.

Sobell, L. C., Sobell, M. B., & Toneatto, T. (1992). Recovery from alcohol problems without treatment. In N. Heather, W. R. Miller, & J. Greeley (Eds.), *Self-control and the addictive behaviours* (pp. 198–242). New York: MacMillan.

Sobell, L. C., Toneatto, T., Sobell, M. B., Schuller, R., & Maxwell, M. (1990). A procedure for reducing errors in reports of life events. *Journal of Psychosomatic Research, 34*, 163–170.

Sobell, M. B., Bogardis, J., Schuller, R., Leo, G. I., & Sobell, L. C. (1989). Is self-monitoring of alcohol consumption reactive? *Behavioral Assessment, 11*, 447–458.

Sobell, M. B., & Sobell, L. C. (1975). A brief technical report on the Mobat: An inexpensive portable test for determining blood alcohol concentration. *Journal of Applied Behavior Analysis, 8*, 117–120.

Sobell, M. B., & Sobell, L. C. (1986/1987). Conceptual issues regarding goals in the treatment of alcohol problems. *Drugs & Society, 1*, 1–37.

Sobell, M. B., & Sobell, L. C. (1987). Conceptual issues regarding goals in the treatment of alcohol problems. In M. B. Sobell & L. C. Sobell (Eds.), *Moderation as a goal or outcome of treatment for alcohol problems: A dialogue* (pp. 1–37). New York: Haworth Press.

Sobell, M. B., & Sobell, L. C. (1993a). *Problem drinkers: Guided self-change treatment.* New York: Guilford Press.

Sobell, M. B., & Sobell, L. C. (1993b). Treatment for problem drinkers: A public health priority. In J. S. Baer, G. A. Marlatt, & R. J. McMahon (Eds.), *Addictive behaviors across the lifespan: Prevention, treatment, and policy issues* (pp. 138–157). Beverly Hills, CA: Sage Publications.

Sobell, M. B., Sobell, L. C., Bogardis, J., Leo, G. I., & Skinner, W. (1992). Problem drinkers' perceptions of whether treatment goals should be self-selected or therapist-selected. *Behavior Therapy, 23*, 43–52.

Solomon, K. E., & Annis, H. M. (1989). Development of a scale to measure outcome expectancy in alcoholics. *Cognitive Therapy and Research, 13*, 409–421.

Solomon, K. E., & Annis, H. M. (1990). Outcome and efficacy expectancy in the prediction of post-treatment drinking behaviour. *British Journal of Addiction, 85*, 659–665.

Spitzer, R. L., Williams, J. B. W., Gibbon, M., & First, M. B. (1988). *Structured Clinical Interview for DSM-III-R—Patient version (SCID-P 6.1.88).* New York: Biometrics Research Department, New York State Psychiatric Institute.

Stockwell, T., Blaze-Temple, D., & Walker, C. (1991). The effect of "standard drink" labeling on the ability of drinkers to pour a "standard drink." *Australian Journal of Public Health, 15*, 56–63.

Stockwell, T., Murphy, D., & Hodgson, R. (1983). The Severity of Alcohol Dependence Questionnaire: Its use, reliability and validity. *British Journal of Addiction, 78*, 145–155.

Straus, R., & Bacon, S. D. (1953). *Drinking in college.* New Haven, CT: Yale University Press.

Thom, B. (1986). Sex differences in help-seeking for alcohol problems—1. The barriers to help-seeking. *British Journal of Addiction, 81,* 777–788.

Tu, G., Kapur, B., & Israel, Y. (1992). Characteristics of a new urine, serum and saliva alcohol reagent strip. *Alcoholism and Clinical Research, 16,* 222–227.

Valle, S. K. (1981). Interpersonal functioning of alcoholism counselors and treatment outcome. *Journal of Studies on Alcohol, 42,* 783–790.

Vuchinich, R. E., Tucker, J. A., & Harllee, L. M. (1988). Behavioral assessment (of alcohol dependence). In D. Donovan & G. A. Marlatt (Eds.), *Assessment of addictive behaviors: Behavioral, cognitive, and physiological procedures* (pp. 51–93). New York: Guilford Press.

Wartenberg, A. A., & Liepman, M. R. (1987). Medical consequences of addictive behaviors. In T. D. Nirenberg & S. A. Maisto (Eds.), *Developments in the assessment and treatment of addictive behaviors* (pp. 49–85). New Jersey: Ablex.

Weissman, M. M., & Meyers, J. K. (1980). Clinical depression in alcoholism. *American Journal of Psychiatry, 137,* 372–373.

Wilkinson, D. A., Leigh, G. M., Cordingley, J., Martin, G. W., & Lei, H. (1987). Dimensions of multiple drug use and a typology of drug users. *British Journal of Addiction, 82,* 259–287.

Wilson, G. T. (1988). Alcohol and anxiety. *Behaviour Research and Therapy, 26,* 369–381.

Woodruff, R. A., Clayton, P. J., Cloninger, R., & Guze, S. B. (1976). A brief method of screening for alcoholism. *Diseases of the Nervous System, 37,* 434–435.

World Health Organization (1987). *Composite International Diagnostic Interview, Core Version, 0.0.* Geneva: Author.

8

Drug Abuse

Jesse B. Milby and Joseph E. Schumacher

Description of the Disorders

Diagnosing drug abuse and dependence is a task complicated by differences among individuals and the compounds used. Although acknowledging these multiple interactions, common behavior patterns and similarities in the development of substance use disorders can be seen. We refer to these developmental phenomena as *stages* in the abuse and dependence process. They need to be thoroughly understood by any clinician who seeks to do diagnostic evaluations. These stages are discussed in detail in this section.

Initiation

Reasons for initiating drug use vary with each person's interests, background, and motivation. There is no common etiological factor for all. Some do it for excitement, some respond to peer pressure, and others do it to satisfy their curiosity or in anticipation of relief from tension. The World Health Organization (1974) has identified seven widely recognized motives for initiating use, and Dohner (1972) has described several others. Initiation is most likely to occur in adolescence or young adulthood. Major risk periods for initiating use of cigarettes, alcohol, and marijuana and other illicit drugs, except for cocaine, typically begin during adolescence and end by age 20–21 (Kandel & Logan, 1984). The most significant phenomenon in first use is that the individual can be strongly reinforced for his or her initial involvement by the effects of the drug itself, by social factors that encourage its repetition, or by both.

Jesse B. Milby • Veterans Administration Medical Center and Behavioral Medicine Unit, Division of Preventative Medicine, University of Alabama School of Medicine, Birmingham, Alabama 35233. Joseph E. Schumacher • Behavioral Medicine Unit, Division of Preventative Medicine, University of Alabama School of Medicine, Birmingham, Alabama 35233.

Diagnostic Interviewing (Second Edition), edited by Michel Hersen and Samuel M. Turner. Plenum Press, New York, 1994.

Increased Dosing and Tolerance

As use of the drug is repeated, typical processes begin. One is tolerance, which refers to the decreased drug effects with repeated administration. Decreased drug effects lead to increased doses in order to experience the same effect. Thus, with repeated use, tolerance develops, and the dose increases.

Drug Preoccupation and Development of Drug-Seeking Behavior

With repeated drug use, drug preoccupation occurs. More time is spent fantasizing about the favorite drug and its effect. Such preoccupation motivates the acquisition of drug-seeking behaviors, including drug knowledge, skills, and language. Young adult drug abusers have more difficulty making a successful transition to adult role responsibilities and engage in more deviant behavior while becoming immersed in a social network supportive of their drug use (Kandel, 1984; Newcomb & Bentler, 1986). As their use increases, these tendencies often lead to family, school, social, health, and occupational problems (Kandel, Davies, Karus, & Yamaguchi, 1986; Schwartz, Hoffman, & Jones, 1987).

Drug Abuse and Dependence

Abuse is the first category that describes patterns associated with maladaptive patterns of substance use. According to DSM-IV (American Psychiatric Association, 1993), abuse is indicated by a continued use (at least 1 month) despite the knowledge of having persistent or recurring problems associated with the drug, or recurrent use in situations in which that use is physically hazardous.

Dependence is a category that describes more pathological drug-use patterns usually characterized by tolerance and withdrawal symptoms. Many experts distinguish between two types of dependence: psychic and physical. *Psychic* dependence occurs when the effects of the substance are pleasing to the individual and a psychological drive develops that motivates the individual to continue using in order to produce pleasure or avoid discomfort. *Physical* dependence is an adaptive state of the body. It is manifested by physical disturbances, known as withdrawal or abstinence syndromes, when drug use is stopped. Both types of dependence are strong motivators of drug-seeking behaviors and prolonged use.

With continued abuse of the drug and tolerance, the consequent decreased drug effects lead to increased doses in order to obtain the same desired experience. Higher and more regular doses are consumed, leading to the establishment of physical or psychic dependence or both. Withdrawal symptoms develop with the reduction or elimination of continued intake of the substance. Adverse physiological signs and cravings are common to the withdrawal experience. The nature and extent of tolerance and withdrawal symptoms vary according to the type of the drug, maximum regular dose levels, and other individual variables, such as metabolism.

During prolonged dependence, dose stabilization is likely to occur. A dose plateau is reached, and dose increases level off. Often, abusers who achieve this "plateau" describe their use pattern as the amount of drug it takes to feel "normal," as they no longer strive for the initial drug effects. Another pattern in dependency involves periods of abstinence, during which the individual stops taking his or her primary drug. He or she may cease drug use altogether or use only drugs that prevent or minimize the withdrawal effects. It is important to note that many who are drug-dependent at some time try to break their dependency. Abstinence may also be caused by other factors, such as drug shortages, lack of money, incarceration, and the like.

Just as there are periods of abstinence, there are also relapses. Many drug-dependent individuals demonstrate a repeated cycle of dependency and abstinence. The unique characteristic of physical dependence is the abstinence syndrome, which occurs soon after the last dose. The syndrome's onset varies with the type of drug being used, but there are many signs and symptoms common to abstinence from various drugs. Common symptoms include headache, irritability, restlessness, cramps, nausea, vomiting, sweating, diarrhea, sleep disturbance, and especially emotional irritability and nervousness. Because of this commonality, it is often difficult to determine which class of drug has been abused on the sole basis of abstinence signs and symptoms.

CHARACTERISTICS ASSOCIATED WITH A DRUG-ABUSE LIFE-STYLE

Because most common mood-altering substances are illegal and abusers must obtain these drugs through illegal means, a frequent characteristic associated with a drug-abuse life-style is criminal involvement. As a consequence of the addiction, the addict may become involved in a subculture of crime, which compounds the risks associated with drug abuse alone. Introduction to the criminal justice system may start in early adolescence with possession or even trafficking charges. Drug-related delinquent or incorrigible behaviors often require the courts to involve extrafamilial controls such as detention centers or residential treatment facilities for children and adolescents. Illegal activities associated with substance abuse during adulthood, such as theft, robbery, prostitution, and illegal sale of drugs, have devastating effects on the user's future. The relationship between illicit drugs and crime is indisputable and should be given significant weight in the assessment of the addiction process.

Another characteristic associated with the drug-abuse life-style is the erosion of non-drug-related interests and family relationships. As the individual becomes physically dependent, he or she must devote increasing amounts of time to procuring the drug supply. This monomania often leads to neglect or loss of interest in the areas of recreation, education, and work that were previously important or rewarding. As this focus on purely drug-related needs increases, time and energy usually directed toward age-appropriate accomplishments become diverted to self-destruction. The egocentric drive to keep the addict's habit satisfied is usually obtained at the expense of self-respect and the respect of others. Job and education are often adversely affected or terminated. Family members and loved ones are often alienated and abused to maintain the addict's habit.

Interview Assessment

The interview is the main diagnostic tool for assessing drug abuse and dependence. Interview content and strategy vary depending on the types of presenting problems and goals of the interviewer and program. For example, the interviewer may work in a screening clinic where referrals for further assessment and treatment are made. In this setting, a good interview would determine the presence of a substance use disorder, what type, associated problems or hypotheses about problems, and treatment options for the client. Additional information, such as family conflict or support, depression, vocational functioning, legal difficulties, and sources of current and future motivation for treatment, should be uncovered. The interview assessment should always include positive client characteristics or strengths on which interventions can be built.

It is appropriate to use for most situations a similar diagnostic interview strategy that would vary only in the degree of focus and amount of detailed information collected. When the interview goals are screening and referral, the interview could terminate before the step of gathering detailed information required to develop a treatment plan. If the interviewer works in a treatment program and provides the main data base for treatment planning, the screening interview format must be extended.

We recommend the use of a structured interview that is guided by a written outline or series of questions in the form of a decision tree. The strategy is analogous to a progressive screen designed to isolate finer and finer particles. The strategy is illustrated in Figure 1. Research has shown that structured interviews produce higher reliability than other assessment procedures, probably by controlling information variance (Helzer, Clayton, Pambakian, & Woodruff, 1978; Hesselbrock, Stabenau, Hesselbrock, & Mirkin, 1982; Mintz, Christoph, O'Brien, & Snedeker, 1980). The interviewer should use this structure as a tool in a flexible manner that allows digressions to follow up leads or get details important for treatment planning. The assessment interview is more likely to be valid and useful when it is broad, idiographic, and detailed enough to make fine discriminations among subtypes of psychopathology and non-drug-related problems.

Information obtained during an interview is often retrospective and based on self-report. Critics have challenged the validity and reliability of this method with substance-abusing populations. Substance abusers are often characterized as being resistant, unreliable, having secondary motivations for seeking help, and using denial. Sobell, Sobell, and Nirenberg (1988) summarized literature reviews on the reliability and validity of self-report data from substance abusers. They concluded that skepticism about self-report is unfounded in situations in which the client is drug-free, the interview is in a controlled setting, rapport is based on confidentiality, jargon and scientific terminology are avoided, and the focus of the interview is on information-gathering rather than social labeling. There is evidence of robust and clinically useful levels of reliability usually obtained using structured interviews (Matarazzo, 1983). Additionally, careful investigations show relatively good correspondence between interview findings and verifiable data. Inconsistencies seem to be due more to faulty memory and inaccurate police records than to

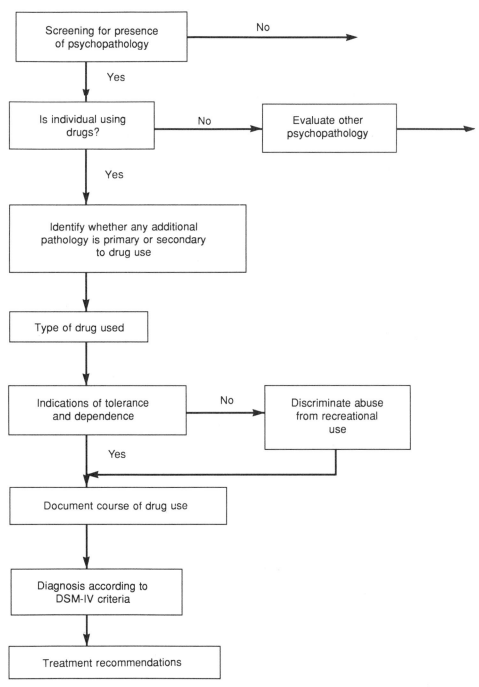

FIGURE 1. Flow chart of major decisions required in interviewing the drug abuse population.

deliberate deception (Amsel, Mendell, Matthias, Mason, & Hocherman, 1976; Bale, Von Stone, Engelsing, Zarcone, & Kuldan, 1981; Bonito, Nurco, & Schaffer, 1976). For a comparison and analysis of the validity of two structured interview formats, see Hasin and Grant (1987).

Despite attempts to avoid it, resistance is encountered in drug-assessment situations due to the sensitivity of the topic being discussed and the denial characteristic of the addictive process. A common interactional approach designed to deal with denial is confrontation. Persons seeking help with drugs or alcohol are often vulnerable, insecure, and ambivalent about admitting they have a problem. However, forceful confrontation is subject to having an unintended effect of creating more resistance and potentially alienating the client. Miller (1983) developed a method of motivational interviewing as an alternative to the confrontational approach. His technique utilizes principles of cognitive dissonance, self-efficacy, and the change theory of Prochaska and DiClementi (1986). The goals of the interview are to affirm the problem as identified by the client, elicit awareness and self-motivation, affirm self-esteem, and cooperatively evaluate treatment alternatives.

Lack of trust in authority figures is a common barrier among adolescents who abuse drugs. The nonconfrontational interview approach can help establish rapport and is a more successful approach with both adolescents and adults. Computerized assessment procedures, as a nonjudgmental way to collect valid substance-abuse information, may also help cope with denial. Paperny, Aono, Lehman, Hammar, and Risser (1990) found that adolescents preferred the computer over a questionnaire or an interview. Bungey, Pols, Mortimer, Frank, and Skinner (1989) found that the computer interview was more acceptable to patients than a face-to-face interview in a general practice reporting drug use.

The format for the interview process we recommend is presented in Table 1. This outline has been developed in order to assist the interviewer in gaining critical information necessary to make appropriate diagnostic decisions and treatment recommendations. The interview process and content derived from the questions are organized to provide information for the decision process illustrated in Figure 1.

Presenting Complaint

As outlined in Table 1, the first level of evaluation is to review the nature of the presenting complaint. Why is the client presenting for evaluation? Many times, clients are responding to some external factor (e.g., legal or family pressure, which may or may not accord with the client's own perceptions). It may be necessary to make contact with the referral source if treatment is a contingency of remaining employed or out of jail. When consent is obtained, it is important to obtain information from a collateral source. A family member or friend can help identify the scope of the problem and assess the reliability of the client's information, particularly if the assessment or treatment is involuntary. Allow the client to voice his or her expectations of treatment, assist the client in setting goals for treatment, and explore preferences for different treatment philosophies and modalities.

TABLE 1.   Assessment Interview Outline

Presenting complaint
1. Who referred the client?
2. Client's view of problem?
3. Collateral's view of the client's problem?
4. Assess the client's living and social environment.
5. What does client want/expect from assessment or treatment?

Psychological and general health assessment
1. Mental status examination.
2. Assess for concurrent emotional problems or dual diagnoses.
3. Any indication of neurological impairment or cognitive deficits?
4. Does client report any related diseases or health problems?
5. Assess risk factors associated with AIDs.
6. Assess psychological assets or strengths to be utilized in treatment planning

History related to drug abuse
1. Are there any pending criminal charges, and does the client have a criminal history related to drug or alcohol use?
2. Prior treatment/recovery attempts, lengths, and modes of intervention?
3. Assess history of drug or alcohol abuse among family members.

Type of drug
1. Identify current drug(s) used.
2. Identify present drug of choice.
3. Assess history of drug use, date of initiation to present time.
4. Amount and frequency of use for each drug?
5. What is the method of intake for each drug?
6. Assess alcohol history and present use.
7. Assess multiple drug use.
8. Identify antecedents, consequences, patterns, and mood states associated with drug and/or alcohol use.

Abuse and dependency
1. Drug taken in larger amounts and longer than intended?
2. Continued use despite knowledge of harm or hazard?
3. Time and effort obtaining the substance?
4. Assess signs of tolerance and withdrawal.
5. Has the client's drug or alcohol use affected educational, recreational, familial, social, or vocational function?
6. Inquire about intoxications, memory loss, flashbacks, urges, cravings, and overdoses.
7. Persistent desire or one or more efforts to quit or cut down?
8. History of attempts to quit or cut down, abstinence, and relapses?

Diagnostic impression
1. Assess for DSM-IV substance-related disorders.
2. Assess and document dual diagnoses (i.e., accompanying psychotic, affective, anxiety, personality, developmental, or organic disorders).

Treatment or referral recommendations
1. Assess the need for detoxification, inpatient, or outpatient treatment.
2. Make appropriate referrals.
3. Operationalize individualized treatment options with short- and long-term goals and monitoring and follow-up procedures.

Psychological and General Health Assessment

A brief mental status examination is needed to rule out the presence of mental disorders and assess the presence of signs and symptoms associated with the drug use. Often, drug abusers do not view their drug use pattern as a "problem," yet readily admit to symptoms of anxiety or depression. It is especially important to recognize the existence of other forms of psychopathology that may be concurrent with the substance-abuse behaviors. The interviewer must also understand the action of various drugs and their relation to presenting psychopathology. For example, depression may predate the use of drugs or be the result of the actions of drugs such as amphetamines (McLellan, Woody, & O'Brien, 1979; Robins, 1974). The significance of detecting such psychopathology will be to qualify any final diagnosis and to assist in the development of an appropriate treatment plan (McLellan, Luborsky, Woody, O'Brian, & Druley, 1983; Woody, et al., 1984).

Cognitive deficits and organic brain syndromes are common in chronic alcohol or polydrug users and should be assessed more thoroughly if indicated. Other forms of health problems are likely to present themselves that may require treatment and referral, e.g., hepatitis and skin lesions among needle users (Milby, 1981; Sapira, 1968). AIDS has been associated with intravenous drug use and is prevalent among the drug-abusing population. Risk factors for AIDS should be addressed and further testing for AIDS recommended if warranted.

History Related to Drug Abuse

Criminal involvement commonly occurs with users of illegal drugs of every socioeconomic stratum. It is important to assess pending as well as prior criminal charges or convictions in order to accurately document the effect of drug use on the client's life. If the client is on probation, then a relapse may be a violation of probation. Coordination of the probation officer, the client, and the professional is in order under these circumstances. Knowledge of prior treatment or recovery attempts is helpful in designing a successful treatment regime. Inquire about the client's response to different treatment philosophies, inpatient vs. outpatient, length of stay, strengths and weaknesses, and history of treatment/recovery success and failures. This information is needed when choosing a treatment model (e.g., Twelve-Step or Community Reinforcement Program) and setting realistic treatment goals. A thorough history of familial drug and alcohol abuse is helpful in identifying potential genetic and learning factors involved in the client's substance-use history.

Type of Drug

Once drug use has been identified, it is important to determine the types of drugs used by the client in the past and present. Clients often progress through use of various drugs, and a complete drug history is often long and complicated. During this interview stage, it is important to identify drug type, when drug use was initiated, frequency, method of intake, usual dosage, and the function the drug seemed to serve. Simply focusing on the current drug of choice may lead to an erroneous diagnosis and inadequate treatment recommendations.

A complete drug history provides information about such elements as duration of drug use, changes in dosages, changes in drug types, periods of self-induced abstinence, overdoses, and previous treatment attempts. In addition to identifying the major drug types, a drug history provides the first opportunity to document evidence of tolerance, degree of drug preoccupation, and dependence. Identification of antecedents and consequences of drug use is particularly important.

Drug Abuse and Dependence

A client is considered to be *abusing* drugs when, at any time within a 12-month period, a maladaptive pattern of substance use leads to clinically significant impairment or distress as manifested by: (1) failure to fulfill major role obligations at work, school, or home; (2) recurrent substance use in situations in which it is physically hazardous; (3) legal problems; or (4) continued use despite persistent or recurrent social or interpersonal problems (APA, 1993). One of the goals of the interview assessment is for the clinician to evaluate the degree of impact drug abuse has had on the client's life and level of functioning. Although they often deny they have a "drug problem" many clients are willing to discuss and can accurately describe their irregular work history, interpersonal conflicts, and legal difficulties. As a result, the clinician should be attentive to interference in normal social and work activities. The interview should also explore signs of dependence and an abstinence syndrome. For example, does the client experience "craving?" Does he or she manifest withdrawal signs when drug availability is blocked? Is daily use needed in order to feel "normal"? This focus is important to determine the extent of dependence or dysfunction or both experienced as a result of drug use patterns.

Substance *dependence* is defined as a maladaptive pattern of substance use leading to significant clinical impairment or distress, as manifested by three or more of the following within a 12-month period: (1) tolerance; (2) withdrawal; (3) the substance is often taken in larger amounts over a longer period of time than intended; (4) a persistent desire or unsuccessful efforts to cut down or control use; (5) a great deal of time spent obtaining, using, or recovering from the substance; (6) social, occupational, or recreational impairment; or (7) continued use despite knowledge of hazards (APA, 1993).

DIAGNOSTIC CONSIDERATIONS

Most diagnostic evaluations should assess for psychoactive-substance-use disorders and psychoactive-substance-induced organic mental disorders as outlined in DSM-IV (APA, 1993). Clients who are seen for possible drug abuse or dependency problems are likely to present concurrent or reactive disorders or both. Emotional, cognitive, and behavioral disorders are most common. Lehman, Myers, and Corty (1989) report that substance abuse and mental illness problems occur together more frequently than chance would predict. Assessment of dual diagnoses can be simplified with a decision tree model (see Woolf-Reeve, 1990).

In dual diagnostic situations, it is important to recognize whether the disorders are primary or secondary to the substance abuse disorder (McLellan et al., 1979, 1983). Primary disorders are those from which other problems such as drug dependence presumably develop (Halikas & Rimmer, 1974). A good example is depression, in which drug dependence may occur when the individual discovers a chemical means of treating dysphoria (Robins, 1974). Another is agoraphobia, in which dependence on hypnotic sedatives may provide escape from intense anxiety and avoid panic attacks. Identifying disorders that can exist before or concurrent with the drug dependence should be a major focus of interview assessment and can contribute greatly to the success of subsequent treatment planning that utilizes these findings (Woody et al., 1984).

Psychopathology can also be secondary to drug dependence. Family estrangement, antisocial behavior, legal difficulties, poor school or work performance, and low self-esteem are problems that often develop from drug dependence. These secondary problems imply a different treatment plan that focuses on the drug dependence and supports reestablishment of old adaptive behavior. Of course, drug dependence can be so entangled with other forms of psychopathology that it plays neither a clear primary nor a clear secondary role. Unfortunately, there are no assessment instruments or procedures by which such inferences can be systematically and reliably derived. They depend on the clinician's judgment after sorting through information available.

Other diagnostic considerations should focus on the use of multiple substances. The synergistic and cross-tolerance effects of some drugs make the use of multiple substances particularly dangerous. Many addicts use secondary substances to regain a state of equilibrium and do not view these drugs or this practice as harmful. Kirsch and Bohnenblust (1990) provide an analysis for the recognition and assessment of multiple dependencies.

With the rise in prevalence of drug abuse among youths, neither assessment nor treatment models for adults have always fit with the characteristics of this population. Nakken (1988–1989) discusses the state of the art in assessment and treatment of substance-abusing adolescents. Blum and Singer (1983) redefine adolescent substance abuse within a social deviance framework and consider the psychological and physical stressors common to this developmental period when assessing rule-violating behaviors such as drug abuse. It is important to give special consideration to developmental factors in the assessment of drug abuse.

Finally, drug abuse can have detrimental short- and long-term neurological effects. Miller (1985) reviews the literature concerning neuropsychological assessment of substance abusers and suggests how such assessment can be incorporated into a multidimensional evaluation and treatment framework.

TREATMENT RECOMMENDATIONS

Assessment and diagnosis of a substance-abuse problem is only the first step in recovery and the maintenance of a drug-free life-style. The assessment is of little value if it does not have implications for treatment. A complete assessment will identify multiple problem areas that result from drug abuse or provide the substrate for the drug problem. It will also indicate strengths, assets, and sources of support that could be utilized to effect change. The development of an individualized treatment plan should be based on the assessment results. An active cycle of reevaluation and revision of treatment goals will keep assessment and treatment updated and provide an empirical basis for evaluation of treatment efficacy.

In most situations, various treatment models are available to the client. It is important to allow the client to choose from various philosophies and models of treatment those that best suit his or her personality, value system, beliefs about drug abuse, and life-style. Many persons are attracted to and work well within a traditional Twelve-Step recovery model; others do not, due to the focus on an external locus of control and reliance on God or a "higher power." Clients who value an internal locus of control may do better in cognitive–behavioral programs, such as a community reinforcement program. Miller (1994) has shown how treatment outcome is improved when client's beliefs about drug abuse and values match the program's philosophy and treatment approach.

SERIAL INTERVIEWING

Diagnostic interviewing often involves several interviews over a span of days or weeks. When interviewing is done in an inpatient detoxification and evaluation unit, clinicians often interview over a 1- to 2-week period. In a methadone maintenance program, an interview is usually done to diagnose the presence and type of drug dependence so that chemotherapy may begin or end, i.e., maintenance or detoxification. Further interviewing is usually carried out over subsequent days to get more detailed information in order to develop psychosocial aspects of the intervention plan.

We recommend serial diagnostic interviewing by more than one clinician if it is possible and consistent with program goals. Spreading the interview process out allows collection of supplemental data using methods previously described. It also allows clients to remember more relevant material and details and to become more objective in evaluating their strengths and problems. We have also found that serial interviewing, when it includes discovery of client strengths and development of realistic personal goals for treatment, increases self-efficacy and general motivation for treatment. To be useful, multiple interviews, especially by more than one clinician, require good record-keeping and communication of findings between interviewers.

USE OF ASSESSMENT INSTRUMENT RESULTS IN INTERVIEWING

Diagnostic interviewing can be enhanced by additional assessment techniques when results are available for the interview. The following methods are typically used: self-report procedures, reports from significant others, direct observation, objective tests, pharmacological procedures to assess tolerance and dependence, biological assays to detect/confirm use, and psychometric procedures. Sobell et al. (1988) review several new and established assessment methods and instruments designed to evaluate the severity of alcohol and drug problems.

Self-report includes self-observation, log-keeping, questionnaires, rating scales, and checklists. A good example of this method is the Addiction Severity Index (McLellan, Luborsky, O'Brien, & Woody, 1980), which is a combined rating scale and structured interview using self-report data. It can be used to provide baseline data on seven areas of functioning, and when readministered in its briefer follow-up form, it provides useful data on changes in functional status.

Reports from significant others can also provide important diagnostic information. They can corroborate self-report, provide new observations and historical detail, and provide important additional diagnostic information. Research has shown, however, that significant others tend to underreport problems and be less aware of dysfunction than clients themselves (Rounsaville et al., 1981). Review of official records, such as prior treatment and arrest reports, can also help corroborate the client's report as well as provide important historical data.

Direct observation of the client's behavior is another useful method of obtaining information. Observation is typically used in research and treatment facilities or other special settings set up for this type of assessment procedure. For a discussion of diagnostic implications of appearance and behavioral factors, see Milby (1981) and Sapira (1968). The unawareness of automatic and habitual behavior makes log-keeping and self-monitoring a useful exercise in the assessment of antecedent and consequential behaviors, mood states, and patterns of abuse. Self-monitoring can also be useful in assessing the efficacy of treatment.

Biological tests and assays can provide further information on the type of drug dependence and validate self-report. Breath alcohol, alcohol dipstick, and urine tests are common tests of recent substance use (Sobell et al., 1988). The same authors identified the sweat patch technique, acute liver function tests, rib fractures and the trauma scale, and taste test and speed of drinking as objective methods of measuring substance use over extended time periods. Blood sampling is more invasive and costly and therefore less frequently used. Pharmacological procedures are used to assess either or both tolerance to and dependence on opiates and barbiturates/hypnotic sedatives. Opiate dependence may be indicated by administration of a narcotic antagonist that precipitates withdrawal symptoms. Tolerance may be determined by timed administration of standard drugs like methadone or pentobarbital until signs of intoxication appear. Because this procedure requires careful medical supervision, it is usually employed in a hospital. A review of the validity and reliability of using biological markers suggests that objective test data can be relatively accurate under certain conditions, but should not be used alone as sole indicators of substance use (Salaspuro, 1986).

Psychometric instruments are widely used to assess substance abuse in both clinical and research settings. A review of instruments designed to assess alcohol abuse was conducted by Lettieri, Nelson, and Sayers (1985) and another by Nehemkis, Macari, and Lettieri (1976) for drug abuse. Paper-and-pencil tests are considered useful for screening purposes and for providing direction for the interview process. Personality tests, such as the Minnesota Multiphasic Personality Inventory and the Millon Clinical Multiaxial Inventory (Millon), are widely used in assessing personality characteristics of substance abusers. They can be helpful in screening for complicating forms of psychopathology (e.g., depression and anxiety-mediated disorders). They also provide the interviewer with hypotheses regarding psychopathology and problems that must be addressed in treatment planning. The Millon test has devised specific scales designed to identify substance-abusing patients (Bryer, Martines, & Dignan, 1990).

CASE ILLUSTRATIONS

In this section, case studies illustrating common diagnostic problems and our recommended interview strategy are provided. We also include excerpts of diagnostic interviews.

Case of Joan: Multiple Drug Dependence

Joan is a 32-year-old nurse who first presented for treatment after being arrested for forging prescriptions. She also had a long history of stealing Demerol from the hospitals in which she worked. She had been terminated from two positions and lost her license as a result of these activities. The court offered her the opportunity to participate in a supervised treatment program with progress monitored by the court system.

I: How did the hospital find out about the drugs?

P: I wrote a script, which I've done before. But, I wrote a script and I went to a pharmacist I didn't know. He called. I don't know why I did that. I just got to the point where I don't think I cared much one way or the other. Yeah, I didn't really care. I think I knew I couldn't ever get away with it. I knew it was a matter of time.

I: How else were you getting Demerol other than prescriptions?

P: I had nurses on the team. They brought it to me for menstrual pain and I'd do it every once in a while. And then when I got on a floor where I had tons of it, I started walking off with it—couldn't waste it. Then it wasn't just the waste, it was, you know, if you were going to give 50, instead of taking out 50, you'd sign out for 100 and waste 50 and take it—you'd give the patient 50 and take the other 50. Then it got to where I was signing out when nobody wanted it. It just got worse and worse. And then your tolerance gets such that it takes more. And my tolerance was high to start with, which didn't help. But I was only doing it at home.

I: You were only taking it at home?

P: I never did it at work. Never did. I don't think I could have functioned on it. For one thing, I don't—some people like to take Demerol and then run up and down the hall and work. I don't. I like to keep laid back. Can't do that at work.

I: How much were you using?

P: I was taking home 800, 900 milligrams at a time which really isn't that—that's a lot I guess for some people. But, it's not for somebody that's doing it all the time. I did it almost every day. When I was off work I didn't do that. When I had a couple of days off, I didn't do it. Which was almost enough to make me want to go back to work, just to get it. I was doing like 2 or 300 milligrams IV when I got home, and then I'd do another 2 or 3 a little later in the evening. I was doing it like that. I was doing a lot at once. Tolerance got so that I was—most of the time I didn't want to do it unless I had at least 350 milligrams. Because I didn't want to just be mellowed out a little. I wanted to be really out of it.

On the basis of this information, it is clear that Joan was opiate-dependent, although she denied having experienced withdrawal. During the interview, Joan casually mentioned use of alcohol and other drugs that needed to be pursued.

I: You mentioned drinking a lot before you began nursing school. How much were you drinking back then?

P: Well, it got to the point, before I started nursing school, where I was drinking all night, 3 or 4 nights a week. I don't know how much alcohol. I spent a lot of money. It was nothing for me to drink a fifth or two, you know. But it wasn't affecting me as much. Then I got to the point where I wasn't remembering what I did. That's when I'd start getting in trouble.

I: Tell me about that.

P: People started telling me about the weird things I was doing and I couldn't remember doing it.

I: Like what?

P: Mainly hostility. People trying to get me to quit drinking and go home and I'd get nasty, which was a little bit out of character at that time. I didn't believe them. At first I didn't believe them, but so many people said something to me about it, I said they can't all be wrong. So I just quit. And part of it, I hated my job, you know—but I loved drinking, I really loved it.

I: What were you drinking?

P: Liquor. Always liquor. But it got to the point where it scared me a little bit, so I just quit, and decided to go back to school. I'd still drink like if I went out to eat or I'd meet somebody for happy hour and have a couple drinks, go eat dinner, and I'd have a couple more. But it wasn't anything like before that—I didn't get drunk. I've been drinking since I was 17. More of a binge drinker though now. It's like it's an occasional thing if I do it, I do it all night or I don't do it at all. There's no such thing as one or two any more. So I just don't do it at all. So I just don't do it because the hangovers are so bad. I don't know if it's age or if it's my body is just tired of it. The drinking's not worth the hangover. They were that bad.

In the following excerpt, the interviewer is assessing Joan's mood and the possibility that depression and low self-esteem are contributing to the drug dependence. One question provides a cascade of important information.

I: During your drug abuse history, how would you describe your mood usually?

P: It varies. I go through periods of depression. It's related to—probably just to things that I've done to myself. It all started, I think, at a young age. I got out of high school, I was very straight, religious, all the way through high school. Typical Baptist background. No sex, no drugs, no nothing, very strict background. When I got out of high school, everybody went haywire, all my friends went nuts. I waited about a year after they did to do the same thing and got married. Then, I think it was a combination of being divorced, sleeping with my boyfriend, and drinking and doing all these things I was taught not to do and not feeling particularly good about it. And when my self-esteem went down, I went into a depression and stayed there. And didn't know what to do about it. And I didn't do anything about it. Instead of changing my life-style, I kept doing the same old things that just reinforced the low self-esteem. It just got worse, and when I first did all of the drugs that summer, LSD and all that, it was right in the middle of the worst period of depression that I had gone through ever, and I didn't particularly care whether I lived or died. So, naturally, I'd do anything. It was a relief you know. The MDA [methylendioxy-amphetamine] was a relief because on MDA you really can't give a hang about anything. It's impossible to care. As a matter of fact, I felt really good on it. I felt so good on it, I didn't ever want to be straight again. That's when I wanted to stay on MDA all the time, which I knew was not possible. We would have ended up in jail sooner or later because in order to do that amount of drugs, you've gotta deal, and sooner or later you'd end up in jail, and I didn't want him in jail. So we quit the drugs, got married, went back to work, and did alright except for drinking. The main problem with the drinking was on weekends. It was your typical, you know, married couple living in an apartment, working 5 days a week, getting drunk on Friday and Saturday.

The interview subsequently revealed that Joan was actually admitted to a hospital and treated with ECT for depression over a 3-week period when she was 22. This is a good case history because it is typical of the kind of substance-use disorders currently extant. Joan abused a variety of substances: hallucinogens, psychostimulants, alcohol, and opiates. She was probably dependent on all of them at different times in her life. She also experienced several different problems that contributed to her substance-use disorder, two of which were probably primary: personality disorder and depression. Additionally, family and marital conflict, low self-esteem, job-related stress, and sex-role confusion all contributed to her difficulties, added to her stress level and depression, and increased her motivation for Demerol use that provided escape.

Case of Suzanne: Crack Cocaine Dependence

Suzanne is a 35-year-old woman serving a 1-year jail sentence for violating probation from a previous rock cocaine possession charge. She is participating in an in-jail relapse prevention oriented substance-abuse treatment program as a substitute for the sentence. Her history is one of significant losses due to drug involvement. This case was chosen to reflect characteristics typical of a crack-cocaine-dependent life-style.

Being involved with the law is commonplace for most crack cocaine users. A complete assessment should include obtaining a history of legal involvement.

I: Tell me what you are doing in jail.

P: I'm here for violation of probation from a charge that stems 3 years ago for a purchase of rock cocaine. Since then I've been avoiding the law and more or less on the run.

I: And how did you get caught?

P: Theoretically, I left the county I was sentenced in and went to live with my mother. I knew they would figure it out and a warrant would be issued and I just decided to let it go. It took them 2½ years to look for me at my mother's house. That was that.

I: What was it like to live your life knowing your freedom could come to an end at any time?

P: I thought to myself, well I might as well get it good now because I'm going to be sitting in a cell somewhere soon. I might as well get real high now and do whatever damage I'm going to do. I'm still waiting to see what a warrant search will bring up during that time. I'm sitting here really not knowing the future right now.

I: Do you have any other previous charges or convictions?

P: Before this present charge, I was arrested for possession of a crack pipe and some pot. When I was busted for the crack, they also charged me with cocaine possession, grand theft auto, possession of marijuana, and child abuse.

Suzanne has a long history of polydrug use. She has been drug-dependent since she was 16 years old. The following excerpt reflects Suzanne's insightful assessment of her own problem with drugs.

I: Suzanne, what is your view of your problem right now?

P: Lack of coping skills. Like I've said, I've been getting high since I was 16 years old. Whenever I had a problem in my life, rather than deal with it, I would get high on drugs.

I: Tell me more about that.

P: I've always turned to drugs. I'm scared to death to be released because now I'm going to have to deal with my problems, emotional problems. I gave up custody of my children when they were young, and I haven't dealt with the death of my grandmother yet. There are things that I never faced in my life. I just killed the pain.

I: What kinds of drugs did you use?

P: It progressed from marijuana to harder drugs, like snorting cocaine. Being born and raised in Miami, it was very easy to get cocaine, for me being a woman.

I: How do you mean that? Being a woman?

P: Well, with all the big dope dealers down here, if you are a woman, young and single, it's easy to get high. I didn't get into prostituting myself until the last year and a half, after I started smoking crack. I did whatever I had to, to get it.

Crack cocaine had a devastating effect on Suzanne's life. Many users report that crack has a particularly powerful influence over their judgment. The following excerpt describes how getting and using crack became her primary reason for existing.

I: When was the first time you started using drugs and alcohol?

P: We were smoking pot in high school. I was about 15 or 16 years old.

I: What about alcohol?

P: Well see, I got hepatitis when I was 15 and it affected my liver so that when I drank I got too loaded. I didn't like the feeling then at all. So, I didn't really use alcohol until I was heavily snorting cocaine and then I drink just to mellow me.

I: When did you start using cocaine?

P: When I got divorced. Prior to that, I had been smoking a lot of pot, about an ounce a week. You see, the position I was in gave me a little control. Like I said, I was in the communications industry in Miami, and at the time drug dealers were into beepers. There were waiting lists and I had the power. A lot was offered to me by these people, both drug wise and money wise, and I took advantage of it. And that's when I starting snorting a lot.

I: How did you get turned on to crack?

P: Well, I had free-based a couple of times with a friend and was sporadic between snorting and smoking for a couple of months. But when I made my crack cocaine connection, that was all she wrote, then I knew crack cocaine was my drug of choice.

I: What is it like to use crack? How is it different from other drugs?

P: How it makes me feel. I have no control over it at all. Snorting, I had some, a little bit of control, as far as time delays in between snorts. But with crack, I had no control at all.

I: How much crack were you using?

P: Ah, three to four hundred dollars a day. That would be as much money as I could make. That's how much I used. There were times where I did use only a hundred or two and then stop. I don't know what caused those special days, but they were few and far between.

I: It sounds like most of your time and money were taken by the drug.

P: Getting money and getting high, yes. Every 3 or 4 days on the street I'd come down and I'd go crash in a motel room or a friend's house and then stuff myself eating because I'd deprive myself of food and then I'd knock off for a bit. After a day or two, with a little money in my pocket, I'd be back at it. I'd go trace the dope man and I'd be back on that vicious cycle again.

In-jail substance-abuse treatment is a unique treatment environment with unique circumstances. The following questions were designed to assess the client's treatment history and expectations for treatment success in an in-jail program.

I: Is this your first drug treatment program?

P: Yes. This is my first attempt to stop doing drugs since, really, since I was 16 years old.

I: How do you feel about being sentenced into treatment, in a jail setting like this?

P: I sit here and I see a lot of girls come back through court and bitching and moaning about being court-ordered into the jail program. I think this program is here to help us. I wanted to quit many times, but I didn't think I ever would have.

I: Is it hard to tell yourself, "I need help?"

P: I think it's rare for people to just say, "I've had it, this is it." They really have to hit rock bottom. I'm looking up. And the jail program, I thought, will let me get help. It's also a stipulation for my release and I might as well, you know, give it a chance.

I: What do you expect to get out of treatment here?

P: I expect it to suddenly change my life. I expect to walk out and push that magic button and everything is going to just be wonderful. I know that's not the way it's going to be. It's going to be a long, hard road dealing with my emotions. I mean I've never cried so much and really soul-searched as much as I have in these past 4 months.

Case of Carl: Amphetamine Dependence

Carl is a 34-year-old white male who has a high school education and is employed as a diesel mechanic for a large trucking firm. He has recently divorced, and his two children are living with his ex-wife. He is living with his mother. He obtained his job 3 years ago, and it represented an opportunity to significantly raise his income because of higher wages and many opportunities for overtime. Since that time, he has raised his income substantially, but his long work hours away from the family, his irritability, and his aggressive behavior associated with job stresses have contributed to his martial conflict and subsequent divorce. Since his divorce, he has worked even longer hours and felt more lonely, withdrawn, and depressed.

He has had stomach symptoms, insomnia, reduced appetite, and weight loss of 15 pounds without intent over the last 3 months. These symptoms reported in the first interview caused him to be admitted to a VA psychiatric hospital with the admission diagnosis of nonpsychotic depression. The excerpt is from a second interview conducted by another staff member and thus illustrates the technique and results of serial interviewing. The interviewer had read the admission note describing the preceding interview and had briefly discussed the case with the staff person who admitted him. The interviewer's objective was to explore reasons for marital conflict and causes of depression and to assess the possibility of alcoholism and drug use.

I: You sure have been through a lot lately, Carl. What do you think contributed to your divorce?

P: Work mostly. Long hours, you know, and not spending time with my wife and family. Sarah was getting frustrated with me 'cause I was never home to help with anything.

I: When you were home, how did you get along?

P: Not so good. She would need help with chores and things, or would ask me to do something with the kids, and I would get irritated with her. She would make me real mad and I'd holler and swear. I also would beat the kids too hard because they'd be so loud and stuff. I slapped her a few times, too, didn't mean to, but I'd just get so mad. I was real irritable because I wasn't sleeping well and I was working a lot of overtime.

I: How did you keep going without much sleep and having to work overtime?

P: Well, one of the mechanics would get some Benzedrine from one of the drivers, and we'd both take them to stay awake and get the jobs done.

I: When did you start to use Benzedrine, Carl?

P: About 3 years ago. Billy and I started working together about 6 months after I began working there, and he started offering them to me. After a while, I started getting "bennies" for myself, and we started using more and more. We could stay awake and work like a son of a bitch. After a while, we got a reputation for really cranking out the work, and our boss would ask us to do more and more special jobs on O.T. We could flat do some work. But we got to the point where we had to take the bennies to keep up the pace, you know.

I: How many did you have to take to keep going?

P: Well, at first one was enough for me, but Billy would keep taking a couple more during the shift, and I started taking more too. Maybe four to five during the whole 14-hour shift. But just before my divorce I was eating them like candy. They was messing me up too.

I: How did they mess you up?

P: Well, they started messing up my mind. I'd get real irritated and suspicious of everything. I'd start thinking Billy was messing with my tools, and I got into it with him a few times. Then, I got to thinking Sarah was stepping out on me, I thought I was going crazy. Then I started to really worry about that and I got down. I'd get so bad I'd want to be left alone all weekend and stay in the bedroom. I'd sleep all weekend. I'd even eat in there. Get Sarah to fix me a tray. I was sorry, I'll tell ya.

Further interviewing established that at the end of his first year on his new job, amphetamine use was routine, and in the following year, use increased to the point where his wife complained about his abuse and the effects the drug had—his sleep disturbance, irritability, and aggressiveness. Despite his wife's complaints, his realization that Benzedrine use was causing him difficulty, and his efforts to cut back his use, he continued the abuse. The year before his admission for treatment, he showed extensive abuse, and had repeated conflicts with his wife, who left him for brief periods several times, two of which involved episodes of psychotic paranoid behavior. Prior to his admission, he reported eating Benzedrine tablets like candy during the week and then "crashing" and sleeping the whole weekend and starting the pattern again the next week whether or not he had to work overtime.

Admission to treatment was motivated by a warning from his employer to get help or be fired and by his ex-wife's repeated urging to get help and his hope that he might get back together with her. He also stated that he did not tell the staff member who did screening about his drug use because he was afraid he would be rejected for treatment or referred elsewhere.

This case is interesting for several reasons. Carl presented for screening to a general psychiatric facility. During screening, he was anxious, dysphoric, and tearful, and he emphasized his recent divorce and sense of loss of his family with consequent loneliness. He reported he was trying to cope with his loss by working and volunteering for overtime so he could lose himself in his work. He also complained of sleep disturbance, weight loss over the past 6 months, and decreased appetite.

The screening diagnostic impression was depression based on the classic symptoms he reported. However, during his first week of admission, serial interviewing revealed the primary role of amphetamine abuse in causing his marital conflict and classic depressive symptoms. More important, serial interviewing uncovered the central role of work for his sense of self-esteem and the basic feelings of inadequacy in most other areas of life. Demands of family responsibility for intimacy and increased socialization from his wife made him feel more inadequate. These challenges to his self-esteem were met by doing more of what he could do best (i.e., work and earn more money). Serial diagnostic interviewing thus yielded a more complete assessment of this man. It sorted out multiple problems and discovered the primary personality disorder and the role of amphetamine abuse in his depressive symptoms and divorce. Thus, serial diagnostic interviewing yielded the most complete and accurate assessment from which a strategic treatment plan was derived.

SOME PRACTICAL DO'S AND DON'T'S FOR INTERVIEWING DRUG ABUSERS

Some practical recommendations for increasing the accuracy and usefulness of the interview are listed next.

Do assess the client's motivation for treatment, especially the court-referred client. If motivation is not assessed, or if wrong conclusions are derived, the usefulness of other interview data may be wasted. It is important here to determine the source and intensity of motivation. Is motivation intrinsic or extrinsic? Is it based on inner factors of dissatisfaction or wanting to improve current status, or is it based on pressure from the court to engage in treatment or suffer immediate incarceration? Timing of presentation for admission often indicates initial motivation. Did the client recently lose his or her job? Is the client under pressure from family or spouse? Usually, whatever motivation is present can be enhanced by the interviewer's emphasizing choices, options, and responsibility for treatment decisions. This tends to build motivation for active participation in the interview process and subsequent treatment. Client motivation can also be enhanced by including an assessment of strengths. This assessment can help devise more realistic treatment plans, but it can also build client self-respect and intrinsic motivation.

Do use a structured interview format. The research clearly shows that structured interviews produce the most reliable and most accurate data (Matarazzo, 1983; Mintz et al., 1980). Do assess the efficacy and usefulness of the interviewing process. Monitor the accuracy of diagnoses by doing occasional dual interviews or comparing information gathered via serial interviewing by different staff members. Request feedback from programs receiving your referrals. It is useful to obtain data on referral show rates, accuracy of referral diagnoses, and viability of recommendations.

Do not assume that drug abuse or dependence is the main or only problem of a client presenting for substance use disorder treatment. Depression, anxiety (such as posttraumatic stress disorder), and personality disorders are prevalent in this group. Clients for whom these and other critical problems are not addressed are prime candidates for treatment failure (McLellan, Woody, Luborsky, O'Brien, & Druley, 1982). However, when these concurrent problems are identified and treatment plans are implemented to address them, results are much better (McLellan et al., 1983).

Do not assume that laboratory data are correct when there is a disparity between self-report and laboratory data (Bernadt, Mumford, Taylor, Smith, & Murray, 1982). Self-report data usually are fairly accurate except for historical details or where there is an obvious reason for distorting certain information (e.g., illegal activities of a client who is court-referred). Unless these circumstances prevail, the assumption that laboratory data are correct can interfere with rapport between the client and the interviewer or other staff and negatively affect the assessment and referral process. Utilize historical information, multiple tests, and collateral information to improve the reliability of your findings.

IMPORTANCE OF THE DIAGNOSTIC INTERVIEW

Establishing a differential diagnosis is not easy. Building rapport, motivation for treatment, and developing a realistic and effective treatment plan is not easy. If reliable and valid differential diagnoses are the only products of the interview process when a treatment plan is needed, the interview is not working. The main point here is that the diagnostic interview is a critical phase in referral and intervention. If it is done poorly, the client may never return. The interview is important enough to command the attention of the most experienced and competent clinicians. It is also important enough to carefully evaluate and use feedback to improve the process.

SUMMARY

This chapter has given a brief overview of common characteristics of drug abuse and dependence that need to be understood in order to do good diagnostic interviewing. These characteristics include initiating use, increased dosing, tolerance, drug preoccupation, development of drug-seeking behavior, and patterns of behavior dependent on societal acceptance of the drug and its type.

In addition to careful attention to a structured interview, its strategies, and format, we have also reviewed other procedures for gathering information that can supplement the diagnostic interview: self-report data sources, reports from significant others, direct observation, breath, saliva, urine, and blood analyses, pharmacological procedures, and psychometrics. We strongly recommend use of serial interviewing. Several cases were discussed to illustrate recommended strategies and procedures. Practical do's and don'ts for interviewing drug abusers were recommended. Last, the importance of the diagnostic interview was underlined, and evaluation of its utility was recommended.

REFERENCES

American Psychiatric Association (1993). *Diagnostic and statistical manual of mental disorders*, 4th ed., draft criteria. Washington, DC: Author.

Amsel, Z., Mendell, W., Matthias, L., Mason, C., & Hocherman, I. (1976). Reliability and validity of self-reported illegal activities and drug use collected from narcotic addicts. *International Journal of the Addictions*, 11, 325–336.

Bale, R. N., Von Stone, W. W., Engelsing, T. M. J., Zacrone, V. P., Jr., & Kuldan, J. M. (1981). The validity of self-reported heroin use. *International Journal of the Addictions*, 16, 1307–1398.

Bernadt, M. W., Mumford, J., Taylor, C., Smith, B., & Murray, R. M. (1982). Comparison of questionnaire and laboratory tests in the decision of excessive drinking and alcoholism. *The Lancet*, 325–328.

Blum, A., & Singer, M. (1983). Substance abuse and social deviance: A youth assessment framework. *Child and Youth Services*, 6, 7–21.

Bonito, A. J., Nurco, D. N., & Schaffer, J. W. (1976). The veridicality of addicts' self-reports in social research. *International Journal of the Addictions*, 11, 719–724.

Bryer, J. B., Martines, K. A., & Dignan, M. A. (1990). Millon Clinical Multiaxial Inventory Alcohol Abuse and Drug Abuse scales and the identification of substance abuse patients. *Psychological Assessment*, 2, 438–441.

Bungey, J. B., Pols, R. G., Mortimer, K. P., Frank, O. R., & Skinner, H. A. (1989). Screening alcohol & drug use in a general practice unit: Comparison of computerized and traditional methods. *Community Health Studies*, 13, 471–483.

Dohner, V. A. (1972). Motives for drug use: Adult and adolescent. *Psychometrics*, 13, 317–324.

Halikas, J. A., & Rimmer, J. D. (1974). Predictors of multiple drug abuse. *Archives of General Psychiatry, 81*, 414–418.

Hasin, D. S., & Grant, B. F. (1987). Assessment of specific drug disorders in a sample of substance abuse patients: A comparison of the DIS and the SADS-L procedures. *Drug and Alcohol Dependence, 19*, 165–176.

Helzer, J. E., Clayton, P. J., Pambakian, R., & Woodruff, R. A. (1978). Concurrent diagnostic validity of a structured psychiatric interview. *Archives of General Psychiatry, 35*, 849–853.

Hesselbrock, V., Stabenau, J., Hesselbrock, M., & Mirkin, M. (1982). A comparison of two interview schedules. *Archives of General Psychiatry, 39*, 674–677.

Kandel, D. B. (1984). Marijuana users in young adulthood. *Archives of General Psychiatry, 41*, 200–209.

Kandel, D. B., & Logan, J. A. (1984). Patterns of drug use from adolescence to young adulthood. *American Journal of Public Health, 74*, 660–666.

Kandel, D. B., Davies, M., Karus, D., & Yamaguchi, K. (1986). The consequences in young adulthood of adolescent drug involvement. *Archives of General Psychiatry, 43*, 746–754.

Kirsch, J. M., & Bohnenblust, S. (1990). The recognition and assessment of multiple dependencies among prospective clients at selected chemical dependency treatment programs. *Addictive Behaviors, 15*, 587–590.

Lehman, A. F., Myers, C. P., & Corty, E. (1989). Assessment and classification of patients with psychiatric and substance abuse syndromes. *Hospital and Community Psychiatry, 40*, 1019–1025.

Lettieri, D. J., Nelson, J. E., & Sayers, M. A. (Eds.) (1985). *Alcoholism treatment assessment research instruments (Treatment Handbook No. 2)*. Rockville, MD: National Institute on Alcohol Abuse and Alcoholism.

Matarazzo, J. D. (1983). The reliability of psychiatric and psychological diagnosis. *Clinical Psychology Review, 3*, 103–145.

McLellan, A. T., Luborsky, L., O'Brien, C. P., & Woody, G. E. (1980). An improved diagnostic instrument for substance abuse patients: The Addiction Severity Index. *Journal of Nervous and Mental Disease, 168,* 26–33.

McLellan, A. T., Luborsky, L., Woody, G. E., O'Brien, C. P., & Druley, K. A. (1983). Predicting response to alcohol and drug abuse treatments: Role of psychiatric severity. *Archives of General Psychiatry, 40,* 620–625.

McLellan, A. T., Woody, G. E., Luborsky, L., O'Brien, C. P., & Druley, K. A. (1982). Is treatment for substance abuse effective? *Journal of the American Medical Association, 247,* 1423–1427.

McLellan, A. T., Woody, G. E., & O'Brien, C. P. (1979). Development of psychiatric illness in drug abusers: Possible role of drug preference. *New England Journal of Medicine, 301,* 1310–1314.

Milby, J. B. (1981). *Addictive behavior and its treatment.* New York: Springer.

Miller, L. (1985). Neuropsychological assessment of substance abusers: Review and recommendations. *Journal of Substance Abuse Treatment, 2,* 5–17.

Miller, W. R. (1983). Motivational interviewing with problem drinkers. *Behavioral Psychotherapy, 11,* 147–172.

Miller, W. R. (in press). Emergent treatment concepts and techniques. In P. E. Nathan, J. W. Langenbucher, B. S. McCrady, & U. Frankenstein (Eds.), *Annual review of addictions and treatment,* (Vol. 1).

Mintz, J., Christoph, P., O'Brien, C. P., & Snedeker, M. (1980). The impact of the interview method on reported symptoms of narcotic addicts. *International Journal of the Addictions, 15,* 597–604.

Nakken, J. M. (1988/1989). Issues in adolescent chemical dependency assessment. Special Issue: Practice approaches in treating adolescent chemical dependency: A guide to clinical assessment and intervention. *Journal of Chemical Dependency Treatment, 2,* 71–93.

Nehemkis, M., Macari, M. A., & Lettieri, D. J. (Eds.) (1976). *Drug abuse instrument handbook (Drug Abuse Research Issues No. 12).* Rockville, MD: National Institute on Drug Abuse.

Newcomb, M. D., & Bentler, P. M. (1986). Cocaine use among young adults. *Advances in Alcohol and Substance Abuse, 6,* 73–96.

Paperny, D. M., Aono, J. Y., Lehman, R. M., Hammar, S. L., & Risser, J. (1990). Computer assisted detection and intervention in adolescent high-risk health behaviors. *Journal of Pediatrics, 116,* 456–462.

Prochaska, J. O., & DiClemente, C. C. (1986). Toward a comprehensive model of change. In W. R. Miller & N. Heather (Eds.), *Treating addictive behaviors: Processes of change* (pp. 3–25). New York: Plenum Press.

Robins, P. R. (1974). Depression and drug addiction. *Psychiatric Quarterly, 48,* 374–386.

Rounsaville, B. J., Kleber, H. D., Wilber, C., Rosenberger, D., & Rosenberger, P. (1981). Comparison of opiate addict's reports of psychiatric history with reports of significant other informants. *American Journal of Alcohol Abuse, 8,* 51–69.

Salaspuro (1986). Conventional and coming laboratory markers of alcoholism and heavy drinking. *Alcoholism: Clinical and Experimental Research, 10(Suppl.),* 5S–10S.

Sapira, J. D. (1968). The narcotic addict as a medical patient. *American Journal of Medicine, 45,* 555–587.

Schwartz, R. H., Hoffmann, N. G., & Jones, R. (1987). Behavioral, psychological and academic correlates of marijuana usage in adolescence. *Clinical Pediatrics, 26,* 264–270.

Sobell, L. C., Sobell, M. B., & Nirenberg, T. D. (1988). Behavioral assessment and treatment planning with alcohol and drug abusers: A review with an emphasis on clinical application. *Clinical Psychology Review, 8,* 19–54.

Woody, G. E., McLellan, A. T., Luborsky, L., O'Brien, C. P., Blaine, J., Fox, S., Herman, I., & Beck, A. T. (1984). Severity of psychiatric symptoms as a predictor of benefits from psychotherapy: The Veterans Administration–Penn study. *American Journal of Psychiatry, 141,* 1172–1177.

Woolf-Reeve, B. S. (1990). A guide to the assessment of psychiatric symptoms in the addictions treatment setting. Special issue: Managing the dually diagnosed patient: Current issues and clinical approaches. *Journal of Chemical Dependency Treatment, 3,* 71–96.

World Health Organization Expert Committee on Drug Dependence (1974). *Twentieth Report.* Geneva: Author.

9

Sexual Dysfunctions and Deviations

Nathaniel McConaghy

Description of the Disorders

In interviewing subjects in order to reach a diagnosis of sexual dysfunction or deviation preliminary to the management of their condition, it is as important to determine the nature of their personalities as it is to diagnose the condition for which they sought help. This information is essential for the second function of the diagnostic interview, the establishment with the subjects of an appropriate therapeutic relationship to maximize their likelihood of remaining in and complying with treatment. Also, the nature of their personality is a major determinant of their response to treatment. In the diagnosis of patients' complaints, the categories provided by the *Diagnostic and Statistical Manual of Mental Disorders*, third edition, revised (DSM-III-R; American Psychiatric Association, 1987) are widely accepted, at least in the published literature, though it is necessary to be aware of their limitations, for which they are undergoing revision (DSM-IV draft criteria; American Psychiatric Association, 1993).

Sexual Dysfunctions

In the DSM-IV draft criteria, the dysfunctions or impairments of sexual functioning were divided into four major categories: (1) Sexual Desire Disorders included Hypoactive Sexual Desire, deficient sexual fantasies and desire for sexual activity; and Sexual Aversion, an extreme aversion to and avoidance of all or almost all genital sexual contact with a partner. (2) Sexual Arousal Disorders included Female Sexual Arousal Disorder, characterized by inability to attain or maintain an adequate genital lubrication–swelling response of sexual excitement until completion of sexual activity; and Male Erectile Disorder, characterized by inability to attain or maintain erection until completion of sexual activity. (3) Orgasm Disorders included Female Orgasmic Disorder (Inhibited Female Orgasm), Male Orgasmic Disorder (Inhibited Male Orgasm), and Premature Ejaculation. Female

Nathaniel McConaghy • School of Psychiatry, University of New South Wales, Kensington 2033 Australia.

Diagnostic Interviewing (Second Edition), edited by Michel Hersen and Samuel M. Turner. Plenum Press, New York, 1994.

Orgasmic Disorder was defined as delay or absence of orgasm following a normal sexual excitement phase. Diagnosis required the clinician's judgment that the woman's orgasmic capacity is less than would be reasonable for her age, sexual experience, and the adequacy of sexual stimulation she receives. Male Orgasmic Disorder was delay or absence of orgasm following a normal sexual excitement phase during sexual activity judged to be adequate in form, intensity, and duration. Premature ejaculation was defined as ejaculation with minimal sexual stimulation before, on, or shortly after penetration and before the person wishes it. (4) The final dysfunction, Sexual Pain Disorders, included Dyspareunia, or genital pain in either males or female before, during, or after sexual intercourse; and Vaginismus, or involuntary spasm of the musculature of the outer third of the vagina that interferes with coitus. In fact, vaginismus usually prevents penetration into the vagina of any object above a certain size, including the subject's finger or a tampon. If intercourse is attempted, vaginismus is commonly accompanied by spasm of the adductor muscles of the thighs, preventing their separation. Vaginismus does not prevent women from experiencing sexual arousal and orgasm with activities other than coitus.

The DSM-IV draft criteria required that all the dysfunctions cause marked distress or interpersonal difficulty, and that they are persistent or recurrent, judgments that are to be made by the clinician, taking into account such factors as the frequency and chronicity of the symptom, subjective distress, and the effect on other areas of the subject's functioning. The lack of criteria for taking these factors into account is a major weakness of this diagnostic categorization, creating difficulty in providing reliable diagnoses for research purposes. As will be discussed subsequently, about 60% of women and 40% of men report occasional episodes of impaired sexual functioning. Without criteria based on their frequency or severity, the decisions of individual clinicians are likely to vary considerably as to which subjects have or do not have sexual dysfunctions.

A further problem with the DSM-IV classification of impairments of sexual function results from its basis in the medical model. It ignores aspects of sexual behaviors that are both more common and more important in determining the sexual satisfaction of couples, or at least of middle-class couples, who are mainly the subjects of investigation. For example, in their classic study, Frank, Anderson, and Rubinstein (1978) investigated the presence of both sexual dysfunctions (that is, problems of performance) and what they termed "sexual difficulties" (problems resulting from the emotional tone of sexual relations) in 100 predominantly white, well-educated, happily married couples. In this study, 63% of the women and 40% of the men reported sexual dysfunctions. The most common in women were difficulty getting excited or reaching orgasm or both, and in men, ejaculating too quickly and difficulty getting or maintaining an erection. In further findings, 77% of the women and 50% of the men reported difficulties. The most common reported by the women were inability to relax, too little foreplay before intercourse, disinterest, and the partner's choosing an inconvenient time. The most common reported by the men were attraction to persons other than their spouses, too little foreplay before intercourse, too little tenderness after intercourse, and the partner's choosing an inconvenient time. In both men and women, the presence of sexual difficulties correlated more strongly with reduced sexual satisfaction than did dysfunctions. In men, the correlation between presence of dysfunctions and reduced sexual satisfaction was insignificant.

Comparable findings were reported in a study of couples presenting with lack of sexual satisfaction (Snyder & Berg, 1983). Sexual dissatisfaction in women did not correlate with the presence of dysfunctions, and in men only with the uncommon dysfunction of failure to ejaculate in intercourse. Sexual dissatisfaction in both sexes correlated strongly with the partner's lack of response to sexual requests and the frequency of intercourse being too low. The nature of sexual difficulties suggests that they often result from poor communication in couples concerning their sexual wishes and needs.

In a study of psychology student couples, Byers and Heinlein (1989) found that the most common initiation of sexual activity was nonverbal, as were the majority of positive responses. In this study, 60% of rejections were verbal, and verbal as compared to nonverbal rejections were resolved more satisfactorily.

It may not be necessary to assess couples' ability to communicate their sexual needs more than impressionistically in the diagnostic interview in order to obtain a good response to treatment, provided establishment of good communication is a major component of the treatment program.

Sexual Deviations

The DSM-IV classification retains from the earlier classification use of the term *paraphilias* for sexual deviations, and the exclusion of the common sex offenses of sexual assault and hebephilia. The term paraphilia was preferred as emphasizing that the deviation (*para*) lay in that to which the subject was attracted (*philia*), namely, sexual objects or situations that are not part of normative arousal–activity patterns. However, in contradiction, the DSM-III-R account pointed out the imagery in paraphilic fantasy is frequently the stimulus for sexual excitement in people without a paraphilia and that the diagnosis is made only if the person has acted on the urges or is markedly distress by them. Investigations of the sexual fantasies of men and women have found that a significant number of normal subjects, and possibly the majority, are attracted to sexual objects or situations that are the stimuli for behaviors regarded as sexually deviant. In addition, evidence has been advanced that a high proportion of adolescents experience such attractions and express them in behaviors (Person, Terestman, Myers, Goldberg, & Salvadori, 1989; Templeman & Stinnett, 1991). It would appear therefore that many normal subjects who would not be classified as paraphiliacs are attracted to the objects and situations involved in paraphilic behaviors, failing to support the justification advanced in DSM-III-R for the introduction of the term paraphilia. The older term, sexual deviation, has the advantage of indicating no more than that the behaviors concerned deviate from those currently socially accepted. In the last few decades, masturbation and homosexuality have ceased to be regarded as deviant.

DSM-IV draft criteria gives diagnostic criteria for exhibitionism, fetishism, frotteurism, pedophilia, sexual masochism, sexual sadism, voyeurism, and transvestic fetishism. Detailed accounts of these behaviors are available (McConaghy,

1991, 1993). Telephone scatologia (lewdness), necrophilia (sex with a corpse), partialism (exclusive focus on parts of the body), zoophilia (sex with animals), coprophilia (feces), klismaphilia (enemas), and urophilia (urine) were listed as examples of paraphilias not otherwise specified. Hebephilia, the attraction of adult men to immediately postpubertal boys, was not included in the DSM-III-R classification, though it has characteristics similar to those of homosexual pedophilia (attraction to prepubertal boys) in that its subjects are usually not sexually attracted to or interested in social relationships with adults, making it very difficult to treat.

The DSM-IV draft criteria abandoned the widely used terms transvestism and transsexualism. The latter condition was included with cross-gender identification in children as Gender Identity Disorder. Transvestism presumably is to be diagnosed as Transvestic Fetishism, although the majority of adult transvestites do not report intense sexual arousal with cross-dressing and many are not distressed by their urges to cross-dress (both requirements of this diagnosis). Alternatively, it may have been decided that cross-dressing in these subjects is not a sexual disorder. DSM-III-R stated that gender identity disorder of childhood was not merely a child's nonconformity to stereotypic sex role behavior—as, for example, in "tomboyishness" in girls or "sissyish" behavior in boys—but rather a profound disturbance of the normal sense of maleness and femaleness. It would appear that no scientific terms have been considered necessary to replace the lay terms *sissy* and *tomboy*. These terms are not restricted to extreme opposite sex-linked behaviors. "Sissy" is applied to boys who avoid rough and tumble play and contact sport and show interest in housework or artistic activities, and "tomboy" to girls who show the opposite behaviors. The degree to which these opposite sex-linked behaviors are shown in childhood correlate in later adolescence and adulthood with the degree to which boys experience homosexual feelings and girls report masculine personality traits (McConaghy & Zamir, in press). Inquiry concerning the presence of these sex-linked behaviors in childhood and adolescence is therefore indicated in some subjects.

Presumably the DSM-IV follows the DSM-III-R in regarding most sexual assaults as not being paraphilias. Sexual sadism is diagnosed in subjects who inflicted suffering on the victims far in excess of that necessary to gain compliance, and in whom the visible pain of the victim was sexually arousing. This was considered true of fewer than 10% of rapists. It was further stated that some rapists were sexually aroused by coercing or forcing a nonconsenting person to engage in intercourse and could maintain sexual arousal while observing the victim's suffering; unlike persons with sexual sadism, however, they did not find the victim's suffering sexually arousing. These subtle distinctions appear to be of little clinical significance and could not be substantiated in sex offenders by Knight and Prentky (1990). The distinctions may have been made to account for the failure in recent studies of penile circumference assessments to distinguish rapists from normal controls, so avoiding the need to confront the evidence that this method of assessment has limited validity (McConaghy, 1989a, 1992).

The distinctions should not mislead the interviewer into regarding as markedly deviant or uncommon the occurrence of sexual arousal in men in response to visual stimuli or fantasies of the infliction of pain or suffering on women (Crepault

& Couture, 1980; Person, Terestman, Myers, Goldberg, & Salvadori, 1989), or in women to fantasies of their having pain or suffering inflicted on themselves or of being raped (Hariton & Singer, 1974; Person et al., 1989). It would seem necessary to investigate the presence of such fantasies in victims of rape, as the acknowledgment and management of these fantasies has been considered of importance in their recovery (McCombie & Arons, 1980).

PROCEDURES FOR GATHERING INFORMATION

Unstructured Clinical Interview

Though little research has investigated how the majority of clinicians obtain information about the sexual disorders of their patients, it would appear that the major method remains the unstructured clinical interview, and, if possible, their partners and other relevant persons. The unstructured interview allows clinicians to vary the nature and order of their questions as seems appropriate in the light of the patient's responses and behavior. Clinicians can decide, possibly intuitively more than consciously, which persona to adopt that is most likely to elicit the patient's trust and enable him or her to feel at ease. This decision requires taking into account the patient's sex, age, appearance, dress, socioeconomic background, intelligence, vocabulary, level of education, ethnic origin, and moral, ethical, and sexual attitudes and values. Though there is little empirical information concerning the individual practice of clinicians in regard to this procedure, it appears from observation that they vary markedly in the extent to which they modify their personalities, including their vocabulary, assertiveness, and apparent ethical structure and social status, to become the person they believe the patient would relate to best.

If the patient shows signs of guilt, embarrassment, or reluctance to talk when particular topics are introduced, the clinician in the unstructured interview can respond with encouragement and support and thus elicit crucial information that may not be obtained if adherence to the rigid format of a structured interview or questionnaire is maintained. Patients are unlikely to reveal such information unless the relationship established by the clinician is such that they are confident that it will not be disclosed, deliberately or inadvertently, without their permission. Clinicians need to determine the policy to adopt concerning behaviors that they are legally mandated to report. Finkelhor (1984) estimated that 36% of case workers in Boston did not report their last case of child sexual abuse. Presumably, clinicians who routinely report such behaviors inform their patients concerning this policy at the beginning of the interview.

Directivity of the Interview

The unstructured interview allows clinicians to continuously modify its directivity, enabling them to obtain information not easily obtained in more structured assessments. A common procedure is to commence the interview nondirectively by adopting a listening approach and asking a minimum of questions, thereby giving the patient the opportunity to take charge. The extent to which this is done allows the patient's confidence, assertiveness, and dominance to be assessed. The unstructured interview in this way allows clinicians to commence determining the nature of the patient's personality while obtaining specific information about his or her sexual behavior. If, as the interview progresses in a nondirective mode, the patient ceases to provide relevant information, the clinician can become more directive. The assumption of a more directive role needs to be done in a manner that does not threaten or antagonize assertive patients, or allow obsessional or paranoid patients, who commonly provide excessive details, to consider that the clinician is dismissing information they consider highly relevant.

Content of the Interview

The unstructured interview is usually commenced by asking patients the nature of their problem or why they have sought help. While assessing how the patient responds to this opportunity to take charge of the interview, it usually is also possible to obtain much of the information necessary to establish the nature of the presenting complaint. The additional necessary information is commonly obtained only after the clinician becomes directive in questioning. This information usually includes any past history of similar problems, other illnesses, previous treatment, childhood and adolescent relationships with parents and siblings, social and sexual relationships and practices including unwanted sexual experiences, education and work history, and current domestic, social, sexual, and occupational situations, including the nature and extent of recreational interests and activities. Use of recreational drugs, including alcohol and tobacco, as well as any medications, needs to be determined.

Establishment of the Relationship

It is the author's practice to attempt to formulate hypotheses concerning the nature of the patient's condition and personality early in the interview and, in light of these hypotheses, to commence to consider the treatment most likely to be effective and to be complied with by the patient. The rest of the interview is then used to obtain data to support or discard these hypotheses. Other clinicians may prefer to continue to collect information without the need of such hypotheses. It is important to remain aware from the beginning of the unstructured diagnostic interview that while one is obtaining the information considered relevant, one is also commencing the process of treatment by establishing a relationship with the patient that will maximize his or her confidence and trust in one's abilities. The degree to which this rapport is successfully established will increase not only the nonspecific effects of the treatment instituted but also the likelihood that the patient will continue to comply with it. Reported dropout rates from treatment for sexual dysfunctions and deviations vary markedly (McConaghy, 1993), and it would seem likely that this variance in part reflects the varying abilities of clinicians to establish appropriate relationships with their patients.

Personality Assessment

Determination of the presence of significant personality disorders in patients seeking treatment for sexual disorders is of major importance clinically because personality disorders markedly influence patients' ability to provide accurate information, their motivation to change their behaviors, and the nature of the relationship they attempt to establish with the clinician. If this relationship is handled inappropriately, lack of compliance with or major disruption of the treatment plan can result, so that the patient is not helped or indeed may be harmed, and the clinician may also suffer considerable distress. The personality features I have found most important to detect in diagnostic interviewing are those indicative of psychopathy, borderline personality, and dependency.

Psychopathy is more prevalent in male than in female patients. Its presence may be suggested early in the interview by the patient's air of confidence, at times reflected in his use, without requesting permission, of the interviewer's first name. When he discusses behaviors or sexual problems that could have harmful effects on others, particularly those emotionally involved with him, he will usually show little evidence of ethical concern or empathy if the interviewer maintains a neutral attitude and shows no evidence of disapproval. Directive questioning is likely to reveal that he was commonly truant in childhood and adolescence, abused drugs, and showed other delinquent behaviors. His subsequent record of educational, occupational, social, and sexual activities demonstrates an instability consistent with an ability to easily form relationships and impress others with his qualities, but an inability to persist once the activities or relationships become demanding or boring. Patients with psychopathic traits are likely to distort their account of their behavior, perhaps unconsciously, minimizing features that show them in a bad light.

They are likely to comply poorly with treatment and frequently miss appointments. Nevertheless, if they can be maintained in treatment by the clinician attempting to establish a relationship with them on the basis of their own values, their continuance in treatment will at times benefit both them and society. The clinician should therefore stress the value of therapy in increasing their life satisfaction or enabling them to avoid unpleasant social consequences or incarceration. Evidence of disapproval from the therapist will result in their being less likely to report behaviors they sense will elicit further disapproval.

Borderline personality disorder, though it occurs in some men, is more likely to be shown by women. Appropriate questioning will usually reveal that, like psychopaths, these patients abused drugs or showed other delinquent behaviors in childhood and adolescence. They were commonly involved in sexual relationships they experienced as destructive due to any combination of their transience, association with emotional turbulence or aggression, or resultant pregnancy. Subjects with this personality commonly report being victims of child sexual abuse, usually in the form of incest. Suicidal attempts, or self-mutilative acts, such as cutting arms or legs, are frequently repeated, consistent with the low self-esteem basic to this personality disorder.

The subjects are likely to present in a manner that can induce the inexperienced therapist to become overinvolved and lose objectivity. These patients may show an initial apathy and withdrawal that the therapist feels challenged to overcome; present a distressed recital of overwhelmingly tragic life events, thus eliciting the therapist's sympathy; or report impulses to carry out aggressive or sexual attacks on children and at times imply that they have acted on such impulses, so that the therapist reacts with shock and alarm. They may respond early in the therapeutic interaction with intense gratitude possibly tinged with sexual seductiveness, stating that for the first time in their lives they have encountered someone who is really concerned for them, who truly understands them, and to whom they have imparted information they have given no one else, a response that the therapist may find difficult to treat with an appropriate degree of skepticism.

The therapist's response to these patients in the diagnostic interview may be crucial in establishing a relationship in which they will improve and the therapist remain comfortable. It is important that the therapist not respond with the overinvolvement that the patients consciously or unconsciously seek. Treatment of these patients is likely to be long and involved, often with an initial honeymoon period when they appear to respond and their relationship to the therapist is positive, followed by relapse and requests for more time and attention. This second stage may prove threatening to an inexperienced therapist who initially becomes overinvolved in response to the patient's mode of presentation, and so gives them a great deal of time and attention. When therapists accept a borderline patient for treatment, they should immediately inform the patient that they will continue to see her for as long as necessary and inform her how much time they can allot to her treatment, thereby avoiding the danger of devoting more time to the initial stages of treatment than they can continue to allow indefinitely. This clarification enables the therapist to continue to see the patient irrespective of her behavior within the limits established at the commencement of therapy. In view of the disturbingly high frequency with which therapists report becoming or are reported to become sexually involved with patients, it is important that therapists be aware that their doing so, which will totally undermine the aims of therapy, is most likely to be reported by patients with borderline personalities (Gutheil, 1989).

Dependent personality disorder is associated with either an inability to tolerate normal anxiety and depression produced by inevitable life stresses or a tendency to react to these stresses with above-average levels of these emotions. It will be suggested in the interview by the patients' lack of confidence and evident anxiety or depression and supported by evidence of their past inability to cope with the stresses that were a part of their education, employment, and emotional relationships. People with this personality will give a history of having performed poorly at school because they found examinations stressful and often avoided them. They are likely to have had several jobs, leaving one after another as they encountered difficulties. Their social relations tend to be limited to those with the few people on whom they are dependent. In my experience, these latter people are commonly supportive or controlling in personality and consciously or unconsciously prefer relationships with dependent persons, so that, like the patients, they may resist the therapist's attempts to change the nature of the patients' dependent relationships.

In the diagnostic interview of patients with dependent personalities, the clinician needs to be sufficiently supportive to engage these patients while encouraging the maximum independence of which they are capable. Particular attention needs to be given to discovering activities that will require some independence but that the patients are likely to enjoy and that can therefore be used to reinforce behavioral changes the therapist wishes to produce. The interviews with their partners and friends should be used to commence to educate and encourage these contacts to gradually cease rewarding the patient's illness behaviors and commence rewarding their healthy behaviors with encouragement and praise.

When it is suspected that patients have a significant personality disorder, it is more imperative that attempts be made to corroborate their history by interviewing relatives and others. It is not unusual for psychopathic and borderline patients to try to prevent this contact—saying, for example, that they dislike their relatives too much to allow any contact. If corroboration is considered sufficiently important, it may be necessary to make treatment conditional on patients' giving permission for such interviews.

The reason for stressing the importance of personality evaluation in the assessment of sexual problems is that in my experience, personality traits are now the major obstacle to successful treatment. Since the 1960s, the development of treatment techniques, particularly behavioral techniques, for most problems has been such that almost all patients who are appropriately motivated can benefit significantly from their application.

Termination of the Interview

Termination of the diagnostic interview requires careful planning, and adequate time must be left to accomplish it. Patients should not leave feeling that they have been asked a lot of questions or been allowed to talk freely but have been given no answers. It is the author's practice at this stage to present the patient with either a treatment plan or an explanation he or she finds satisfying as to why the clinician requires further information before the treatment plan can be formulated. Other therapists prefer to interview the patient on a number of occasions before making a decision about treatment. When a treatment plan is proposed, the clinician should ensure that patients are fully aware of what it entails and why the particular plan rather than an alternative, has been selected. Any reservations patients have concerning the plan should be fully dealt with, so that following its discussion, they commit themselves either to accept the plan or to make a decision concerning acceptance within the next week, possibly in consultation with the person who referred them.

RELIABILITY AND VALIDITY OF DIAGNOSTIC INTERVIEWS

Unstructured Interview

The accuracy of the information obtained in an unstructured clinical interview depends on the clinician's ability to correctly assess the extent to which the patient's self-report can be accepted without modification and the extent to which it should be regarded as distorted and in need of further confirmation. Determination of the patient's personality is of value in this regard. Patients who are attention-seeking are likely to exaggerate their symptoms, those with antisocial personalities may lie concerning them, and those who are depressed or have the high ethical standards commonly associated with obsessional features may present them in a somewhat negative light. Though most clinicians feel confident of their ability to utilize the clinical interview to obtain information that is at least sufficiently accurate for them to effectively treat their patients, little research has been carried out to justify this confidence. Furthermore, in their own practice, clinicians tend to modify the diagnostic categories they were taught to use during their apprenticeship with their teachers. This tendency for the diagnoses of clinicians to be somewhat idiosyncratic probably does not significantly alter the type of treatment all but a few patients receive. However, in the few cases in which it does, it could be expected that the clinician believes the treatment indicated by his or her diagnosis will be more effective than the alternative treatment a colleague making a different diagnosis would use. Again, virtually no research has been carried out to justify this belief, though in my experience if clinicians are asked to identify colleagues who have much higher than average diagnostic and treatment skills, they tend to nominate the same few people.

Lack of research evidence of the accuracy of the information produced by unstructured interviews stimulated criticism by academics. This criticism did not lead to investigation of the efficacy of treatments chosen on the basis of diagnoses made in such interviews, the so-called "treatment validity" of the diagnoses (Nelson & Hayes, 1981). Rather, workers took the easier research option of investigating the reliability of the diagnoses made by different clinicians. Studies in the 1950s and 1960s revealed that the agreement between the diagnoses made independently by two clinicians on the same group of subjects varied from 49% to 63% for specific diagnoses (Matarazzo, 1983). These findings stimulated the development by academics of methods of assessment that could ensure high reliability, provided the same method was used by different interviewers. In the absence of evidence that the low level of reliability of diagnoses based on unstructured interviews significantly affected treatment outcome, it would appear that few clinicians have adopted these highly reliable methods of assessment. In the area of sexuality, evidence to be discussed below indicates that this was also true of researchers, suggesting that at least in this area, some problems remain to be solved concerning these methods of assessment.

STRUCTURED INTERVIEW

The methods advanced to obtain diagnoses with high reliability were the development, first, of structured interviews with which all interviewers asked the same questions in the same order and manner and, second, of sets of criteria for each diagnostic condition, which were applied to the patients' responses to the structured interviews. The aim was that the diagnostic criteria would be defined sufficiently clearly that different interviewers would experience no uncertainty as to whether the criteria were present or absent in a particular patient. Diagnoses resulting from the use of this procedure were termed *operational diagnoses*, as each operation involved in reaching the diagnosis was defined in a manner that aimed to be totally objective, requiring no judgment from the diagnosticians that could be influenced by their subjectivity.

Two operationally defined assessment procedures have been widely used in the 1980s to diagnose patients with psychological disorders. One was developed in the United States—the structured interview termed the Diagnostic Interview Schedule (DIS; Robins, Helzer, Croughan, & Ratcliff, 1981)—to be used with the diagnostic criteria specified by the earlier edition of DSM-III-R, DSM-III. The other, developed in England, was the Present State Examination (PSE), the information from which was analyzed by the Catego computer program (Wing & Sturt, 1978). As stated above, the diagnoses reached by appropriately trained clinicians using either of these procedures were highly reliable. However, it could be considered that a fairer test of their reliability in comparison with that of the diagnoses of different clinicians using unstructured interviews would be the determination of the reliability of the diagnoses reached with one operational procedure as compared with those reached using the other. One study investigating the reliability of diagnoses reached using the two procedures was carried out by van den Brink et al. (1989). The PSE was modified so that the same interview could be used to obtain both DSM-III and Catego diagnoses for 175 nonpsychotic, nonaddicted psychiatric outpatients. Agreement between the diagnoses made by the two systems was 58% for cases of depression and 46% for cases of anxiety. It will be noted that the reliability of the diagnoses made by the two systems was of the same order as that cited above for unstructured clinical diagnoses by different clinicians that the systems were developed to replace.

Though diagnoses cannot be more valid than they are reliable, high reliability does not guarantee validity. An attempt was made to investigate one aspect of the validity of operational diagnoses by comparing them with more traditional psychiatric diagnoses in a population sample of 370 subjects (Helzer et al., 1985). The subjects were first interviewed by trained lay people using the DIS and subsequently by psychiatrists who were unaware of the subjects' responses to the lay-administered DIS. The psychiatrists also used the DIS interview, but were free to pursue clinical hunches and follow up on leads in an unstructured fashion. Subjects' responses to both procedures were examined to determine whether they conformed to the DSM-III-R diagnostic criteria. The number of subjects whom the psychiatrists considered to show a condition diagnosed as present by lay-administered DIS varied from a low of 3 (10%) of 29 subjects diagnosed as having obsessive–compulsive disorder to a high of 42 (74%) of 57 diagnosed as having major depression. For most diagnoses, the agreement was between 40% and 50%. It is likely that this relatively low level of agreement is significantly greater than the agreement between lay-administered DIS diagnoses assessed by DSM-III criteria and the diagnoses reached by psychiatrists using totally unstructured clinical interviews would have been had the latter agreement been investigated. It is possible that operational diagnostic procedures have sacrificed some degree of this validity of unstructured clinical diagnosis without obtaining a higher degree of reliability between different operational procedures. This question could be answered if the two types of diagnoses were compared to determine which produced a better outcome with treatment. No studies have as yet compared the treatment validity of operational and clinical diagnoses.

Clearly, highly reliable diagnostic procedures are of value for research workers. It is important that workers can be confident, for example, that schizophrenic patients studied in the United States are comparable to schizophrenic patients studied in Europe. This concordance would be highly likely if the workers in the two countries are prepared to use the same operational procedure. However, operational procedures can present a problem to therapists because they exclude a percentage of patients as not able to be diagnosed. In his review of psychiatric and psychological diagnosis, Matarazzo (1983) praised as destined to become as classic a study (Helzer et al., 1977) of the reliability of operational diagnostic criteria that investigated 101 first admissions to a medical school psychiatric service. Of these admissions, 18% were unable to be diagnosed. In the comparison study of the PSE and DIS/DSM-III assessments discussed above (van den Brink et al., 1989), all 175 outpatients had been referred by their general practitioner or medical specialist, and 80% had complaints of 6 months' or more duration. In this group, 55 (31%) were unable to be diagnosed as having a current mental disorder by the PSE, 23 (13%) by the DIS/DSM-III, and 17 (10%) by both. Of course, patients who cannot be diagnosed pose no problem in a research study, as they can be excluded. This option is not available to clinicians.

Special Problems with Sexual Disorders

It may be that the operational diagnosis of sexual problems and disorders presents special problems as compared to other psychiatric conditions. For the reason discussed above, it is becoming common practice in research publications to report that diagnoses of patients with schizophrenia or affective psychoses were made using standardized interviews such as the DIS or the Structured Clinical Interview for DSM-III-R (SCID; Spitzer, Williams, Gibbon, & First, 1990).

Such interviews do not appear to have been used in sexuality research. In none of the studies from 1989 to 1993 in the *Archives of Sexual Behavior*, a major academic sexuality research journal, were structured interviews used to reach diagnoses, and only a minority of those investigating sexual disorders made reference to the employment of DSM-III or DSM-III-R criteria in diagnosis. In review studies of hormonal replacement therapy, Walling, Andersen, and Johnson (1990) commented that though the most common sexual dysfunction noted was dyspareunia, a DSM-III-R definition was never cited.

This failure to use DSM-III-R definitions may be due in part to the lack of objectivity of some of the criteria that were discussed earlier. It was pointed out that to give the diagnosis of sexual dysfunction by the DSM-III-R criteria, the clinician must make the subjective judgment of taking into account such factors as the frequency and chronicity of the symptom, subjective distress, and the effect on other areas of the subject's functioning. In some studies in the issues of the *Archives of Sexual Behavior*, the authors developed their own criteria. Anorgasmia was diagnosed as present in women if they reported that orgasm resulted from 5% or less of all sexual activities with their partners and absent if orgasm resulted from 70% or more of such activities (Kelly, Strassberg, & Kircher, 1990). Premature ejaculation was diagnosed as present in subjects who estimated ejaculation latencies of 2 minutes or less on at least 50% of intercourse occasions and in addition perceived lack of control over the onset of orgasm (Strassberg, Mahoney, Schaugaard, & Hale, 1990).

A further problem with structured interviews could result from the marked reluctance of many subjects to reveal aspects of their sexual behavior. A number of studies in the issues of the *Archives of Sexual Behavior* examined stated that for this reason, anonymous questionnaires were employed. Reluctance of this nature was responsible for the failure of a high percentage of adolescents to report the presence of homosexual feelings to experienced sex researchers (McConaghy, 1989b). Such reluctance also led to the recommendation by Wyatt and Peters (1986) that face-to-face interviews in which multiple probing questions were asked about specific types of abusive sexual behaviors should be conducted by interviewers given special training in ideologically correct attitudes if women who had been sexually abused in childhood were to be correctly identified. Studies using such interviews found much higher prevalence rates. Structured interviews are unlikely to be useful in obtaining information concerning sexual behaviors from patients who are illiterate, schizophrenic, depressed, or brain-damaged. To establish and maintain a relationship with these patients in which adequate information can be obtained requires the more flexible approach of the unstructured interview. Also, these patients are rarely able or motivated to complete self-rating scales or questionnaires. This limitation is particularly relevant to the assessment of sex offenders, a moderate percentage of whom are intellectually impaired, brain-damaged, or psychotic (McConaghy, 1993).

In relation to the frequent use of self-report questionnaire interview methods in estimations of the incidence and prevalence of sexual dysfunctions, Spector and Carey (1990) commented that while questionnaires had the advantage of anonymity, interviews could be used to probe for more detailed and perhaps more accurate data. While pointing out this advantage, which would require a somewhat unstructured format, they also pointed out the existence of a number of structured interviews that they recommended. They were critical of the failure of many studies to provide clear operational definitions and recommended the use of a common system that classified dysfunctions by failure rate, lifelong vs. acquired disorders, and situational concomitants that would allow multiple diagnoses along desire, arousal, and orgasm axes.

Reluctance to use operational diagnostic procedures with sexual disorders has also been evident in epidemiological studies. It would appear that only one of the National Institute of Mental Health Epidemiological Catchment Area Program studies of the prevalence of psychiatric disorders investigated the prevalence of specific sexual dysfunctions. That one, carried out in St. Louis using the DIS administered by lay interviewers, reported a prevalence of 24% for all psychosexual dysfunctions (Robins et al., 1984). No further information was provided, so that the validity of the procedure cannot be commented on.

In view of the infrequent use of structured interviews for diagnostic purposes in research on sexual disorders, it is unlikely that clinicians treating patients with sexual disorders will in the near future use them in place of the unstructured clinical interviews they have been trained to administer. Further empirical evidence of the advantages of structured interviews would appear necessary to motivate clinicians to cease to utilize the skills they have developed to use the interview flexibly to investigate patients' personalities and to establish the relationships with patients that maximize the likelihood of the patients' remaining in and complying with treatment.

RATING SCALE AND QUESTIONNAIRE INVESTIGATIONS

In addition to the criticism of unstructured interviews on the basis of their low reliability, with the emergence of behaviorism as a major influence on clinical practice in the 1960s, they were also criticized as being based on self-report rather than observation of behavior. As evidence demonstrated the limited validity and relevance of behavioral observation, self-report as a source of information was rehabilitated (McConaghy, 1988). However, some behaviorally oriented researchers preferred that subjects' self-reports be elicited by the interviewer using rating scales, in the expectation that this procedure would increase the reliability of the information obtained. Also, questionnaires completed by patients were considered to have the added advantage of being less influenced by the interviewer. Again, it is necessary to consider the possibility that the reliability and possible increase in objectivity obtained may be at the sacrifice of some degree of validity. Research investigating this possibility appears to have been rarely undertaken in recent years. Earlier studies investigated the validity of psychiatrists' global assessments of patients' clinical response to treatment made in unstructured interviews by asking the psychiatrists to judge which patients were being treated with placebo and which the active medication. Their judgments proved highly valid in comparison to most of the objective methods of assessing treatment response that were used including psychological tests, rating scales, and physiological measures (Lipman, Cole, Park, & Rickels, 1965; Paredes et al., 1966). Paredes and co-workers pointed out that in making global assessments in unstructured interviews, clinicians were sensitive to a multitude of factors. When they were limited to rating behavior on scales, they narrowed their perspective, reducing their ability to make valid intuitive judgments.

A similar narrowing of perspective may occur with patients' assessments of their own responses. Women reported increased satisfaction in their sexual relationship by global assessment, but decreased satisfaction when specific activities were measured by the Sexual Interaction Inventory (De Amicis, Goldberg, LoPiccolo, Friedman, & Davies, 1985). In an investigation of female victims of rape or incestuous assaults, Becker, Skinner, Abel, and Treacy (1982) used a Sexual Arousal

Inventory developed to discriminate sexually functional from dysfunctional sub-jects. It did not discriminate those who on clinical assessment reported no sexual problems from those who reported one or more problems related to the assault. The authors accepted the clinical assessment finding and concluded that the inventory lacked discriminative capability. Such findings suggest that until ques-tionnaires or rating scales are demonstrated to have this capability, it would seem wise when they are used to also use unstructured clinical assessment.

A rating-scale method commonly used to assess sexual behaviors is to ask subjects to rate on diary cards, daily or more frequently, the frequency with which they engage in the behaviors. The validity of this method was found to be low when investigated by an innovative technique designed to assess patient recording behavior. Patients were asked to record on diary cards their home use of relaxation audiotapes. Their use of the tapes was independently monitored, without the patients' knowledge, by incorporation of electronic devices in the tape recorders with which they were provided (Taylor, Agras, Schneider, & Allen, 1983). Compari-son of the diary cards and monitoring devices revealed that 32% of patients falsely reported their use of the tapes on the cards. Wincze, Bansal, and Malamud (1986) found no difference between the responses of pedophilic sex offenders receiving placebo as compared to the male-sex-hormone-reducing chemical medroxyproges-terone when the reduction in frequency of their urges for sexual contacts with children was assessed by diary card ratings they made daily and submitted weekly. However, in addition to the clinical evidence of the value of medroxypro-gesterone in reducing the likelihood that sex offenders will act on their deviant impulses (McConaghy, 1993), sex offenders' global assessments of the degree of reduction in their deviant sexual urges, self-reported at interview, were validated by the high correlations found with the degree of reduction in their serum levels of the male sex hormone testosterone produced by medroxyprogesterone (Mc-Conaghy, Blaszczynski, & Kidson, 1988). Both patients and interviewer were unaware of the testosterone levels at the time of the assessment.

Methodological features of studies may also influence self-reports. AuBuchon and Calhoun (1985) asked 18 women to record their moods on a 16-item adjective checklist twice weekly for 8 weeks. Nine were randomly selected and informed that the study was investigating a possible relationship of mood to their menstrual cycles. Their self-report scales demonstrated a relationship between negative mood and menstruation. The scales of those not so informed did not. The authors attributed the relationship found to the social expectancy and demands charac-teristics resulting from the information.

Just as academics appear to have shown somewhat greater tolerance in regard to the variable degree of reliability and lack of evidence of validity of structured clinical and behavioral assessments compared to unstructured interview assess-ments, they have shown similar tolerance in regard to rating scales. Conte (1983), in his review of self-report scales for rating sexual function, found a number to have test–retest reliabilities in the range of $r = 0.5$. Apart from this evidence of reliability in the range of that of different clinicians' diagnoses, he pointed out the need for studies to establish their validity. In addition, most of the scales provided no measures of important aspects of sexual function such as the frequency of sexual behaviors or of subjects' satisfaction with their current sexual functioning. A review of 51 objectively scored, mainly self-rated assessments of sexual function and marital interactions reported little evidence of their validity (Schiavi, Derogatis, Kuriansky, O'Connor, & Sharpe, 1979). When validity was referred to, it was usually described as adequate or as demonstrated by the test's ability to discriminate two groups of subjects, a criterion that can be achieved by tests that misclassify a number of individuals in the groups.

Clearly, in research studies of particular sexual behaviors, the use of questionnaires is essential to ensure that the relevant information concerning the behaviors is obtained from all subjects investigated. Also, as stated earlier, anonymous questionnaires can be used to obtain information that subjects will not provide when interviewed individually. At the same time, it is necessary to be aware that the use of structured procedures additional to the diagnostic interview can reduce patient compliance with treatment. Reading (1983) randomly allocated paid male volunteers to report details of their sexual behavior either by interview after 1 and 3 months; by interview after 1, 2, and 3 months; or by the latter procedure plus diary cards completed daily and returned every 3 days. In this group, 34% allocated to the last form of assessment discontinued it, as compared to 14% with the first and 16% with the second. Another 3 subjects dropped out from the diary card assessment prior to the first month, considering that it was causing them difficulty maintaining their sexual potency. These findings as well as those of Taylor et al. (1983) and Wincze et al. (1986) reported earlier, which demonstrated lack of validity of reports by diary cards, indicate that it cannot be assumed that structured self-reports provide assessments superior to those obtained by unstructured clinical interviews. Whatever assessment measures are employed in research studies, it would seem that their validity should be demonstrated for the particular subjects being investigated.

OBSERVATIONAL ASSESSMENT

Intuitive interpretation of observations of subjects' nonverbal behaviors plays a major role in assessment in the unstructured clinical interview. Observations of sexual behaviors are rarely reported, though such assessments of sexual behaviors either directly or by videotape were briefly popular in the more explorative climate of the 1970s (LoPiccolo, 1990). LoPiccolo believed there were convincing arguments against their use. These arguments included that the effect of observation on patients with sexual dysfunctions would make it unlikely that their observed behaviors would be similar to their private behaviors, that the procedure would be unacceptable to the majority of couples, and that it allowed the exploitation of patients by the therapist. These issues were certainly relevant to the "sexological exam," described by LoPiccolo, in which sex therapists stimulated the breasts and genitals of the opposite sex partner to assess and demonstrate physiological responsiveness. However, it would seem possible to provide adequate ethical safeguards to allow videotaped observational assessment of couples' sexual interactions. With the use of preliminary sessions to allow the couples to adjust to the procedure, it would seem possible that their observed behavior would be sufficiently related to their private behavior for its assessment to be of value. This is accepted to be the case with the observational assessment of nonsexual behaviors such as phobias and the laboratory assessment of physiological evidence of sexual arousal, both of which remain widely used. It is likely that taboos concerning sexuality remain the major obstacle to observational assessment of sexual activity. This assessment, of course, plays a major role in surrogate sex therapy. Observation of erections occurring during sleep or produced by masturbation remain recommended (Karacan, 1978; Wasserman, Pollak, Spielman, & Weitzman, 1980).

Maletzky (1980) used observational assessment of exhibitionists. A comely actress with whom the subjects were unacquainted placed herself in situations in which they had previously committed frequent offenses. The subjects had been informed that experimental and unusual procedures would be employed. Observational assessment of the effeminate behavior of boys has also been reported, either by clinicians (Rekers & Lovaas, 1974), by teachers (Kagan & Moss, 1962), or by parents (Bates, Bentler, & Thompson, 1973). The therapists observed boys playing with boys' and girls' toys through a one-way mirror. The teachers and parents were requested to complete inventories reporting the effeminate behaviors shown by their pupils or sons. Observation and quantification of the effeminate behavior of adult males has also been reported (Schatzberg, Westfall, Blumetti, & Birk, 1975), but does not appear to have been widely used, possibly because of its complexity.

Case Illustrations

Indications of Trustworthiness

William was a 23-year-old man whose dress and manner reflected his middle-class background and somewhat introverted though warm personality. The referral letter from his general practitioner stated he had had an impotence problem before performing the sexual act for about 4 months, that he had had a similar problem 3 years ago, and that he had a satisfactory libido. I used this information when commencing the initial interview:

T: Your doctor's letter says you have a problem in regard to erections in sexual situations?
P: Yes. Three years ago when I attempted to have sex in a relationship I lost my erection. . . . It put my confidence down a bit.
T: Was that the first time you attempted intercourse?
P: Yes.
T: When did you start dating?
P: Three or four years ago. I suppose I'm an old fashioned guy. I didn't go out with a different girl every week.

It was obvious that William was markedly diffident and the interview would need to be conducted directively. Questioning revealed that he had attempted intercourse 5 months after his first serious relationship, and though full penetration was not achieved, he subsequently developed a urinary infection, causing urination to be painful for a week or so. No cause for the infection was identified. He did not attempt intercourse again, and the relationship was gradually terminated by both parties. Subsequently, he spent an enjoyable year traveling alone, backpacking in Europe and the United States. He avoided any sexual relationships.

His current relationship commenced 9 months ago with a woman of his age whom he met at a business conference, and who lived in another state, so that they usually were only able to spend alternate week-ends together, and the longest time they had had together was 3 days. They had commenced to attempt intercourse in the last 5 months. He volunteered the statement, "Going without sex doesn't worry me." He thought he never got a full erection when with his girlfriend, though he did on his own. He didn't masturbate in the periods between seeing his girlfriend, saying, "I sort of lack the desire." However, it seemed that he may have always had this lack of desire, as he had masturbated very infrequently in adolescence.

Asked about the frequency of his shaving, he said he shaved daily but probably did not need to shave that often. When asked about his life-style, he stated that he wasn't enjoying the inner-city area where he was living, stating it was "claustrophobic . . . there were a lot of alternative people. I feel I don't fit in." This attitude supported his history that he didn't smoke or use soft or hard drugs, and only occasionally drank a few beers.

He volunteered the statement concerning his girlfriend that "she's going through the stage that she thinks it's her. She's wanting to lose a bit of weight. . . . I keep telling her that she's got nothing to do with it." Subsequently, he said of his sexual difficulty that "it's the only thing we have hang-ups about." His manner of presentation made his sincerity and strong feelings for his girlfriend apparent. When asked his main source of enjoyment in life, he said "Our relationship," and he appeared near to tears when discussing his fear that his condition could threaten it. This was explored:

T: It's getting to you emotionally?

P: Yes.

T: Is it interfering with your sleep?

P: When I'm with her I can't get to sleep thinking about it.

T: Do you find it causes you to cry at times?

P: [nodded] . . . At times when I'm thinking about it I try and fight back the tears.

T: At times do you feel hopeless about it?

P: It really hits me when I'm going to bed . . . the rest of the time you're busy.

Further questioning revealed that his sleep and appetite were not affected and he was continued to meet friends from school once or twice a week. It was considered that his depression was probably reactive, but that the possibility of a biological element that could require antidepressant medication would need to be kept in mind when assessing his progress, and I would remain alert to any indication of suicidal impulses.

To deal with some of his depressive ideation, I explained that it was to be expected that his impotence would not have improved when he and his girlfriend could spend only short periods of time together in sexual activity. Anxiety about his ability to perform sexually had become conditioned to this activity by his earlier experiences and, for this anxiety to be inhibited, he would need prolonged regular experiences of sexual activity without pressure to perform. I then explained the modified Masters and Johnson procedure (McConaghy, 1993) I use for couples when the male partner has impotence. A further complication consistent with his personality was that he had not told his girlfriend he was seeking treatment because she had said they would work it out on their own. I encouraged him to tell her, as this would mean I could treat them as a couple. The alternative was that he discuss the treatment program with her as something he had read about. In view of the indication in his history of a possible constitutional low sexual drive, his hormonal status was investigated.

Indications of Unreliability

Peter was a 33-year-old man about whose treatment with medroxyprogesterone I had been consulted by phone 2 months previously following his admission to a Sydney psychiatric hospital. He had a long history of psychiatric treatment and had been variously diagnosed as suffering from schizophrenia, borderline personality disorder, alcohol and benzodiazepine addiction, and panic attacks. His admission had followed the last of many presentations to a rural district hospital near where he lived with his parents. Previously, he had sought treatment for alcoholism and drug abuse, but on this occasion he reported impulses to strangle children, a fear of masturbation associated with fantasies of sexual and violent acts, and auditory hallucinations of a critical and insulting nature. On admission to the Sydney hospital, he had been put on a withdrawal regime for alcohol and benzodiazepines, medicated with the antipsychotic thioridazine, and commenced on the low-dosage 6-month medroxyprogesterone program used for the treatment of compulsive sexuality (McConaghy, 1993).

In his letter to me, the referring doctor at the hospital where Peter was still an inpatient stated that Peter reported loss of libido following the medroxyprogesterone and no more "whacky" thoughts. His testosterone level had dropped from 19 mmoles/liter prior to the first medroxyprogesterone injection to 6.3 mmoles/liter prior to the third. The letter continued: "We remain deeply concerned over his paraphilia. He has strangled women to the point of unconsciousness during intercourse, and has at another time derived sexual pleasure from placing a plastic bag over a child's head. Your opinion re ongoing treatment would be greatly appreciated. . . . He too is keen to see you." Records of admission to hospitals outside Sydney in the past few years were attached.

In the interview, Peter talked freely and confidently, revealing that he had been having daily interviews with his doctor since his admission except for a short period when the doctor had holidays, during which time Peter became depressed and expressed thoughts of committing suicide. Asked about the nature of the problem, he referred to acts of self-abuse, which commenced when he started to masturbate when he was aged 15 and was using "pot and LSD."

T: What form did the acts take?

P: I used rubber bands to cut off the blood supply to my penis. Also, I would try and hang myself.

T: How?

P: With a rope. When I climaxed I'd grab something. In the last 6 months, this was getting dangerous. I felt I had no control. It stopped once I started on the injections. Now I don't masturbate or get crazy thoughts.

T: How frequently was it happening?

P: When I was in the psychiatry unit in Queensland last year, it stopped for a month, when I was given Largactil, plus being in the hospital. Since then it's been a couple of times a week.

T: Would you do anything else apart from attempt to strangle yourself when masturbating?

P: No.

T: Tell me about the crazy thoughts.

P: I had fantasies of the strangling being done to me by a man or a woman. They were the dominant one.

T: Did you have other thoughts?

P: No, just having sexual intercourse. I wanted help because I couldn't live that way any more. About 5 years ago I put a plastic bag over a little boy's head.

T: Who was the boy?

P: My stepson.

T: How did he react?

P: He was asleep at the time. I put it on for 8 seconds. In my sick mind I got off on it.

T: In what way?

P: I think it was a sexual feeling . . . sexual aggressive. After that I got obsessed with the thought, I couldn't get rid of the obsession, the guilt, fear and anger, but I'd still masturbate over it. Whatever I'd fantasize I'd do it, be disgusted, sick, but I'd masturbate over it again. I slept with a man about six months ago.

T: Did you have fantasies of that before?

P: Yes, for years.

T: Were there any other sexual behaviors or acts you were involved in?

P: None other than self-abuse—the strangulation was the most extreme.

T: Did you ever attempt to strangle anyone?

P: I did strangle women at times when having intercourse with them, and they seemed to enjoy it.

T: They never complained?

P: No.

T: Were they women you were having a regular relationship with?

P: Yes.

T: Would you do it regularly?

P: Fairly regularly. Yes.

Prior to his admission to hospital, he had been living with his parents, and his references to them suggested a dependent attitude. When asked about his childhood, he reported it was not happy, continuing:

P: We moved to Australia from England when I was 8. I got stirred because of my accent. Everyone threw insults at me.

In response to questioning, he reported that his brother, who was a few years older, adjusted much better. Asked how he got on with his parents, he said, "I was happy with them *when* they were at home," strongly emphasizing the "when." Asked to elaborate on this, he said they were both out working, adding, "So I lacked emotional support." He started to drink when he left school at age 15 and said he was introduced to Alcoholics Anonymous at age 19, following which he didn't drink for 2 years, the longest time he ever did not drink. He married at age 20 when he wasn't drinking and said the sexual relationship with his wife was normal. His alcoholism led to their divorce when he was 24, but they are still friendly. When he was 26, he married a woman who also drank heavily, but they stopped living together 2 weeks after the marriage. "It was an unbelievable personality clash . . . we stopped and started for two years. Then I ended it." Subsequently, he traveled around Australia, being able to obtain certificates from doctors every 3 months to remain on sickness benefits, which he supplemented with casual work. During this time, he had a 12-

month relationship with a third woman. When asked if he attempted to strangle this woman or either of his wives, he said, "No. Only other women. If they didn't want me to, I wouldn't . . . if they pushed my hands away."

In regard to previous treatment, he couldn't give an account of dates, but stated that he had been in treatment on and off over the years since he was admitted to the psychiatry ward of the local hospital a few times for alcohol abuse when he was 19. Subsequently, he had been in alcoholism programs, hospitals, and detoxification units. He was critical of the previous treatments he received:

P: They weren't getting to the root of the problem, only chipping away at the edges.

T: When did you reveal your sexual problems?

P: I only let the cat out of the bag last year. They scheduled me for a month, but then transferred me. If I'd stayed on, I would have had to pay rent. They reckoned I was O.K. to go. I hadn't been treated for my sexual problem, and it started again after I left the hospital. The only thing they gave me was Largactil.

T: Would they have gone on seeing you as an outpatient?

P: No.

T: What help do you feel you need?

P: I just want some sort of stability. Getting depressed and anxious is no way to live. I'm absolutely ecstatic about the effect of the injections. There's no urge to masturbate.

T: Do you get erections at all?

P: No. I'm not complaining. It makes me feel better that I don't have to think about those things and I'm in control.

T: But you still got depressed recently.

P: I wanted to go home. The doctor was away. I just wanted to die. If I could go home now I would be O.K. You really get sick of being in the hospital.

Peter presented his history in a dramatic manner using exaggerated expressions ("unbelievable personality clash," "absolutely ecstatic") and with at times an apparent attempt to shock and to emphasize the seriousness of his problem and at times to stress that he had responded to treatment and could safely return home. His dependency and his ability to manipulate people into helping him were suggested by his being able to stay on sickness benefits for some years, even though he was physically well and his psychological state would not have prevented him from working if he wanted to do so, as well as by his continuing to live with his parents and clearly feeling the need to return to them for support.

He showed no appreciation of the help of any of the therapists of the many previous programs to which he had been admitted, though available records indicated that at least some of them were very dedicated. Report of his previous medical treatment revealed that Androcur (another chemical that reduces testosterone level) was recommended, but he declined this drug, stating that the Largactil he was taking enabled him to withstand his sexual impulses. In the interview with me, he dismissed this offer with the misleading statement, "The only thing they gave me was Largactil." The report also stated, "On occasions he hangs himself, cutting himself down before he loses consciousness," suggesting that he did not report the frequency of a couple of times a week that he reported to me. He did not mention cutting himself down to me. In the interview with me, he initially said that he strangled his regular sexual partners, but later that the women were those he was not involved with. The report contained the information that he described occasions on which he had carried out violent fantasies toward children and had been violent to his sexual partners, adding that there was no history of his being charged with violence. Such charges would have been likely if he had actually carried out the behaviors, and the report continued with the comment that "his glibness reinforced the opinions that many of his problems were fabricated." In regard to his statement that he didn't get erections at all, in my experience virtually all men whose testosterone levels are reduced by medroxyprogesterone in the dosage employed in his treatment continue to obtain erections. Emphasis on having an unhappy childhood and not receiving sufficient parental love is frequently reported by subjects with personality disorders associated with attention-seeking.

This patient's tendency to present information in a manner designed to elicit from the interviewer an emotional response of increased involvement and sympathy caused me to consider that much of the information could be false and that he had used this technique successfully in the past to obtain attention, maintain a sick role, and obtain sickness benefits. This tendency combined with the inconsistency of aspects of his account with the report of his previous treatment caused me to conclude that it was more necessary than usual to corroborate the information he gave. When I interviewed him, he wished to be discharged from the hospital in order to return home. This could have accounted for his reporting symptoms less suggestive of potential dangerousness than his earlier description, which obviously impressed the doctor who interviewed him at the time he was seeking admission. It would also account for his claim of an excellent response to treatment.

INFORMATION CRITICAL TO MAKING THE DIAGNOSIS

The major problem in the diagnosis of sexual disorders is not so much obtaining the information concerning the exact nature of the dysfunction or deviation as the significance to attach to it. No criteria have been accepted to establish the degree of deficiency of sexual fantasies and desire to justify the diagnosis of Sexual Desire Disorder, of reduction of lubrication with sexual arousal to justify the diagnosis of Sexual Arousal Disorder in women, or of reduction in frequency of erection to justify the diagnosis of Male Erectile Disorder. Premature ejaculation was defined in DSM-III-R as ejaculation with minimal sexual stimulation before, upon, or shortly after penetration and before the person wished it. However, some men consider that they suffer from premature ejaculation when they ejaculate several minutes after penetration but before their partner reaches orgasm. As pointed out earlier, DSM-III-R recommended that to diagnose sexual dysfunction, the clinician was to judge that the condition be persistent or recurrent, taking into account such factors as the frequency and chronicity of the symptom, the subjective distress caused, and the effect on other areas of the subject's functioning. This procedure must almost certainly result in low reliability of the diagnoses made by different clinicians and hence limit the ability to compare research findings using these DSM-III-R criteria.

At the same time, in clinical practice, the patient's subjective distress is a major factor influencing the patient's conclusion that he or she has a problem that justifies treatment. This conclusion may have little relationship to whether or not a dysfunction is diagnosed. Osborn, Hawton, and Gath (1988) investigated a community sample of 436 women in the United Kingdom and concluded that 142 showed at least one of four operationally defined dysfunctions: impaired sexual interest

(17%), vaginal dryness (17%), infrequency of orgasm (16%), and dyspareunia (8%). Only 32 of the 142 considered they had a sexual problem, as did a further 10 who showed no dysfunction. Of the total of 42 who considered they had a problem, 16 said they wished treatment if it was available. As stated earlier, sexual difficulties (problems related to the emotional tone of the patients' relationships) were more important determinants of their sexual satisfaction than were their dysfunctions (Frank et al., 1978; Snyder & Berg, 1983).

When it is concluded that the patient has a sexual dysfunction, it is necessary to exclude the presence of organic causes requiring physical investigation. Ruling out organic causes is particularly relevant in older men with erectile problems and in women with vaginal dryness or tenderness following menopause. If men give a history of obtaining adequate erections in nonstressful situations such as private masturbation, or with some partners but not with others, organic factors can be excluded, apart from that which produces the uncommon "pelvic steal syndrome." This syndrome results from iliac artery pathology that leads to blood being shunted from the pelvic region to the musculature of the lower extremities when these muscles become active in coital thrusting. The resultant loss of erection occurs only following penetration. It is therefore necessary to determine whether erectile failure occurs only at this stage of coitus and does not occur if intercourse is carried out with the patient lying on his back without thrusting. Understandably, as Segraves, Schoenberg, and Segraves (1985) pointed out, clinicians unaware of the syndrome are likely without further investigation to attribute impotence occurring at this stage to psychological factors.

Though isolated sexually deviant acts may be shown by the majority of adolescent males (McConaghy, 1993), considerations of frequency are not taken into account, and any such acts reported or detected are usually diagnosed as sexual deviations or paraphilias. Sexually deviant fantasies are common in both men and women, so the DSM-III-R criterion that the subject be distressed by them is the usual indication for accepting that they warrant treatment. Probably many workers would consider fantasies of sexual activity with children to justify a diagnosis of sexual deviance, although such fantasies also may not be uncommon. About 15% of male and 2% of female university students in the United States and Australia reported some likelihood that they would engage in sexual activity with a prepubertal child if they could so without risk (Malamuth, 1989; McConaghy, Zamir, & Manicavasagar, 1993). A significant percentage of apparently otherwise normal men demonstrate penile volume arousal to pictures of nude young girls (Freund, McKnight, Langevin, & Cibiri, 1972). Freund and colleagues concluded that for the nondeviant adult male, the female child—at least from her 6th year— was biologically a more appropriate surrogate sexual object than a male person, and that many heterosexual pedophilic offenses may be carried out by men who are not truly pedophilic in their sexual preference. If so, these offenses express urges that are deviant not sexually but socially. Markedly harmful sadistic fantasies may also be commonly regarded as sexually deviant. Yet over 30% of men reported sexual fantasies of tying up and of raping a woman and 10–20% of torturing or beating up a woman (Crepault & Couture, 1980; Person et al., 1989). When sexual fantasies are investigated, any tendency for the subject to experience urges to carry them out should be determined. If such urges are present, the subject's ability to control them needs to be assessed.

When, at the initiation of the diagnostic interview, the information as to why the patient sought treatment is being obtained, the reason he or she did so at that particular time should also be established. This reason can be valuable in determining the patient's conscious or unconscious motivation for treatment. Reasons could include pressure from the partner or legal requirements. A woman seeking treatment to become orgasmic in intercourse may reveal, possibly only when interviewed with her partner, that she is quite content with their sexual life; it is the partner who is distressed that she is not reaching orgasm in their sexual relationships, as he finds this incompatible with his concept of himself as a lover.

Do's and Don't's

Sexual therapists who are commencing their practice should not be inhibited by being aware that they feel somewhat diffident or embarrassed at questioning subjects about the details of their sexual activity, normal and deviant. Most patients will not react negatively if the therapist shows some signs of this diffidence. Many of them will also be diffident and may feel more comfortable with a therapist who is not a model of total assurance. However, therapists must not let these feelings stop them from asking all the appropriate questions or cause them to use technical language rather than selecting words they can be sure the patient will understand. For some patients, these words will be the colloquial words other patients would regard as crude or obscene.

Do continuously hold in mind that while assessing patients, you are also establishing the relationship that will ensure their continued attendance and compliance with treatment. An attitude of detached inquiry will make the establishment of such a relationship less likely.

Do ask older patients about their sexual activity. As they are aware of the still prevalent belief that older people don't or shouldn't have any sexual activity, many are reluctant to seek help if they are having sexual problems. Most clinicians appear equally reluctant to inquire concerning them. Slag et al. (1983) found that 401 of 1080 men attending a medical outpatient clinic reported having erectile dysfunction when specifically questioned. Prior to the inquiry, only 6 had been identified as having the dysfunction. Slag and associates commented that the subjects were reluctant to call attention to their dysfunction, but were eager to discuss and seek evaluation for it when the physicians broached the topic.

Don't provide patients with the information you are trying to elicit, particularly if there is evidence that they may be motivated to distort their history. Asking a series of leading questions can encourage suggestible patients or those who wish to provide evidence that they suffer from a significant disorder to confirm the suggestions implicit in such questions. Questions that specify symptoms that characterize a particular condition allow the patient to answer in the affirmative and thereby give the false impression that he or she shows all the typical symptoms. For example, when questioning Peter about his self-strangulation, an approach such as the following, by which the questioner reveals the nature of sexual asphyxia, should be avoided:

T: How did you attempt to strangle yourself?

P: I used a rope.

T: Did you look at pornography while you were doing it?

P: Sometimes.

T: Did you try and hurt yourself in other ways—like using nipple-clamps?

P: I did at times.

T: Would you ever cross-dress in women's clothes and underwear?

P: I used to do that.

If this approach is used, patients with no knowledge that these behaviors commonly accompany sexual asphyxia can convince the interviewer they have the condition. Open questions in which the subject is asked to reveal the nature of his sexual activity avoid this possibility.

Don't allow your sympathy for subjects reporting sexual victimization to cause you to treat them as special patients so that you depart from your usual practice. Your usual practice is the result of your training and experience. Any departure from it is likely to produce a less satisfactory result. Treating victims as requiring extra concern can convey the message that their competence to cope with the trauma is suspect, so that they require more than your usual attention. In particular, it is important, while being supportive of appropriate distress, not to reinforce illness behaviors such as regression, as McCombie and Arons (1980) pointed out in regard to the counseling of victims of sexual assault. Such illness behavior could account for the findings of Burgess and Holmstrom (1985) that "rape-work" following the treatment of the acute phase of the reaction to sexual assault could last months or years and of Courtois and Sprei (1998) that the therapy of adult victims of childhood sexual abuse could take years and that patients were likely to be discouraged or enraged by the length of treatment.

In this regard, it would seem advisable that reports of sexual victimization should not be given more credence than reports of other sexual behaviors. Given the current emphasis on the prevalence and significance of such victimization, it would seem not impossible that some subjects in need of attention could respond to unconscious reinforcement on the part of the therapist by coming to believe that innocent activities in their childhood were forms of abuse. Yet it has been suggested that not believing subjects' reports of sexual victimization is itself a form of victimization (Armsworth, 1989).

From my experience, I have concluded that failure to be skeptical of such reports when skepticism is appropriate could also be regarded as a form of victimization. I have seen a number of patients with marked dependent personality disorders who became permanent victims, chronically incapable of living a normal life or working, after receiving prolonged treatment for sexual victimization. Frequently, the victimization was remembered by them only after a series of probing interviews by therapists convinced of the severe and persistent effects of such experiences. In view of the marked suggestibility of some of these patients, it would seem likely that in some instances the experience as it was remembered had not occurred. Whether it did or not, in these patients it became an event that dominated their thinking about themselves and served to explain all their inabilities. They no longer experienced any necessity to accept responsibility for their behavior and lost all motivation to change, while remaining prepared to discuss their experience of and response to the victimization indefinitely. Concern for patients must be accompanied by awareness that ultimately if they are to enjoy life again, they must cease to be victims. Therapists must not overreact to the possibility or indeed the reality of their patients' past traumatic experiences, but rather award them respect for their ability to survive, respect that will enable them to recover from the effects of the experiences.

SUMMARY

In diagnostic interviews of patients with sexual dysfunctions, it is necessary to investigate the nature of any sexual difficulties, i.e., the problems resulting from the emotional tone of their relationships, as these are more important in determining sexual dissatisfaction. Little significance need be attached to deviant sexual fantasies unless the patient is distressed by or feels urges to express them. For clinical purposes, diagnostic information is obtained by most therapists in an unstructured interview that also allows investigation of the presence of personality disorders and the establishment of a relationship with the patient that will maximize the likelihood that he or she will remain in and comply with treatment. The high reliability of structured interviews, provided the same one is used, is likely to encourage their use in research studies, particularly when diagnostic criteria for sexual disorders are operationalized. Case illustrations were given to illustrate patient characteristics that make the information they give more or less credible. The marked prevalence of sexual dysfunctions and deviations makes their diagnosis dependent not so much on the presence of the behaviors as on their frequency and intensity or the degree to which they distress the subject. Organic causes need to be excluded, particularly in sexual dysfunctions in the middle-aged and elderly, who commonly will not volunteer that they suffer from dysfunctions, so that they must be specifically asked concerning them.

REFERENCES

American Psychiatric Association (1987). *Diagnostic and statistical manual of mental disorders*, 3rd ed., revised. Washington, DC: Author.

American Psychiatric Association (1993). *Diagnostic and statistical manual of mental disorders*, 4th ed., draft criteria. Washington, DC: Author.

Armsworth, M. W. (1989). Therapy of incest survivors: Abuse or support? *Child Abuse and Neglect, 13*, 549–562.

AuBuchon, P. G., & Calhoun, K. S. (1985). Menstrual cycle symptomatology: The role of social expectancy and experimental demand characteristics. *Psychosomatic Medicine, 47*, 35–45.

Bates, J. E., Bentler, P. M., & Thompson, S. K. (1973). Measurement of deviant gender development in boys. *Child Development, 44*, 591–598.

Becker, J. V., Skinner, L. J. Abel, G. G., & Treacy, E. C. (1982). Incidence and types of sexual dysfunctions in rape and incest victims. *Journal of Sex and Mental Therapy, 8,* 65–74.

Burgess, A. W., & Holmstrom, L. L. (1985). Rape trauma syndrome and post traumatic stress response. In A. W. Burgess (Ed.), *Rape and sexual assault* (pp. 46–60). New York: Garland Publishing.

Byers, E. S., & Heinlein, L. (1989). Predicting initiations and refusals of sexual activity in married and cohabitating heterosexual couples. *Journal of Sex Research, 26,* 210–231.

Conte, H. R. (1983). Development and use of self-report techniques for assessing sexual functioning: A review and critique. *Archives of Sexual Behavior, 12,* 555–576.

Courtois, C. A., & Sprei, J. E. (1988). Retrospective incest therapy for women. In L. E. A. Walker (Ed.), *Handbook on sexual abuse of children* (pp. 270–308). New York: Springer.

Crepault, C., & Couture, M. (1980). Men's erotic fantasies. *Archives of Sexual Behavior, 9,* 565–581.

De Amicis, L. A., Goldberg, D. C., LoPiccolo, J., Friedman, J., & Davies, L. (1985). Clinical follow-up of couples treated for sexual dysfunction. *Archives of Sexual Behavior, 14,* 467–489.

Finkelhor, D. (1984). *Child sexual abuse: New theory and research.* New York: Free Press.

Frank, E., Anderson, B., & Rubinstein, D. (1978). Frequency of sexual dysfunction in "normal" couples. *New England Journal of Medicine, 299,* 111–115.

Freund, K., McKnight, C. K., Langevin, R., & Cibiri, S. (1972). The female child as a surrogate object. *Archives of Sexual Behavior, 2,* 119–133.

Gutheil, T. G. (1989). Borderline personality disorder, boundary violations, and patient–therapist sex: Medicolegal pitfalls. *American Journal of Psychiatry, 146,* 597–602.

Hariton, E. B., & Singer, J. L. (1974). Women's fantasies during sexual intercourse. *Journal of Consulting and Clinical Psychology, 42,* 313–322.

Helzer, J. E., Clayton, P. J., Pambakian, R., Reich, T., Woodruff, R. A., & Reverley, M. A. (1977). Reliability of psychiatric diagnosis: II. *Archives of General Psychiatry, 34,* 136–141.

Helzer, J. E., Robins, L. N., McEvoy, L. T., Spitznagel, E. L., Stoltzman, R. K., Farmer, A., & Brockington, I. F. (1985). A comparison of clinical and diagnostic interview schedule diagnoses. *Archives of General Psychiatry, 42,* 657–666.

Kagan, J., & Moss, H. A. (1962). *Birth to maturity.* New York: John Wiley.

Karacan, I. (1978). Advances in the psychophysiological evaluation of male erectile impotence. In J. LoPiccolo & L. LoPiccolo (Eds.), *Handbook of sex therapy* (pp. 137–145). New York: Plenum Press.

Kelly, M. P., Strassberg, D. S., & Kircher, J. R. (1990). Attitudinal and experiential correlates of anorgasmia. *Archives of Sexual Behavior, 19,* 165–177.

Knight, R. A., & Prentky, R. A. (1990). Classifying sexual offenders. In W. L. Marshall, D. R. Laws, & H. E. Barbaree (Eds.), *Handbook of sexual assault* (pp. 23–52). New York: Plenum Press.

Lipman, R. S., Cole, J. O., Park, L. C., & Rickels, K. (1965). Sensitivity of symptom and nonsymptom-focused criteria of outpatient drug efficacy. *American Journal of Psychiatry, 122,* 24–27.

LoPiccolo, J. (1990). Sexual dysfunction. In A. S. Bellack, M. Hersen, & A. E. Kazdin (Eds.), *International handbook of behavior therapy and modification,* 2nd ed. (pp. 547–564). New York: Plenum Press.

Malamuth, N. M. (1989). The attraction of sexual aggression scale: Part two. *Journal of Sex Research, 26,* 324–354.

Maletzky, B. M. (1980). Assisted covert sensitization. In D. J. Cox & R. J. Daitzman (Eds.), *Exhibitionism: Description, assessment, and treatment* (pp. 289–293). New York: Garland STPM Press.

Matarazzo, J. D. (1983). The reliability of psychiatric and psychological diagnosis. *Clinical Psychology Review, 3,* 103–145.

McCombie, S. L., & Arons, J. H. (1980). Counselling rape victims. In S. L. McCombie (Ed.), *The rape crisis intervention handbook* (pp. 145–171). New York: Plenum Press.

McConaghy, N. (1988). Sexual dysfunction and deviation. In A. S. Bellack & M. Hersen (Eds.), *Behavioral assessment,* 3rd ed. (pp. 490–541). New York: Pergamon Press.

McConaghy, N. (1989a). Validity and ethics of penile circumference measures of sexual arousal: A critical review. *Archives of Sexual Behavior, 18,* 357–369.

McConaghy, N. (1989b). Psychosexual disorders. In L. K. G. Hsu & M. Hersen (Eds.), *Recent developments in adolescent psychiatry* (pp. 334–366). New York: John Wiley.

McConaghy, N. (1991). Sexual disorders. In M. Hersen & S. M. Turner (Eds.), *Adult psychopathology and diagnosis* (pp. 323–359). New York: John Wiley.

McConaghy, N. (1992). Validity and ethics of penile circumference measures of sexual arousal: A response. *Archives of Sexual Behavior, 21,* 187–195.

McConaghy, N. (1993). *Sexual behavior, problems, and management.* New York: Plenum Press.

McConaghy, N., Blaszczynski, A., & Kidson, W. (1988). Treatment of sex offenders with imaginal desensitization and/or medroxyprogesterone. *Acta Psychiatrica Scandinavica, 77,* 199–206.

McConaghy, N., & Zamir, R. (in press). Sissiness, tomboyism, sex role, identity and orientation. *Australian and New Zealand Journal of Psychiatry.*

McConaghy, N., Zamir, R., & Manicavasagar, V. (1993). Non-sexist sexual experiences survey and scale of attraction to sexual aggression. *Australian and New Zealand Journal of Psychiatry, 27,* 686–693.

Nelson, R. O., & Hayes, S. C. (1981). Nature of behavioral assessment. In A. S. Bellack & M. Hersen (Eds.), *Behavioral Assessment,* 2nd ed. (pp. 3–37). New York: Pergamon Press.

Osborn, M., Hawton, K., & Gath, D. (1988). Sexual dysfunctions among middle age women in the community. *British Medical Journal, 296,* 959–962.

Paredes, A., Baumgold, J., Pugh, L. A., & Ragland, R. (1966). Clinical judgment in the assessment of psychopharmacological effects. *Journal of Nervous and Mental Disease, 142,* 153–160.

Person, E. S., Terestman, N., Myers, W. A., Goldberg, E. L., & Salvadori, C. (1989). Gender differences in sexual behaviors and fantasies in a college population. *Journal of Sex and Marital Therapy, 15,* 187–198.

Reading, A. E. (1983). A comparison of the accuracy and reactivity of methods of monitoring male sexual behavior. *Journal of Behavioral Assessment, 5,* 11–23.

Rekers, G. A., & Lovaas, O. I. (1974). Behavioral treatment of deviant sex-role behavior in a male child. *Journal of Applied Behavioral Analysis, 7,* 173–190.

Robins, L. N., Helzer, J. E., Croughan, J., & Ratcliff, K. (1981). National Institute of Mental Health Diagnostic Interview Schedule: Its history, characteristics and validity. *Archives of General Psychiatry, 38,* 381–389.

Robins, L. N., Helzer, J. E., Weissman, M. M., Orvaschel, H., Gruenberg, E., Burke, J. D., & Regier, D. A. (1984). Lifetime prevalence of specific psychiatric disorders in three sites. *Archives of General Psychiatry, 41,* 949–958.

Schatzberg, A. F., Westfall, M. P., Blumetti, A. B., & Birk, C. L. (1975). Effeminacy 1: A quantitative rating scale. *Archives of Sexual Behavior, 4,* 31–41.

Schiavi, R. C., Derogatis, L. R., Kuriansky, J., O'Connor, D., & Sharpe, I. (1979). The assessment of sexual function and marital interaction. *Journal of Sex and Marital Therapy, 5,* 169–224.

Segraves, R. T., Schoenberg, H. W., & Segraves, K. A. B. (1985). Evaluation of the etiology of erectile failure. In R. T. Segraves & H. W. Schoenberg (Eds.), *Diagnosis and treatment of erectile disturbances* (pp. 165–195). New York: Plenum Press.

Slag, M. F., Morley, J. E., Elson, M. K., Trence, D. L., Nelson, C. J., Nelson, A. E., Kinlaw, W. B., Beyer, H. S., Nuttall, F. Q., & Shafer, R. B. (1983). Impotence in medical clinic outpatients. *Journal of the American Medical Association, 249,* 1736–1740.

Snyder, D. K., & Berg, P. (1983). Determinants of sexual dissatisfaction in sexually distressed couples. *Archives of Sexual Behavior, 12,* 237–246.

Spector, I. P., & Carey, M. P. (1990). Incidence and prevalence of the sexual dysfunctions: A critical review of the empirical literature. *Archives of Sexual Behavior, 19,* 389–408.

Spitzer, R. L., Williams, J. B. W., Gibbon, M., & First, M. B. (1990). *Structured Clinical Interview for DSM-III-R.* Washington, DC: American Psychiatric Press.

Strassberg, D. S., Mahoney, J. M., Schaugaard, M., & Hale, V. E. (1990). The role of anxiety in premature ejaculation: A psychophysiological model. *Archives of Sexual Behavior, 19,* 251–268.

Taylor, C. B., Agras, W. S., Schneider, J. A., & Allen, R. A. (1983). Adherence to instructions to practice relaxation exercises. *Journal of Consulting and Clinical Psychology, 51,* 952–953.

Templeman, T. L., & Stinnett, R. D. (1991). Patterns of sexual arousal and history in a "normal" sample of young men. *Archives of Sexual Behavior, 20,* 137–150.

van den Brink, W., Koeter, M. W. J., Ormel, J., Dijkstra, W., Giel, R., Slooff, C. J., & Wohlfarth, T. D. (1989). Psychiatric diagnosis in an outpatient population. *Archives of General Psychiatry, 46,* 369–372.

Walling, M., Andersen, B. L., & Johnson, S. R. (1990). Hormonal replacement therapy for postmenopausal women: A review of sexual outcomes and related gynecologic effects. *Archives of Sexual Behavior, 19,* 119–137.

Wasserman, M. D., Pollack, C. P., Spielman, A. J., & Weitzman, E. D. (1980). Theoretical and technical problems in the measurement of nocturnal penile tumescence for the differential diagnosis of impotence. *Psychosomatic Medicine, 42,* 575–585.

Wincze, J. P., Bansal, S., & Malamud, M. (1986). Effects of medroxyprogesterone acetate on subjective arousal, arousal to erotic stimulation, and nocturnal penile tumescence in male sex offenders. *Archives of Sexual Behavior, 15,* 293–305.

Wing, J. K., & Sturt, E. (1978). *The PSE-ID-Catego system: Supplementary manual.* London: MRC Social Psychiatry Unit.

Wyatt, G. E., & Peters, S. D. (1986). Issues in the definition of child sexual abuse in prevalence research. *Child Abuse and Neglect, 10,* 231–240.

10

Eating Disorders

JOHN P. FOREYT AND G. KEN GOODRICK

DESCRIPTION OF THE DISORDERS

The disorders of anorexia nervosa and bulimia nervosa are referred to as *eating disorders* because the most observable symptoms involve pathological binging, purging, and self-starvation. These disorders may develop as the result of developmental processes that cause the patient to place undue importance on physical appearance as a way to obtain love and to feel in control. The emphasis on appearance is part of our modern culture and is often reinforced by parents, especially mothers. The need to obtain love may have been exaggerated by the patient having been a member of a rigid or nondemonstrative family. The need for control may have been exaggerated by the emphasis on control in a rigid family or by the inability to control other aspects of life due to a dysfunctional family.

The resulting focus on appearance leads to a fear of becoming fat. Along with this fear, a distorted body image may develop, so that the patients perceive themselves to be fatter than they really are. The fear of fat and body image distortion usually leads to dieting. Dieting may lead to binging. Binging may lead to obesity with binging (binge eating disorder) or to a more normal weight with binging and purging (bulimia nervosa). Some dieters may be able to achieve a state of self-starvation with some binging (anorexia nervosa).

Thus, while observable eating and purging behaviors remain objective criteria for diagnosis, the dynamics of the disorder involve self-esteem and body image. To complicate matters, the pathological behaviors may alter physiological functions, which in turn may affect emotional and cognitive functioning. Thus, while interviewers will want to uncover the diagnostic criteria, they should keep in mind the dynamics of the disorder so that the behavioral, cognitive, affective, and social manifestations of the disorder can be put into a conceptual whole. An awareness of the underlying dynamics of eating disorders will also help the interviewer to establish the rapport needed to motivate the patient to reveal the aspects of eating

JOHN P. FOREYT AND G. KEN GOODRICK • Nutrition Research Clinic, Baylor College of Medicine, Houston, Texas 77030.

Diagnostic Interviewing (Second Edition), edited by Michel Hersen and Samuel M. Turner. Plenum Press, New York, 1994.

disorders that involve feelings of shame and self-disgust. A comprehensive conceptualization will help form the treatment strategy and must be gradually communicated to the patient as part of the therapeutic process.

This chapter will concentrate on anorexia nervosa, bulimia nervosa, and "binge eating disorder," the last of which has been proposed for DSM-IV (American Psychiatric Association, 1993) under the category "Eating disorder not otherwise specified."

Anorexia Nervosa

Of the three disorders described in this chapter, anorexia nervosa is the one most noted for its severe course and consequences. It is the eating disorder that can result in death, most often from the complications arising from the state of starvation.

Anorexia nervosa is a perplexing condition, for its most notable characteristic is self-imposed starvation in a country and culture blessed with an abundance of food. However, for anorectics, the apparent illogic of their actions is overridden by a psychological framework ruled by two powerful contingencies: the reward of weight loss and a morbid fear of fatness (Garner, Garfinkel, & Bemis, 1982).

The DSM-IV (APA, 1993) diagnostic criteria for anorexia nervosa are presented in Table 1. Anorectics of the binge/eating purging type tend to be heavier, with more lability of mood, impulsivity, and drug abuse.

There is an increased comorbidity of the affective and anxiety disorders with anorexia nervosa, and alcoholism and other psychiatric diagnoses including eating disorders are more likely in first-degree relatives (Halmi et al., 1991). Additional symptomatology includes low metabolic rate, low blood pressure, cold intolerance, insomnia, bradycardia, pathological EEG patterns, alopecia, and dry skin (Bemis, 1978; Williamson, 1990).

TABLE 1.   DSM-IV Diagnostic Criteria for Anorexia Nervosa[a]

A. Refusal to maintain body weight at or above a minimally normal weight for age and height (e.g., weight loss leading to maintenance of body weight less than 85% of that expected; or failure to make expected weight gain during period of growth, leading to body weight less than 85% of that expected.

B. Intense fear of gaining weight or becoming fat, even though underweight.

C. Disturbance in the way in which one's body weight or shape is experienced; undue influence of body weight or shape on self-evaluation, or denial of the seriousness of the current low body weight.

D. In postmenarchal females, amenorrhea, i.e., the absence of at least three consecutive menstrual cycles. (A woman is considered to have amenorrhea if her periods occur only following hormone, e.g., estrogen, administration.)

Specify type:

Restricting type: During the episode of anorexia nervosa, the person does not regularly engage in binge eating or purging behavior (i.e., self-induced vomiting or the misuse of laxatives or diuretics).

Binge eating/purging type: During the episode of anorexia nervosa, the person regularly engages in binge eating or purging behavior (i.e., self-induced vomiting or the misuse of laxatives or diuretics).

[a]From American Psychiatric Association (1993).

It is notable that 95% of anorectics are female (American Psychiatric Association, 1987). Such disproportionate representation of females indicates the strong cultural influences in its etiology (Brownell, 1991). In the United States and many of the other Western nations, slenderness has become synonymous with attractiveness, and it is apparent that the achievement of both is an expectation more of women than of men.

A number of psychological traits characterize the anorectic, including shyness, anxiety, and obsessive–compulsive behaviors (Bemis, 1978). These characteristics, although the source of much inner turmoil, are frequently manifested in outward behaviors that are viewed positively by family and friends. In many families, the presymptomatic anorexic child is frequently perceived as the pride and joy of the brood, often characterized by parents as being well-behaved, high-achieving, and perfectionistic (Halmi, Goldberg, Eckert, Casper, & Davis, 1977). Some authors (e.g., Bruch, 1978; Rosman, Minuchin, Baker, & Liebman, 1977), however, suggest that many of the anorectic traits are engendered by the particular interactional patterns and values of the families involved. Bruch (1977) noted that among anorectic families, parents tended to be overprotective, overconcerned, and overambitious. Within this setting, she noted that expectations of obedience and superior performance of the children were a concomitant observation.

Other psychological characteristics associated with anorexia included distorted thoughts and beliefs (Garner et al., 1982), distorted body image (Crisp & Kalucy, 1974), and fears about matters of self-control (Bruch, 1977). These characteristics, in combination with the familial setting, peer influences, particular experiences, and even the child's physiology, may lead to anorexia nervosa.

Bulimia Nervosa

In recent years, bulimia nervosa has gained increasing attention as the extent of its occurrence and the severity of its symptomatology have become known. Although bulimia is literally translated to mean *ox hunger*, for most who have this condition, their eating has little association with the fulfillment of normal biological hunger. Binging seems to be more a result of voluntary dietary restriction and distorted perceptions of body size and the need to have a perfect body. The purging behavior is learned as a way to rid the body of excess calories from a binge; however, purging and subsequent dietary restriction lead to the next binge, thus continuing the vicious cycle.

The DSM-IV (APA, 1993) diagnostic criteria for bulimia nervosa are presented in Table 2.

Data from available literature and a survey of professionals concerned with eating disorders failed to show a requirement for rapid consumption of food during a binge, or a requirement that the binge consist of a large amount of food, or that the minimal binge frequency in criterion C (Table 2) be met before a diagnosis of bulimia nervosa was made (Wilson, 1992). Thus, bulimics may binge slowly, a "binge" may consist of only a few potato chips, and binging may occur only once per week. The important psychological factors of feeling that the eating was out of control, that the food was "forbidden," and the resulting purging response seem to be the critical features for the diagnosis. These variations from

Table 2.   DSM-IV Diagnostic Criteria for Bulimia Nervosa[a]

A. Recurrent episodes of binge eating. An episode of binge eating is characterized by both of the following:
  1. Eating, in a discrete period of time (e.g., within any 2-hour period), an amount of food that is definitely larger than most people would eat during a similar period of time and under similar circumstances.
  2. A sense of lack of control over eating during the episode (e.g., a feeling that one cannot stop eating or control what or how much one is eating).
B. Recurrent inappropriate compensatory behavior in order to prevent weight gain, such as: self-induced vomiting; misuse of laxatives, diuretics, or other medications; fasting; or excessive exercise.
C. The binge eating and inappropriate compensatory behaviors both occur, on average, at least twice a week for 3 months.
D. Self-evaluation is unduly influenced by body shape and weight.
E. The disturbance does not occur exclusively during episodes of anorexia nervosa.
Specify type:
  Purging type: The person regularly engages in self-induced vomiting or the misuse of laxatives or diuretics.
  Nonpurging type: The person uses other inappropriate compensatory behaviors, such as fasting or excessive exercise, but does not regularly engage in self-induced vomiting or the misuse of laxatives or diuretics.

[a]From American Psychiatric Association (1993).

bulimia nervosa are listed under "Eating disorder not otherwise specified" in DSM-IV (APA, 1993).

There is controversy as to whether the modality of purging is more important diagnostically than the psychological motivation to rid one's body of calories. For example, a patient of ours habitually "corrected" her binge episodes with 20-mile bike rides. The excursions were marked by their compulsive and urgent quality; they sometimes occurred at odd hours in the morning, during inclement weather, or even during the course of a social gathering. This patient was revulsed by the idea of vomiting, but she nevertheless had an extreme purgative reaction to binging.

Bulimia, like anorexia nervosa, is a problem primarily of young women. In this regard, it is probable that some of the sociocultural dynamics that result in anorexia operate to influence the onset of bulimia. White and Boskind-White (1981) theorized that this condition occurs because of the need for some women to fit into the role of "stereotyped femininity." In fulfilling this stereotyping, these researchers suggest, the basis for bulimia is also developed and reinforced; this basis includes a need to please others, tendencies toward passivity, and an excessive concern for appearance and thinness.

The physical toll taken by the practice of bulimia is not so great as the one experienced by the anorexic; however, it can be severe. Among the physical sequelae are esophageal rupture and hiatal hernias from frequent vomiting, urinary infections, impaired kidney function, irregular menstrual cycles, dental problems, electrolyte disturbances, and metabolic and endocrine changes (Neuman & Halvorson, 1983; Mitchell, Specker, & de Zwaan, 1991). Because many bulimics maintain a normal weight and appear healthy, the damage done by their compulsion often goes unrecognized, even by the closest of contacts, until medical intervention is required.

For most bulimics, there is a psychological cost of their practice that parallels the physical ones. Our culture promotes standards of acceptable behavior concerning ingestion and elimination (including vomiting). Bulimic behavior, with its sometimes prodigious consumption and forced elimination, crosses the boundaries of acceptability. Most who engage in this practice are exceedingly aware of its unacceptability; some are ashamed of it. Such awareness is associated with the low self-esteem, feelings of inadequacy, and self-derogation observed among many. The shame that accompanies this practice is probably the primary reason this problem remained in the closet for so long and continues to remain there for many sufferers.

Binge Eating Disorder

Some individuals have problems with recurrent binge eating, but do not engage in compensatory vomiting or use of laxatives. In recognition of this disorder, the proposed DSM-IV (APA, 1993) draft criteria include Binge Eating Disorder, as an "otherwise unspecified" eating disorder, with the following criteria: recurrent episodes of binge eating in the absence of the inappropriate compensatory behaviors characteristic of bulimia nervosa.

About 2% of the general population, and about one third of those presenting for weight control treatment, may have this disorder, which is more common in females and is associated with severity of obesity and a history of marked weight fluctuations (Spitzer et al., 1992). The diagnostic criteria indicate that this disorder shares the same psychodynamics found in bulimia nervosa. Research is needed to determine what the differences are; perhaps the distinction is that one group learned to purge as a successful weight-control strategy, while the other failed to learn this coping method, or is revulsed by regurgitation.

Overview of Conditions

The diagnostic interview process will want to touch on the specific criteria set forth in DSM-IV to achieve an official diagnosis. While probing for specifics, the interviewer should keep in mind the psychological themes of eating disorders. These themes may involve:

1. The extreme fear of being fat, or the disgust at being fat.
2. Low self-esteem exacerbated by a hypercritical body image, and failure to control eating habits and weight.
3. The belief that self-worth hinges on bodily appearance.
4. The perceived blocks to developing interpersonal relationships due to negative self-image; the feeling of isolation associated with eating disorders.
5. The intrapunitive nature of exercise and other abusive purging techniques; the feeling that self-punishment is deserved for failure to control eating or weight.

Procedures for Gathering Information

Our procedure for gathering information is generally to incorporate this process into treatment as naturally and comfortably as possible. The initial meeting has more of the elements of an interview than subsequent ones. It is not our general practice to use structured scales or questionnaires. Issues suspected to have relevance to the client's eating problem are explored and investigated. Their validity is determined by the manner in which the client is affected (i.e., "treatment validity"); if they bring insight or change or both, then relevance is verified.

The multifactorial etiology of eating disorders often requires a multidisciplinary approach to treatment. In such cases, it is important for the therapist to be aware of the diagnoses of the other caregivers involved, as they may have relevance. For example, in anorexia nervosa, weight must be returned to a medically determined minimum before effective work can begin on the psychological issues (Bruch, 1973). In cases of bulimia, the client may seek psychotherapeutic help without prior consultation with a physician. It is incumbent on the therapist to insist on medical examination early in treatment as well as during its course if any form of purging is involved. As indicated previously, the continual practice of vomiting and abuse of diuretics or laxatives can lead to serious physical consequences. Our experience has been that the participation of a physician and dietitian is essential in the treatment of an eating disorder. An exercise physiologist is also needed to prescribe sensible exercise.

It is not our expectation that the initial diagnostic meeting (usually the first treatment session) will reveal much of the client's difficulties. Eating disorders and the associated practices (e.g., vomiting) are considered aberrant in our society, and most clients are acutely aware of this proscription. Thus, it is common for information to be purposely withheld, "forgotten," or distorted in the early interviews. This pattern is especially typical of anorectics, who frequently deny the existence of a problem and do not see the necessity for their presence in treatment. Obtaining accurate information is a *process* based on many of the factors that make for effective treatment: a good therapeutic relationship, trust, and the client's sense that the therapist is working with and for his or her benefit. We find that as our relationship with the client solidifies, the diagnostic picture becomes concurrently richer.

Considering the shame involved in these disorders, it may be helpful with a female patient if the interviewer is a female who has had personal experience with eating disorders and can self-disclose that fact. At least the interviewer can reveal that she has at times overeaten after being on a diet and felt somewhat out of control at times. She might also discuss how vomiting brings a feeling of relief in the case of stomach flu, and how she can understand how this can become a habit.

Sensitivity is another important aspect of the process of diagnosis. The therapist needs to be aware of the client's sensitive areas in probing for information and, at times, be willing to delay seeking the information until readiness on the client's part is apparent. A good example of this necessity occurs with the use of food records. Although we find food records to be invaluable tools for diagnosis and treatment, some react to our use of them with considerable resistance. Food records require individuals to document patterns that they have frequently denied or suppressed. Their accurate utilization would be tantamount to a personal confrontation with the problem. The therapist needs to be aware of the client's readiness for such confrontation in suggesting the use of food records.

A particularly sensitive area for many patients is that of the effect their disturbed eating patterns and real or imagined body image have on their sexual relations. A recent patient of ours, Beth, had lost a substantial amount of weight in treatment and found that one of its concomitants was a deteriorating relationship with her husband. Symptomatic of this deterioration was his growing sexual impotence. This problem, needless to say, created stress in both parties. In terms of Beth and her treatment, these occurrences were viewed in terms of their possible utilization as a rationale for returning to the prior state (i.e., overweight and disordered eating). From the standpoint of diagnosis, Beth revealed these problems and saw their possible pertinence to treatment.

As implied in the example of Beth, we feel that diagnosis and treatment need to occur with the active involvement of both therapist and client. Clients often enter therapy with a perspective that they will be treated and that their role is essentially passive. Our approach is to emphasize the clients' active role: that they can find the bases of their problems and make the necessary changes and that the control is in their hands as much as it is in the therapist's hands. Bruch (1973) conveyed a similar thought when she noted (p. 338):

> For effective treatment, it is decisive that a patient experience himself as an active participant in the therapeutic process. If there are things to be uncovered and interpreted, it is important that the patient makes the discovery on his own and has a chance to say it first.

If clients are to be participants in the diagnostic process, they need to be taught that they *can* do this, and they need to be shown *how*. Thus, we see part of our role in treatment as educators. Much treatment time is spent helping our clients understand their disorders, the many things that can influence their occurrence, and the importance of their collaborative involvement. This education is eclectic and is oriented to the disorder and individual. Some of the things we have used include bibliotherapy, modeling, role-playing, and problem-solving methodologies.

CASE ILLUSTRATIONS

Case 1

Linda is an attractive, normal-weight 32-year-old female employed at a temporary services agency. She is living with her husband Bill, an accountant who has little understanding of or tolerance for the psychology of eating disorders. He apparently has no ability to express warmth or sympathy for her problem. When Linda came to her first session, she was binging and purging about 5 times per week. Binges were quite variable in amount, and purging consisted of vomiting, taking 10 or more laxative and stool softener pills each day, and engaging in at least 2 hours a day of intense aerobic exercise and swimming.

Linda's father was an alcoholic who verbally abused her. She had very traumatic dating experiences in high school and had dabbled in drugs and alcohol after graduating. Her self-esteem was near zero. She had two small children and felt very guilty about being an inadequate mother.

The following are extracts from her initial interviews:

T: What is the main reason you have come to this clinic?

P: Well, I guess it's because I'm too fat.

T: What parts of your body are too fat?

P: My legs are really too thick. I am wearing loose pants. If you could see my legs, you would see the legs of an elephant. [Her legs appear normal.]

T: How did your legs get thick? Have they always been thick? [Therapist leads the patient to elaborate on body image distortion.]

P: Ever since I was a teenager. They got thick because I eat too much. I can't stop eating.

T: What do you mean, you can't stop eating? [Explore sense of lack of control.]

P: Well, when I am home by myself I get to eating whatever I can find. Like a bag of potato chips or any leftover food in the fridge. Once I get going, I really look for all the food I can find that can be eaten.

T: Don't you stop eating when you are full?

P: I really don't realize I am full, my eating just keeps going until I just can't eat any more. I worry about choking to death.

T: What do you do after you eat all you can?

P: For a few minutes, I just seem to blank out mentally. Then I go to the bathroom.

T: What do you do in the bathroom?

P: You know, I get rid of it.

T: Get rid of the food? [Not probing for intimate details of method at this early stage.]

P: Yes.

T: How do you feel then?

P: I feel weak, but I'm glad the food didn't stay in my body.

T: So without getting rid of the food you would be fat, given the amount of food you eat?

P: I can't imagine how fat I would be. Like the fat lady of the circus.

T: But you feel your legs are too fat? [Probe for body image.]

P: Yes. I wish I could just take a knife and carve them down to decent size. They have fat surgery now for that, don't they?

• • •

T: Tell me about your last problem with food.

P: I was at a restaurant. I was having a salad with nonfat dressing since I really can't eat any fat in my food. [dietary rigidity] My neighbor was with me and she told me to try a bite of her apple turnover because she said it was so good. So I did.

T: What happened then?

P: I started to feel nauseous right away. I could feel the fat from that turnover inside my throat and I could see in my mind's eye the fatty food in my stomach. It was like I swallowed a spider, something I wanted to get rid of right away, so I went to the restroom and did it.

T: Did you feel O.K. after getting rid of it?

P: No, of course not. I knew I was getting out of control in my eating since I had eaten the turnover. So I went home and jogged slowly in the park for about 1 hour. I think the calories from 1 hour of jogging would burn up the turnover. I need to jog to get back into control.

T: You must be in really good shape to be able to jog for an hour.

P: I guess so. But I plan to increase my jogs to 2 hours on weekends because I think that will help burn up the fat on my legs. I see marathon runners and they have nice legs, I mean the women who run all the time.

Case 2

Karen is a 24-year-old female who came into treatment for bulimia. She had been married for 2 years to Dennis, a 27-year-old attorney. Her bulimia had become increasingly worse during the past year, and she had become frightened. Her husband called to make the appointment and accompanied her to the first session. Karen was later seen individually in therapy, and a pattern became increasingly clear. After graduating from college, Karen took a job as a filing clerk at a large oil company at her father's insistence. She was still in the same job when we began meeting. She was clearly overqualified, hated it, but she had not attempted to leave. Second, Karen had been a skilled organist at her local church, where she was respected and in great demand on Sundays and for special occasions. She also had many close friends there. When she married, her husband insisted that she join his church, one of Houston's largest, where he was deacon and active on many church committees. Because the church had many talented organists, she played only once there in almost 2 years. Third, Dennis's mother, who lived close by, called or visited daily. Her calls were frequently like, "Put Channel 13 on right now. There's a program I want you to see," or, "Look at the advertisement on page 6 of today's paper. There is a dress there you should buy."

T: These examples we have been discussing over the past few sessions seem to be related.

P: I have not seen the connection previously, but it is as if I do not have any control over my life any more.

T: Tell me more about that.

P: Well, my father got me my job which I cannot stand, but I seem to be afraid to leave. I attend my husband's church and no longer play the organ, which I love to do. My husband's mother tells me what I should watch, read, and wear. Who is running my life? About the only part of my life I control is my weight, by binging and purging.

Through problem-solving and some assertive training, Karen decided to change jobs, attend her husband's church once a month with him and play the organ at her church the rest of the time, and take a more direct stance with her mother-in-law. With the control shifted to Karen, her bulimia decreased dramatically.

STANDARDIZED INTERVIEW FORMATS

Structured interview formats ensure that all the diagnostic criteria are covered in an orderly fashion during the interview process. This structure is important for research projects and may be necessary in clinics with a large volume of patients and limited resources. The Eating Disorder Examination (EDE; Cooper & Fairburn, 1987) consists of 62 items asking about symptoms of bulimia over the preceding 4 weeks. This instrument was designed more for assessing therapeutic progress than for detailed initial diagnosis.

The Interview for Diagnosis of Eating Disorders (IDED; Williamson, 1990) was designed to evaluate the core psychopathology of bulimia nervosa, anorexia nervosa, and obesity. It also assesses diagnostic criteria proposed by Williamson (1990) for "compulsive overeating," which is similar to binge eating disorder. This instrument covers historical, medical, and family information as well as current behavior and cognitions regarding eating and food. The IDED has rating scales for each disorder, which allow the evaluator to rate each DSM-IV symptom on a 7-point scale.

Information Critical to Making the Diagnosis

Strong evidence suggests that the eating disorders are influenced by physiological factors, familial food habits, sociocultural influences, self-perception, familial interaction patterns, and emotional status. The following discussion highlights information that we, from our research and experience, consider important in the diagnosis of eating disorders. This information is applicable to all the eating disorders, though the extent of applicability may differ with the disorder and individual.

Prior to an elaboration of *what* is required for diagnosis, a reiteration of the *how* of this process is important. For some patients, there is considerable shame, guilt, and pain associated with their problem. In this regard, the revelation of the particulars of their difficulty is often an emotionally trying task. Hence, we feel that sensitivity and tentativeness are essential in obtaining information. No information is worth risking the impairment of the therapeutic relationship. Information is obtained most readily and comfortably when it is obtained in the context of therapy, and not apart from it. That is, inquiries regarding behavior, interpersonal relationships, and feelings are made as part of a treatment session when appropriateness is obvious and the client is judged ready.

Medical and Physical Status

For almost all the eating disorders, the point of departure for treatment is information concerning the state of the client's physical health. As noted earlier, the practices regularly engaged in by some clients can cause varying degrees of physical damage and even death. Therefore, medical assessment is a necessary first step to ensure the client's physical welfare. In cases in which the disorder has severe physical ramifications, it is highly recommended that periodic medical evaluation be incorporated into the treatment plan. It should be noted that the individual's physical appearance may belie the physiological imbalances that are not always obvious. Many bulimics maintain a normal weight while in the throes of extensive purging practices. The electrolyte imbalances that result from this behavior may not become observable until clients have fallen into a severe state of distress.

In anorexia nervosa, the client's physical condition is sometimes intimately associated with readiness for therapy. If the disorder has progressed to its more advanced stages, the consequences of the starvation will make any attempts at therapy fruitless. Such clients must achieve a medically prescribed weight and strength before such efforts can begin.

Because of the potentially severe consequences of anorexia, we suggest that treatment of a client begin even if all the diagnostic criteria have not been met. In particular, the criterion of 15% below expected weight (APA, 1987) must be viewed with flexibility. For some clients, original body weight represents a degree of overweight; for others, normal or even underweight. In the latter cases, 15–20% weight loss may yield severe emaciation.

Who Wants the Treatment?

This question is an important one in processes that require personal change. When treatment has been sought by the *client*, the motivation implied provides the basis for effective therapeutic work. On the other hand, when the impetus for treatment derives from another, greater difficulties can be expected. This difficulty is typified in anorexia, in which it is frequently the case that the client is brought to treatment by concerned parents. The client is generally unable to comprehend the existence of a problem and is therefore disinclined to enter treatment.

The matter of who wants the treatment is most problematic in cases of binge eating disorder with obesity. We occasionally find that a client has come for treatment because of the insistence or at least strong encouragement of another. The source of this encouragement is often the family physician, spouse, or close relative. In such instances, the matter of client motivation is explored in detail at the beginning of treatment. If it is apparent that the client does not desire treatment, it is usually recommended that treatment be delayed until a more appropriate time.

Behavior

Behaviors are the external manifestation of the eating disorder; their nature and frequency largely define the severity of the problem. Examples of these behaviors include binge eating, vomiting, limited food intake, excessive exercise, and strange food-related rituals (e.g., order of food consumption, insistence on a specific place setting, lists of forbidden foods, and regular departures to the bathroom after meals). It is helpful for both diagnosis and treatment that such behaviors be quantified. By so doing, the client and therapist have a baseline with which to compare later progress.

For the nonhospitalized client, self-report is the only practical way to obtain information on behavior. This self-reporting can be done through use of either food records or a short-term dietary and behavioral recall. It is our preference to use food records, though both techniques have value. Because of the sensitive nature of these behaviors, we place no insistence on these records if the client shows resistance to their completion.

The client's behavioral patterns may assist in the development of a more specific definition of the disorder and enhance the possibility of using appropriate interventions. This usefulness of behavioral patterns is exemplified by the bulimic and nonbulimic variations of anorexia. Some investigators defined a *bulimic anorectic* as an anorectic who purged. Strober (1981), however, studied the etiology of bulimia in anorexia nervosa and found significant differences. Primarily, his results indicated that the family life of the bulimic anorexic is more tumultuous, conflict-ridden, and negative in comparison to that of the nonbulimic. Bulimics also seem to have greater tendencies to impulsive behaviors: drug use, alcoholism, stealing, and self-mutilation (Casper, Eckert, Halmi, Goldberg, & Davis, 1980; Garfinkel, Moldofsky, & Garner, 1980; Wilson, 1991). In contrast to the typical view of the anorectic as introverted, the bulimic variation is likely to be more socially and sexually active (Casper et al., 1980; Johnson, 1982; Russell, 1979). The symptom complexes that differentiate the bulimic and nonbulimic anorectic suggest disorders of substantially different etiological and psychological nature.

There appears to be a significant comorbidity of the affective and anxiety disorders with anorexia nervosa (Halmi et al., 1991). Although personality disorders, especially borderline personality disorder, have been thought to be associated with bulimia nervosa, the relationship is not clear, since personality trait scores may change so that an Axis II diagnosis cannot be made after treatment for bulimia (Ames-Frankel et al., 1992).

Cognitive and Emotional Factors

Most, if not all, who suffer from an eating disorder have a structure of dysfunctional cognitions that exists in association with their aberrant eating behaviors. It is our view that many of the emotional difficulties encountered by clients derive from distorted cognitive processes (Beck, 1976; Ellis, 1979). Thus, assessment of the predominant thought patterns and the factors that lead to their development is important in the understanding and subsequent treatment of the problem.

Body image in anorexia is one of the most powerful examples of how distorted cognitions can influence the cause and course of an eating disorder. The anorectic perceives her body as too large regardless of how thin she becomes (Warah, 1989). Because this distortion of perception does not diminish with weight loss, it persists as a relentless incentive. Bruch (1973) noted that this disorder is not "cured" until the body image misperception has been corrected, even if substantial weight gain has been achieved in therapy.

Examples of cognitive distortions have been reported for anorexia nervosa (Garner et al., 1982), binge eating (Loro & Orleans, 1981), and obesity (Mahoney & Mahoney, 1976). We have found that certain of these distortions are present in all eating disorders, indicating the possibility of a cultural pattern gone awry. In some, for example, staunch perfectionism is the cause of much distress and sometimes failure. These individuals proceed with substantial success on a diet until the first infraction occurs, no matter how minor. The inability to maintain a perfect record sends many into a binge that ends with self-recrimination and guilt. Perfectionism in the anorexic takes on an even more extreme form. Some carry this trait in all aspects of their life as well as in their anorexia. As indicated earlier, parents often characterize the ill child as the "perfect one."

Familial Factors

The eating disorders are the products of multiple influences. One of the most important influences is the family, for it has impact on the individual's development of self-concept, values, food and eating patterns, and personal standards. Specific ways in which the family may have impact on the eating disorders have been suggested by various clinicians and theorists (e.g., Bruch, 1973, 1977; Rosman et al., 1977; White & Boskind-White, 1981; Pike & Rodin, 1991).

The therapist needs to find patterns of interactions and behaviors that appear to have relation to the client's difficulties. The works of Bruch (1973) and Rosman et al. (1977) provide insight into the characteristics of the obese and anorexic families. Of the two, the latter has been the subject of more research, and therefore more is known. Research on the familial factors associated with bulimia has been sparse. In a clinical investigation, Strober (1981) reported a number of significant differences between families of bulimic and nonbulimic anorectics. Families of bulimics, in comparison to those of nonbulimics, were found to have less structure, less cohesion, and more conflict and negativity.

In cases in which the client remains in the care of the parents, diagnosis and treatment of the entire family is frequently necessary. A child or adolescent is little able to discern the familial complexities that have contributed to the problem, much less change them. For adults with an eating disorder, diagnosis of possible family contributions to causation is integral to treatment, though their direct involvement is determined on an individual basis.

Social Factors

For many who have an eating disorder, social factors have association to both the etiology and the perpetuation of their problem. From a sociocultural perspective, eating disorders are likely to be a product of contemporary American society (i.e., a society that places inordinate value on slimness while simultaneously emphasizing the consumption of our abundant food supply). At the personal level, these societal traits are translated into interpersonal transactions that lead the susceptible into an eating disorder. For many of the youthful, the most important social influence is the family, but others are important as well.

In some cases of bulimia, for example, the idea of purging is obtained from an acquaintance or friend as an action to avoid the consequences of excessive eating. For the susceptible, it begins as a logical and apparently socially acceptable way to have your cake and eat it too. Unfortunately, this rather innocent beginning can progress into a disturbing, all-encompassing compulsion. For anorectics, it is not unusual to find that their social activities or work or both have association to their disorder. Those involved in ballet, gymnastics, modeling, or cheerleading seem to have particular pressures to maintain sylphlike figures. A local high school, for example, has eligibility requirements for the cheerleading squad that include rather stringent height–weight standards.

One of the phenomena we frequently observe with individuals who suffer from an eating disorder is difficulty with interpersonal relationships. Among bulimics, problems in this area are the frequent cause of a binge. For obese young children, their self-imposed isolation impedes their social development. Lacking the rewards of social interaction, some may seek solace in a way that only exacerbates their problem: eating. The ways in which social factors may contribute to an eating disorder are varied and often complex. Discerning them is an important part of the diagnostic process.

DO'S AND DON'T'S

Do try to lessen the stigma of eating disorders so that the patient may be more willing to disclose symptomatology. This can be done by explaining the prevalence of eating disorders in the population, by explaining how eating disorders are caused by unrealistic cultural norms for body shape and size, and the mistaken idea that diets are effective in weight management, and by self-disclosure. For example:

T: I understand that you are here because you feel out of control in your eating. How do you feel about this problem?

P: I guess I have an addictive personality. I am the kind of person who can't control myself.

T: Almost every patient tells me what you have just said. But I want you to know that there are hundreds of thousands of people in this country who have exactly the same problem that you have. The problem is caused by the body's natural response to dieting. If you try to breathe really shallowly for a long time, soon you will be gasping uncontrollably for air. Would you blame yourself, or feel like you had an "air addiction?"

P: You mean, if I gasped for air after breathing shallowly?

T: Yes.

P: No, I guess not, since anybody would gasp for air.

T: O.K. So you shouldn't blame yourself for "gasping for food" after being on a diet, right?

P: I guess not.

· · ·

T: One thing you need to realize is that you dieted because there is a widespread belief that dieting works to control weight. So you shouldn't blame yourself for dieting. I mean, everybody does it. But now we know that almost everyone who develops an eating disorder, a problem with controlled eating, has a history of serious dieting. Scientists are fairly sure that this is caused by physiological processes, not psychological. In other words, you shouldn't blame yourself for dieting, and once you have dieted, you shouldn't blame yourself for your eating-control problems. Now our task is to find out all about your eating control problems so that we can help you do what you need to do to change those physiological processes so you can eat normally.

· · ·

T: I should tell you that I have never been officially diagnosed with an eating disorder, but I *can* tell you that sometimes when I have to skip breakfast, and have a hectic day at work, that sometimes when I go home I really pig out on bad stuff, like pizza and chips. And I should know better, since I am the doctor! So I think I have some of the symptoms of eating disorder, but not quite as serious as most people who come in to the clinic. But I can identify with what you are going through. I mean, I am like you in some ways. You know, we're all in the same boat as women trying to cope with the weird ideas about what we should look like and what we should eat in this society!

Don't imply that the patient may have an eating disorder because of some unresolved past sexual trauma, such as incest. There is no evidence for such causality (Pope & Hudson, 1992; Waller, 1991), and bringing up such subjects in the evaluation phase may only add to the patient's burden of guilt and shame associated with eating disorders. It may be best to stick to cultural/physiological explanations of eating disorders and let patients reveal any history of abuse later in therapy.

Don't reinforce the notion that the patient has a disease and that family members will be consulted to help the patient. In eating disorders, it may be best to explain the problem as a cultural/physiological problem in which the patient and family members are equally involved as victims.

SUMMARY

The diagnosis of eating disorders is far more complex than simply checking the criteria listed in the *Diagnostic and Statistical Manual of Mental Disorders*. Their complex nature, multiple etiologies, family dynamics, and highly refractory nature make them exceedingly challenging clinical problems.

ACKNOWLEDGMENT.   Preparation of this manuscript was supported in part by Grant 1RO1 DK43109-01A1 from the National Institute of Diabetes and Digestive and Kidney Diseases.

REFERENCES

American Psychiatric Association (1987). *Diagnostic and statistical manual of mental disorders*, 3rd ed., revised. Washington, DC: Author.

American Psychiatric Association (1993). *Diagnostic and statistical manual of mental disorders*, 4th ed., draft criteria. Washington, DC: Author.

Ames-Frankel, J., Devlin, M. J., Walsh, B. T., Strasser, T. J., Sadik, C., Oldham, J. M., & Roose, S. P. (1992). Personality disorder diagnoses in patients with bulimia nervosa: Clinical correlates and changes with treatment. *Journal of Clinical Psychology, 53*, 90–96.

Beck, A. T. (1976). *Cognitive therapy and the emotional disorders*. New York: International Universities Press.

Bemis, K. M. (1978). Current approaches to the etiology and treatment of anorexia nervosa. *Psychological Bulletin, 85*, 593–617.

Brownell, K. D. (1991). Dieting and the search for the perfect body: Where physiology and culture collide. *Behavior Therapy, 22*, 1–12.

Bruch, H. (1973). *Eating disorders*. New York: Basic Books.

Bruch, H. (1977). Psychological antecedents of anorexia nervosa. In R. A. Vigersky (Ed.), *Anorexia nervosa* (pp. 1–10). New York: Raven Press.

Bruch, H. (1978). *The golden cage*. Cambridge, MA: Harvard University Press.

Casper, R. C., Eckert, E. D., Halmi, K. A., Goldberg, S. C., & Davis, J. M. (1980). Bulimia: Its incidence and clinical importance in patients with anorexia nervosa. *Archives of General Psychiatry, 37*, 1030–1035.

Cooper, Z., & Fairburn, C. G. (1987). The eating disorder examination: A semistructured interview for the assessment of the specific psychopathology of eating disorders. *International Journal of Eating Disorders, 6*, 1–8.

Crisp, A. H., & Kalucy, R. S. (1974). Aspects of the perceptual disorder in anorexia nervosa. *British Journal of Medical Psychology, 47*, 349–361.

Ellis, A. (1979). Rational emotive therapy. In R. J. Corsini (Ed.), *Current psychotherapies* (pp. 167–206). Itasca, IL: F. E. Peacock.

Garfinkel, P. E., Moldofsky, H., & Garner, D. M. (1980). The heterogeneity of anorexia nervosa: Bulimia as a distinct subgroup. *Archives of General Psychiatry, 37*, 1036–1040.

Garner, D. M., Garfinkel, P. E., & Bemis, K. M. (1982). A multidimensional psychotherapy for anorexia nervosa. *International Journal of Eating Disorders, 1*, 3–46.

Halmi, K. A., Eckert, E., Marchi, P., Sampugnaro, V., Apple, R., & Cohen, J. (1991). Comorbidity of psychiatric diagnoses in anorexia. *Archives of General Psychiatry, 48*, 712–718.

Halmi, K. A., Goldberg, S. C., Eckert, E., Casper, R., & Davis, J. P. (1977). Pretreatment evaluation in anorexia nervosa. In R. A. Vigersky (Ed.), *Anorexia nervosa* (pp. 43–54). New York: Raven Press.

Johnson, C. (1982). Anorexia nervosa and bulimia. In T. J. Coates, A. C. Peterson, & C. Perry (Eds.), *Promoting adolescent health: A dialogue on research and practice* (pp. 397–412). New York: Academic Press.

Loro, A. D., & Orleans, C. S. (1981). Binge eating in obesity: Preliminary findings and guidelines for behavioral analysis and treatment. *Addictive Behaviors, 6*, 155–166.

Mahoney, M. J., & Mahoney, K. (1976). *Permanent weight control*. New York: W. W. Norton.

Mitchell, J. E., Specker, S. M., & de Zwaan, M. (1991). Comorbidity and medical complications of bulimia nervosa. *Journal of Clinical Psychiatry, 52 (Suppl.)*, 13–20.

Neuman, P. A., & Halvorson, P. A. (1983). *Anorexia nervosa and bulimia: A handbook for counselors and therapists*. New York: Van Nostrand Reinhold.

Pike, K. M., & Rodin, J. (1991). Mothers, daughters, and disordered eating. *Journal of Abnormal Psychology, 100*, 198–204.

Pope, H. G. & Hudson, J. I. (1992). Is childhood sexual abuse a risk factor for bulimia nervosa? *American Journal of Psychiatry, 149*, 455–463.

Rosman, B. L., Minuchin, S., Baker, L. & Liebman, R. (1977). A family approach to anorexia nervosa: Study, treatment, and outcome. In R. A. Vigersky (Ed.), *Anorexia nervosa* (pp. 341–348). New York: Raven Press.

Russell, G. (1979). Bulimia nervosa: An ominous variant of anorexia nervosa. *Psychological Medicine, 9*, 429–448.

Spitzer, R. L., Devlin, M., Walsh, B. T., Hasin, D., Wing, R., Marcus, M., Stunkard, A., Wadden, T., Yanovski, S., Agras, S., Mitchell, J., & Nonas, C. (1992). Binge eating disorder: A multisite field trial of the diagnostic criteria. *International Journal of Eating Disorders, 11*, 191–203.

Strober, M. (1981). The significance of bulimia in juvenile anorexia nervosa: An exploration of possible etiological factors. *International Journal of Eating Disorders, 1*, 28–43.

Waller, G. (1991). Sexual abuse as a factor in eating disorders. *British Journal of Psychiatry, 159*, 664–671.

Warah, A. (1989). Body image disturbance in anorexia nervosa: Beyond body image. *Canadian Journal of Psychiatry, 34*, 898–905.

White, W. C., & Boskind-White, M. (1981). An experiential–behavioral approach to the treatment of bulimarexia. *Psychotherapy: Theory, Research and Practice, 18*, 501–507.

Williamson, D. A. (1990). *Assessment of eating disorders: Obesity, anorexia, and bulimia nervosa*. New York: Pergamon Press.

Wilson, G. T. (1991). The addiction model of eating disorders: A critical analysis. *Advances in Behavioural Research and Therapy, 13*, 27–72.

Wilson, G. T. (1992). Diagnostic criteria for bulimia nervosa. *International Journal of Eating Disorders, 11*, 315–319.

11

Psychophysiological Disorders

Donald A. Williamson, Susan E. Barker,
and Kevin J. Lapour

Description of the Disorders

It is generally presumed that there are biological bases to the psychophysiological disorders and that stress, emotional, and behavioral habits contribute to the occurrence of the physical symptoms. This conceptualization is reflected in the most recent editions of the *Diagnostic and Statistical Manual of Mental Disorders*, DSM-III (American Psychiatric Association, 1980), DSM-III-R (American Psychiatric Association, 1987), and DSM-IV (American Psychiatric Association, 1994). Beginning with DSM-III, the diagnosis psychophysiological disorders was subsumed under Psychological Factors Affecting Medical Conditions. The types of somatic conditions that might be affected by stress or other environmental factors are quite diverse, including dermatological, cardiovascular, musculoskeletal, gastrointestinal, and central nervous system functioning (Ferguson & Taylor, 1981).

It is important in evaluating psychophysiological disorders that the diagnostician evaluate antecedents and consequences of somatic symptoms (Williamson, Labbé, & Granberry, 1983). Also, it is important to integrate biological and behavioral variables into a comprehensive formulation of each case (Russo & Budd, 1987). For the purposes of illustrating the process of diagnostic interviewing for psychophysiological disorders, we have selected four disorders for discussion: headache, insomnia, essential hypertension, and irritable bowel syndrome. These disorders were selected because they represent the diversity of psychophysiological disorders and because structured diagnostic interviews have been constructed for each disorder.

Donald A. Williamson, Susan E. Barker, and Kevin J. Lapour • Department of Psychology, Louisiana State University, Baton Rouge, Louisiana 70803.

Diagnostic Interviewing (Second Edition), edited by Michel Hersen and Samuel M. Turner. Plenum Press, New York, 1994.

HEADACHES

Description

The most common types of headaches are migraine and muscle-contraction headaches (Williamson, 1981). Headache is a widespread problem, occurring in about 60–80% of adults (Waters, 1974). Severe headaches, which affect one's daily activities, are reported in about 15–30% of women and 7.5–15% of men (Blanchard & Andrasik, 1985).

Migraine headache is described as a severe, throbbing pain that is often located on one side of the head (i.e., unilateral location). The most common locations of pain are the temple, forehead, or occipital regions of the head. Migraine headaches frequently radiate to affect the entire head. Nausea and vomiting often accompany the headache, and many migraineurs report that vomiting relieves the headache. Sensitivity to bright lights during headache, which is called *photophobia*, is also symptomatic of migraine. In cases that are diagnosed as *classic* migraine, patients report reliable warning signs, or prodromal symptoms, which precede the headache by about 30 minutes. Common prodromal symptoms are visual disturbances (e.g., flashing lights or blind spots in the visual field) and somatosensory disturbances (e.g., numbness in fingers, and disorientation). Migraine headaches that are not preceded by prodromal symptoms are diagnosed as *common* migraine. It is generally presumed that both types of migraine are caused by vasoconstriction of intracranial arteries, which causes prodromes in some cases, and rebound vasodilation of the extracranial arteries, which causes the throbbing pain associated with migraine. For a more complete description of the pathophysiology and diagnosis of headache, the reader may refer to Diamond and Dalessio (1982), Williamson (1981), and Williamson, Davis, and Kelley (1989).

Muscle-contraction or tension headaches are described as a dull steady ache or a tension like that of a hat that is too tight. Muscle-contraction headache pain is usually bilateral, involving the following regions of the head: forehead, top half, or back and neck/shoulders. Nausea, vomiting, and photophobia are generally not associated with muscle-contraction headache. Also, prodromal symptoms are not reported in these headaches. It is generally presumed that muscle-contraction headache is primarily caused by sustained contraction of facial or neck/shoulder muscles, often as a result of stress (Williamson, 1981).

Some headache sufferers report a combination of migraine and muscle-contraction headache symptoms. These patients may report symptoms indicative of two distinct types of headache or may describe the co-occurrence of symptoms associated with migraine and muscle-contraction headache. These patients are diagnosed as combined or mixed headache (Blanchard & Andrasik, 1985).

Procedures for Gathering Information

Diagnosis of headache is best accomplished using an interview such as that described by Blanchard and Andrasik (1985). The diagnostic interview should attempt to identify the type(s) of headaches experienced by the patient and the symptom cluster(s) associated with head pain. Also, the frequency and pattern of headache over a short period of time (e.g., a month) can provide a good index of frequency of head pain. History of headache and family history of headache should be assessed. Finally, antecedents of headache and behavioral consequences of reporting headache can be used to formulate a functional analysis of each case. The headache interview format described by Blanchard and Andrasik (1985) was found to yield 86% agreement with the diagnosis of a neurologist (Blanchard, O'Keefe, Neff, Jurish, & Andrasik, 1981).

Interview data can be supplemented by information derived from headache questionnaires and self-report inventories. Also, psychological testing may be helpful in certain cases (Blanchard & Andrasik, 1985). Two headache question-naires have been reported in the literature (Arena, Blanchard, Andrasik, & Dudek, 1982; Williamson, Ruggiero, & Davis, 1985). Both questionnaires have been par-tially validated (Williamson et al., 1989). Self-monitoring of headache usually follows a format similar to that described by Williamson et al. (1985).

Case Illustration

Ann was a 42-year-old woman who had suffered from headache since childhood. She had never sought specialized treatment for headache, but in recent months head pain had worsened, resulting in a referral for comprehensive evaluation. Excerpts from the diagnostic interview of Blanchard and Andrasik (1985) are presented to illustrate key features of this case of classic migraine.

I: Describe your headache for me in detail.

P: It feels like a sharp, pulsating pain, like someone was stabbing me in the head with an ice pick.

I: Where on your head do they seem to start?

P: They usually start in my right temple, but the pain generally spreads to the entire right side of my head.

I: Does the pain ever occur on the left side of your head?

P: Very seldom; occasionally my whole head hurts, but that's usually a bad one.

I: How long do they last?

P: Usually for at least 3 to 6 hours; sometimes for 2 days or more.

I: How often do they occur?

P: They are kind of variable, but usually at least one per week.

I: In the last month, how many have you had?

P: I would say at least 6, but last month they were even worse, probably 8 or 10.

I: Do you have any kind of warning signs that a headache is about to start?

P: Yes, about 20 to 30 minutes before a headache begins, I start to see black spots in front of things. Then I know I'm going to get a headache.

I: Do the spots move when you move your eyes?

P: Yeah, but if I focus on something, they generally stay still.

I: Do you ever feel nauseous before, during, or after a headache?

P: Sometimes, and if I can throw up, sometimes the headache goes away faster.

From this information, it was learned that the patient was experiencing classic migraine and that the headaches were quite severe. The next set of questions were intended to evaluate potential antecedents of headache.

I: Now I need some information on your current life situation. How would you describe your marriage?

P: Well, we get along pretty well. My husband is a recovering alcoholic and now he's a workaholic.

I: Are you getting along well?

P: Well, we argue some.

I: Can you tell me a little more?

P: He kind of avoids me.

I: Do you know why he avoids you?

P: He says that I'm controlling.

I: How are you getting along on the job?

P: My boss loves me.

I: Are there any problems?

P: I'm kinda stressed out.

I: Does your boss give you a lot of work to do?

P: No, I just can't seem to get it done.

From further interview data, it was learned that Ann was experiencing severe problems related to obsessive–compulsive disorder, which had never been diagnosed. Headaches reliably followed becoming upset because she "made an error" or "couldn't get tasks done on time" or her husband "was too messy." Much later in therapy, it was learned that she had been repeatedly sexually traumatized in her first marriage and had developed posttraumatic stress disorder. Using the diagnostic procedures described in DSM-IV, this case would be diagnosed as a mental disorder (posttraumatic stress disorder) affecting migraine headache. While most migraine headache patients do not have psychological problems of this magnitude, it is of utmost importance to evaluate this possibility. We are happy to report that after lengthy treatment, this patient is doing quite well; her obsessive–compulsive and sexual trauma problems are very much improved, and headaches are reduced by 75%.

Critical Information

Migraine and muscle-contraction headaches must be differentiated from a variety of other conditions. Table 1 summarizes the primary symptoms required for differential diagnosis of migraine, muscle-contraction, and mixed headache. For a diagnosis of classic or common migraine, patients presenting with unilateral headache should report throbbing pain that is located in the temple, above one eye, or in the occipital region.

If pain is located near the temporomandibular joint (TMJ), which connects the jaw to the skull, the diagnostician should evaluate further for a diagnosis of TMJ pain. The primary symptoms of TMJ pain are summarized in Table 1.

Migraine and muscle-contraction headache are best distinguished by unilateral vs. bilateral locus of pain and the description of pain as constant vs. pulsating. Many patients report a mixture of migraine and muscle-contraction headache.

TABLE 1. Guidelines for Differential Diagnosis of Headaches

Headache diagnosis	Presenting symptoms for diagnosis	Symptoms contraindicated for diagnosis
Classic migraine	Unilateral locus of pain. Description of pain: severe and throbbing or pulsating. Prodromal symptoms, e.g., visual disturbances before headache. Possible nausea and vomiting. Episodic attacks. Family history of migraine. Ingestion of foods containing tyramine (e.g., cheese, sea foods) often initiates headache. For women, headaches often increase during menses, reduce or disappear during pregnancy and menopause. Relief after sleep. Tenderness in affected areas for several days after the headache.	Description of pain: constant with bandlike tightness. Bilateral locus of pain. Pain locus near jaw or ear, with bruxism (teeth grinding) or jaw popping.
Common migraine	Locus of pain is more often bilateral than unilateral. No clearly defined prodromal phase. All other symptoms similar to those of classic migraine.	Prodromal symptoms. Description of pain: constant bandlike tightness. Pain locus near jaw or ear with bruxism or jaw popping.
Muscle-contraction headache	Diffuse or bilateral locus or pain that usually begins in either suboccipital or frontal areas of the head. Description of pain: constant bandlike tightness or pressure around the head or stiffness or soreness in the neck. Possible tinnitus, vertigo, and lacrimation occurs when pressure is applied. Pain intensity: mild to severe. Frequency varies widely	Prodromal symptoms. Description of pain: pulsating or throbbing. Unilateral locus of pain. Pain locus near jaw or ear with bruxism or jaw popping. Nausea and vomiting.
Mixed headache	Pulsating or throbbing pain and, or at other times, bandlike tightness or pressure. Bilateral or unilateral locus of pain. Other symptoms of both migraine and muscle-contraction headache.	Pain locus near jaw or ear with bruxism or jaw popping. Clearly migraine or clearly muscle-contraction headaches
TMJ pain	Locus of pain over masseter muscles near ear. Pain may extend over the face, head, and neck. Often associated with jaw dysfunction. Bruxism may occur at night, occasionally during the day. Chronic pain and hypomobility of the mandible. Tension of masseter muscles with increasing tightness or tension; may also throb or pulsate. Muscle spasms. Jaw popping.	Unilateral or bilateral head pain only in frontal or temporal areas of head. Nausea and vomiting. Prodromal symptoms. Spontaneous or traumatic dislocation of joint. Chronic mandibular hypomobility—painless restriction of jaw movement.

For a more complete description of the diagnosis of these mixed-headache cases, the reader is referred to Bakal (1982).

INSOMNIA

Description

Chronic insomnia can be simply defined as an inability to initiate and maintain adequate sleep. Whereas almost everyone experiences occasional nights of sleeplessness, chronic insomnia produces impairment that interferes with one's daily functioning. The complaint of insomnia is frequently subjective; there is no standard definition of insufficient sleep because the amount of sleep needed by different individuals varies widely. The DSM-IV diagnostic criteria for primary insomnia disorders (APA, 1994) require a complaint of "difficulty in initiating or maintaining sleep, or of nonrestorative sleep," that lasts for a minimum of 1 month and results in daytime fatigue, irritability, or impaired daytime functioning.

The classification system published by the Association of Sleep Disorders Centers (1979) includes insomnia in its category of Disorders of Initiating and Maintaining Sleep (DIMS). The DIMS category is further divided into nine subtypes (Table 2). The first subtype, psychophysiological DIMS, is viewed as the result of chronic somatized tension and negative conditioning (i.e., emotional arousal prevents sleep, which leads the individual to try harder to sleep, which produces more arousal and causes further sleeplessness). Primary insomnia is usually diagnosed by excluding the other categories of DIMS, in which sleep disturbance is attributed to other factors. These factors will be discussed in more detail below.

Epidemiological studies disagree on the prevalence of chronic insomnia, with estimates ranging from 10% (Kripke, Simons, Garfinkel, & Hammond, 1979) to over 30% (Bixler, Kales, Soldatos, Kales, & Healey, 1979) of the adult population. In a more recent survey, Mellinger, Balter, and Uhlenhuth (1985) reported from a sample of 3161 adults that 18% complained of serious sleep problems and another 18% reported mild to moderate difficulties. Complaints of insomnia appear to be

TABLE 2.   Subtypes of the Disorders
of Initiating and Maintaining Sleep (DIMS)

1. Psychophysiological DIMS
2. DIMS Associated with Psychiatric Disorders
3. DIMS Associated with the Use of Drugs and Alcohol
4. DIMS Associated with Sleep-Induced Respiratory Impairment
5. DIMS Associated with Nocturnal Myoclonus and "Restless Legs"
6. DIMS Associated with Other Medical, Toxic, and Environmental Conditions
7. Childhood-Onset DIMS
8. DIMS Associated with Other Conditions
9. No DIMS Abnormality

more frequent in the elderly (Bixler et al., 1979), in women (Kripke et al., 1979), and among individuals of lower socioeconomic status (Kales & Kales, 1983).

The most common way to categorize complaints of insomnia is according to the time of night when sleep is most disturbed. On this basis, three types of insomnia are usually described. About 75% of poor sleepers experience "sleep onset" insomnia (Lacks, 1987), or difficulty in falling asleep. The second most common type of disrupted sleep is "sleep maintenance" insomnia, which consists of intermittent awakenings during the night. A third type is "terminal" insomnia, or early morning awakening with an inability to return to sleep.

Procedures for Gathering Information

Complaints of sleep disturbance are often complex and require a thorough, individualized assessment of relevant physiological, environmental, and psychological factors. Ideally, assessment should include careful interviewing of the patient and significant others, a medical examination, all-night sleep recordings, and daily self-monitoring of sleep and daytime activity.

An indispensable part of the assessment of insomnia is a comprehensive diagnostic interview with the patient and his or her bedmate and significant others. The interview is important not only to ensure that a correct diagnosis is made but also to aid in treatment planning. Lacks (1987) has developed the Structured Sleep History Interview, which provides for a thorough assessment of sleep disturbance, along with its antecedents and possible maintaining consequences. This diagnostic interview will be discussed in more detail below.

Another important step in diagnosis is the completion of a thorough medical examination to rule out sleep disturbance as secondary to a physical disorder (i.e., "secondary" insomnia). Many medical conditions, such as thyroid dysfunction, pain, CNS disorders, cardiovascular disorders, and renal insufficiency, can cause or contribute to sleep problems (Parkes, 1985). Interviews with the patient and others can also help to rule out the existence of medical problems.

All-night sleep recordings through polysomnography are widely regarded as the most reliable and valid measure of sleep. Polysomnography allows monitoring of electrical activity in the brian, as well as eye movements and muscle tension during sleep. Unfortunately, the procedure is expensive and time-consuming to perform and typically must be conducted in a laboratory setting. Recently, however, portable polysomnography equipment has been developed that permits sleep data to be collected in the patient's natural environment. Sleep recordings can be particularly useful in distinguishing "subjective" insomnia (previously called "pseudoinsomnia"), in which a person complains of insomnia but EEG readings reflect normal sleep. Several studies have shown that people complaining of insomnia often overestimate the latency of sleep onset and underestimate total sleep time (Bootzin & Engle-Friedman, 1981).

Self-monitoring procedures such as daily sleep diaries provide a quick and easy way to assess complaints of insomnia, both for diagnostic purposes and for assessment of treatment outcome. Lacks (1987) developed a Daily Sleep Diary to monitor sleep continuously, patients being required to mail in the diaries each morning. However, this and other sleep diary questionnaires [e.g., Daily Sleep

Questionnaire (Turner & Ascher, 1979)] are subject to the same problems of bias (i.e., reactivity, reliability, and validity) that affect self-monitoring in general (Kazdin, 1974). Several studies have shown, however, that sleep diaries are reliable and valid assessment measures (Bootzin & Engle-Friedman, 1981).

Case Illustration

The following dialogue is an excerpt from a diagnostic interview for insomnia. The interviewer's questions are drawn from the Structured Sleep History Interview developed by Lacks (1987).

The patient, Janet, was a 44-year-old married white female who presented at a psychology clinic with complaints of insomnia and daytime irritability. Prior interview established that her sleep-onset latency was about 1–2 hours and that she awakened about 3 times during the night, but required less than 5 minutes to return to sleep with each awakening. She reportedly started to have problems sleeping when she was experiencing a high amount of stress at work and had had problems with sleep for approximately 4 months before presenting for treatment.

I: Do you wake up early in the morning, before your scheduled wake up time, and are unable to return to sleep?

P: No, I usually don't wake up until my alarm goes off—and then I don't want to get out of bed. In the mornings and throughout the day, I have no energy because of my lack of sleep the night before. I'm really worried about what effect this is going to have on my physical health.

I: You've said that your daytime energy level is lower. Have you noticed any changes in your mood, appetite, sex drive, or level of concentration?

P: Well, my mood is irritable sometimes, but usually only when I know I haven't gotten enough sleep the night before. Also, I am probably not concentrating as well as I should, because people need a normal amount of sleep to be able to concentrate. I try to sleep as late as I can in the morning, and sometimes I take naps during the day to catch up on sleep. The funny thing is, I can fall asleep easily when I'm napping.

I: How long would you like to be able to sleep each night?

P: I've read that people need 8 hours of sleep to be able to function properly—I'd like to get about that much.

I: What do you do when you can't sleep?

P: Mostly I just lie there and watch the clock. I know that doesn't help because it just makes me worry more about not being able to go to sleep. I've tried all kinds of things to make me sleep—warm milk before bedtime, counting sheep, planning what I'm going to do the next day. I'm afraid to take any kind of sleeping pills; I don't want to get addicted to them.

I: Are you the kind of person who tends to worry a lot?

P: My husband and kids tell me that I am—I just like things to be right. That's why it bothers me so much to not be able to go to sleep. I just know that I'm going to get sick or something if I don't start sleeping better.

Although this illustration presents only a small part of a thorough diagnostic interview, the information provided by this patient suggests that she presents with a case of primary insomnia in which her initial sleeplessness was precipitated by stress and was exacerbated by unrealistic ideas about one's need for sleep, emotional arousal caused by performance anxiety, and changes in the sleep–wake cycle.

Critical Information to Make the Diagnosis

In order to properly diagnose primary insomnia and to differentiate it from other disorders of initiating and maintaining sleep, the interviewer should ask specific questions regarding the presence or absence of particular symptoms. Table 3 summarizes the symptoms that should be present and those that must be ruled out when making a diagnosis of primary insomnia. The "presenting symptoms for diagnosis" are taken from criteria proposed by Lacks (1987) and the American Psychiatric Association (1994).

When a diagnosis of primary insomnia is made, further assessment of the patient's alcohol and drug use history is vital, because these substances are frequently used as sleeping aids. Alcohol shortens sleep latency, but causes subsequent sleep disturbances; for example, chronic alcoholics have fragmented sleep and decreased rapid eye movement (REM) and deep sleep periods (Johnson, Burdick, & Smith, 1970). Hypnotic drugs, which are frequently prescribed to treat insomnia, can lead to the development of tolerance, disruption of natural sleep patterns, and suppression of REM sleep with rebound on withdrawal from the drug. These drugs often lead to insomnia of greater severity than before their administration (Parkes, 1985).

Knowledge of a patient's sleep hygiene is also important. Several factors, including the patient's sleep environment (e.g., level of noise and light in the room, room temperature, presence of a bedmate), can affect his or her ability to sleep. Sleep scheduling may also play a role. For example, poor sleep one night may prompt the patient to nap the next day, which may in turn disrupt sleep that night. Changes in the sleep–wake cycle (e.g., shift work) may easily interfere with one's

TABLE 3.   Guidelines for Differential Diagnosis of Disorders
of Initiating and Maintaining Sleep

Presenting symptoms for diagnosis of primary insomnia	Symptoms contraindicated for diagnosis of primary insomnia
Sleep onset latency of more than 30 minutes. *or* More than 30 minutes spent awake during the night. *or* Less than 6½ hours of sleep in a night	Diagnosis of physical illness that causes sleep disturbance. Diagnosis of other symptoms of depression. Diagnosis of symptoms of other psychiatric condition, such as schizophrenia or anxiety disorder.
Daytime fatigue accompanied by decreases in mood and performance.	Use of CNS stimulants such as caffeine or other drugs.
Symptoms that occur at least 3 nights per week.	Myoclonus (repetitive twitching of the leg muscles during sleep).
Symptoms that occur for at least several months.	Sleep apnea (respiration disorder in which breathing is repeatedly interrupted for more than 10 seconds during sleep). Narcolepsy. Parasomnias (sleepwalking, sleep terrors, enuresis, bruxism).

ability to sleep. Daytime and presleep activities should also be examined. It has been shown that exercise during the day can promote better sleep, but exercise at night may actually hamper it (Horne & Porter, 1976). Also, attempts to lose weight may cause insomnia; dietary intake of lower caloric levels has been associated with shorter and more fragmented sleep (Lacks, 1987).

ESSENTIAL HYPERTENSION

Description

Perhaps the most potentially dangerous of all psychophysiological disorders is hypertension, or high blood pressure. Estimated to affect as many as 15% of Americans (e.g., Garrison, Kannel, Stokes, & Castelli, 1987), hypertension puts one at risk for coronary heart disease, renal failure, stroke, and other cardiovascular dysfunction. The disorder strikes a disproportionate number of African-American males for reasons that are yet unclear (Ernst, Rupert, & Enwonwu, 1990). The term *essential* denotes those 90% of cases in which etiology is unknown. The remaining cases occur secondary to known medical pathology.

Hypertension is defined in terms of diastolic and, less frequently, systolic blood pressure. Blood pressure is a function of total cardiac output and peripheral vascular resistance, which operate together in a complex system (Hollandsworth, 1986). A diagnosis of mild hypertension is warranted when diastolic pressure is greater than 90 mm Hg, or systolic pressure is greater than 160 mm Hg, or both. Moderate hypertension is defined as diastolic pressure in the range of 105–115 mm Hg, while an individual with diastolic pressure above 115 mm Hg is considered severely hypertensive.

Procedures for Gathering Information

Unlike patients with other psychophysiological disorders, many patients who present to the mental health practitioner for treatment of hypertension have already received a diagnosis (Blanchard, Martin, & Dubbert, 1988). If a medical evaluation has not been completed, a mandatory first step is referral of the patient to a physician for a complete medical evaluation. Assessment by the mental health practitioner usually emphasizes identification of behaviors that could elevate blood pressure (e.g., consuming excessive amounts of cholesterol, sodium, or alcohol; cigarette smoking; or lack of exercise).

Also, assessment of coronary-prone behavior or the Type A personality style (Jenkins, Rosenman, & Friedman, 1967) is usually conducted. The Type A behavior pattern is described as being overly ambitious, competitive to the point of hostility, and having a constant sense of urgency and pressure. This behavior pattern has been associated with both hypertension and coronary heart disease (Review Panel on Coronary-prone Behavior and Coronary Heart Disease, 1981). The most recent research in this area has focused on the interaction between hostility and hypertension. Data suggest that overt and covert manifestations of anger and hostility may adversely affect blood pressure reactivity (e.g., Ernst et al., 1990; Jorgensen & Houston, 1988; Suarez & Williams, 1990). Hence, assessment of angry or hostile affect is particularly relevant for hypertensive patients.

Questionnaires, checklists, and interview are useful for gathering data on behaviors that may contribute to chronic hypertension. Self-monitoring is an excellent assessment tool when the patient has been trained to record blood pressure with a home measuring device. Instructions are given to keep a record of stress and anxiety level, diet and sodium intake, and exercise, or a combination of these. Blood pressure is recorded at regular intervals and when symptoms such as flushed skin or pounding heart are present. Blanchard et al. (1988) have noted that blood pressure is a highly reactive physiological response, and procedures for measuring blood pressure should be as standardized as possible. These authors have provided detailed procedural guidelines for the patients when recording blood pressure in the natural environment.

A number of objective psychological tests are available for measurement of stress, anxiety, and hostility in hypertensive patients. Among the more commonly used are the State–Trait Anxiety Inventory (Spielberger, Gorsuch, & Luschene, 1970), the State–Trait Anger Scale (Spielberger et al., 1985), the Buss–Durkee Hostility Inventory (Buss & Durkee, 1957), and the Novaco Anger Scale (Novaco, 1975). The Jenkins Activity Survey (Jenkins et al., 1967) was designed to measure Type A behavior pattern.

Several interview formats are available for assessment of coronary-prone behavior and Type A personality (Jenkins, 1978). For example, Rosenman (1978) has published a structured interview loosely based on items of the Jenkins Activity Survey. The interview assesses coronary-prone behaviors, rather than hypertension. The interviewer is instructed to note the patient's behavior (e.g., strength of handshake, speech patterns, motor pace) and questions the patient about these behaviors and traits such as drive and ambition, speed of work, feelings of pressure, especially time pressure, and visible displays of anger and irritability. The purpose of the interview is to classify the patient as to his or her temperament (Type A, Type B, mixed).

To our knowledge, only one structured interview specific to hypertension and related behaviors has been published (Blanchard et al., 1988). It is comprehensive in nature, containing sections regarding blood pressure history, medical regime, consequences of hypertension for both the patient and others, life concerns (work, marriage, and social), exercise, diet, smoking, and a section that screens for other psychopathology.

Case Presentation

The case presented below uses the interview format presented by Blanchard et al. (1988).

The patient was a 46-year-old, normal-weight black male referred by his general practitioner for psychological treatment of mild hypertension to supplement the patient's pharmacological regimen.

I: What's the highest your blood pressure has ever been?

P: About 165 over 105.

I: Are there any sensations you become aware of when your blood pressure is higher than usual?

P: Sometimes I'll get a headache, and my heart will pound.

I: When you realize your blood pressure is higher than usual, do you do anything?

P: I try to relax, but it makes me angry that I have to deal with this sometimes.

I: Does your hypertension interfere with your daily life?

P: Yeah, a lot. My doctor says I have to take it easy because of it, so I can't get all the things done that I need to do in a day.

Note that this exchange, though abbreviated, provides the interviewer with information on affective and behavioral consequences of the patient's hypertension. This provides a starting point for further exploration of Type A behavior pattern. Information should also be gathered on diet, activity, and other life-style variables following the format developed by Blanchard and his colleagues.

Critical Information

Abnormally high blood pressure not due to organic etiology is the sole criterion for the diagnosis of essential hypertension. We have emphasized a number of other psychosocial variables that require assessment by the clinician. This information is presented in Table 4.

IRRITABLE BOWEL SYNDROME

Description

Irritable bowel syndrome (IBS), which is estimated to affect 15% of people in industrialized nations (Almy & Rothstein, 1987), has the primary symptoms of abdominal pain and bowel habit alternating between constipation and diarrhea. Pain can range from mild to severe discomfort, although rarely do mild cases present for treatment (Sandler, Drossman, Nathan, & McKee, 1984). The typical patient is female, in her 30s or 40s, and has had gastrointestinal (GI) symptoms for at least 5 years prior to referral to a mental health practitioner (Ford, 1986). Many

TABLE 4. Guidelines for Differential Diagnosis of Essential Hypertension

Presenting symptoms for diagnosis	Contraindicated for diagnosis	Associated symptoms
BP ≥ 160 mm Hg systolic BP ≥ 90 mm Hg diastolic	Hypertension to organic cause	Dizziness Nosebleed Pounding heart/head Perspiration Type A personality characteristics

IBS patients present with a concomitant psychiatric disorder. Anxiety, depressive, and somatization disorders are seen most frequently (Ford, McMiller, Eastwood, & Eastwood, 1987).

The etiology of IBS is unknown, but the diagnosis is not made in the presence of an established organic GI disorder. A number of factors may exacerbate symptoms, including diet, medication, and stress. The latter may be an especially important component, as IBS is usually considered a functional disorder. Associated symptoms may include headache, nausea, avoidance of eating, weakness, and insomnia.

Procedures for Gathering Information

Symptoms of IBS can mimic or hide signs of GI pathophysiology, ulcer, inflammatory bowel disease, esophageal motility disorders, intolerance to some foods, and medication side effects (Tunks & Bellissimo, 1991). As with other psychophysiological disorders, a complete physical examination by a physician is required to rule out organic etiology. In many cases, the patient will present to the mental health clinic only after repeated trips to a medical specialist or the emergency room.

IBS has been conceptualized within a multidimensional framework, with physiological, emotional, cognitive, and behavioral factors each playing an important role in the development and maintenance of the syndrome (Latimer, 1981). Thus, it is important to assess each of these biopsychosocial domains. Abnormality of physiological functioning of the gut or colon must be detected by a physician. However, interview and a myriad of questionnaires are used in the mental health setting to assess for depression, anxiety, and dysfunctional cognitions that may be related to the symptoms of IBS. It must be noted that GI distress is found in a number of psychiatric disorders, and care must be taken to distinguish between somatic symptoms, secondary psychiatric disorder, and the comorbidity of IBS and another diagnosable disorder. Behavioral interview and self-monitoring serve to gather critical information on symptomatology, diet, bowel habits, and functional behaviors related to IBS.

Case Illustration

The patient, a 31-year-old white female, was referred by her physician after a series of diagnostic tests could find no medical cause for her complaints of abdominal pain. Her records indicated that she had been experiencing GI symptomatology for over 3 years. Interview questions were taken from an unpublished history/interview form by Blanchard (1991).

I: Do you have abdominal pain?

P: Yes. It's kind of a sharp pain, on the left side. [Points to lower abdomen.]

I: Is the pain relieved by bowel movements?

P: Yeah, usually that helps, but not always.

I: Do you have diarrhea?

P: Some weeks. I kind of alternate between having diarrhea for a while, and then I won't be able to go at all for a few days.

I: Does your GI problem prevent you from engaging in certain activities?

P: Yes, especially when I have diarrhea. I don't like to go to work when I have diarrhea because I might have an accident or something. It's embarrassing.

I: Would your life be significantly different if you never had this GI problem?

P: Definitely. I hurt all the time, and I'm always missing work. I'm starting to worry that I might lose my job, but I just can't go in to work when my stomach hurts so bad. It makes me nauseous just thinking about how much work I've missed. My stomach is starting to hurt right now.

Here, the interviewer has elicited description of the patient's IBS symptoms and begins to detail the effect her GI distress has had on her life. The patient notes a relationship between symptoms and her ability to work. She is aware of her avoidance of work and is distressed by this behavior. Note also that her anxiety over work absenteeism brings about GI symptoms. Hence, preliminary information suggested that there was a positive relationship between mood state and IBS symptoms. At this point, the interviewer would continue to explore this relationship, gathering data on the frequency, severity, and duration of IBS symptoms as well as fluctuations in the patient's mood state. If stress was found to be a primary antecedent of IBS symptoms the case would be diagnosed as stress-related physiological response affecting irritable bowel syndrome (APA, 1994).

Critical Information

Information on the patient's diet, bowel movement schedule, and occurrence of pain is highly pertinent in establishing the presence of IBS. For example, Manning, Thompson, Heaton, and Morris (1978) reported that for IBS patients, onset of pain results in more frequent bowel movements, loose stools, and often a relief of pain after defecation. Other considerations in making the diagnosis include whether the patient experiences distention of the stomach, passing of mucus in the stool, and a sensation of incomplete evacuation (Manning et al., 1978). Positive response to any of these symptoms is common in IBS. However, abdominal pain and intermittent or alternating episodes of diarrhea and constipation are the only symptoms necessary to establish a diagnosis of IBS.

As illustrated in the case presentation, it is very important to investigate functional aspects of IBS. The unpredictability some patients feel about their bowel control makes avoidance of work, school, or social activities a possibility. The effect the patient's IBS has had on family members and friends should also be assessed, as some IBS patients are reinforced for illness behavior by having those around them take over responsibilities. Table 5 summarizes information critical for a diagnosis of IBS.

SOME DO'S AND DON'T'S

Do consider the possibility of a somatoform disorder.

Don't take the patient's explanation of his or her somatic complaints at face value.

TABLE 5.   Guidelines for Differential Diagnosis of Irritable Bowel Syndrome

Presenting symptoms	Symptoms contraindicated	Associated symptoms
Abdominal pain	Symptoms are of organic etiology.	Pain is eased by bowel movement.
Diarrhea	Symptoms are of other psychiatric etiology.	Mucus is present in stool.
Constipation	Pain is relieved by ingestion of food.	Feeling of distention.
Alternation between diarrhea and constipation		Feeling of incomplete evacuation. Headache, weakness, lethargy. Avoidance behavior due to GI symptoms.

Do ask about a few symptoms unrelated to the suspected disorder in order to rule out a response bias of reporting virtually any somatic symptom asked about by the interviewer.

Don't rely exclusively on interview data for a diagnosis.

Do define the presenting problem in behavioral or biological terms when possible.

Don't assume that the patient's report of medical information is accurate.

Do gather medical records to document the diagnostic workups and treatment by other health care professionals.

Don't assume that somatic complaints are exclusively determined by antecedents such as stress or emotion.

Do evaluate the potential for secondary gain for the expression of physical complaints.

Don't assume that the patient's report of frequency and severity of episodic somatic is an accurate representation, since patients often remember periods of acute distress rather than a more balanced sample of symptoms.

Do supplement interview data with information derived from daily self-monitoring of symptoms and environmental events.

SUMMARY

Diagnostic interviews for headache, insomnia, essential hypertension, and irritable bowel syndrome have been constructed in recent years. This chapter summarized the information that is critical for diagnosing these psychophysiological disorders.

The format for diagnosing psychological factors in any such disorder is similar to those described in this chapter. First, the diagnostician must establish whether a complex of somatic symptoms is being described. This complex of symptoms should be consistent with established knowledge about the physiology of the biological symptoms that are implicated (e.g., the cardiovascular system in the case of hypertension). The second step involves determining environmental,

sion of somatic symptoms. From this process, a treatment program tailored to the individual patient can be established.

References

Almy, T. P., & Rothstein, R. I. (1987). Irritable bowel syndrome: Classification and pathogenesis. *Annual Review of Medicine, 38,* 257–265.

American Psychiatric Association (1980). *Diagnostic and statistical manual of mental disorders,* 3rd ed. Washington, DC: Author.

American Psychiatric Association (1987). *Diagnostic and statistical manual of mental disorders,* 3rd ed., revised. Washington, DC: Author.

American Psychiatric Association (1994). *Diagnostic and statistical manual of mental disorders,* 4th ed. Washington, DC: Author.

Arena, J. G., Blanchard, E. B., Andrasik, F., & Dudek, B. C. (1982). The headache symptom questionnaire: Discriminant classifactory ability and headache syndromes suggested by a factor analysis. *Journal of Behavioral Assessment, 4,* 55–69.

Association of Sleep Disorders Centers (1979). Diagnostic classification of sleep and arousal disorders. *Sleep, 2,* 1–137.

Bakal, D. A. (1982). *The psychobiology of chronic headache.* New York: Springer.

Bixler, E. O., Kales, A., Soldatos, C. R., Kales, J. D., & Healey, S. (1979). Prevalence of sleep disorders in the Los Angeles metropolitan area. *American Journal of Psychiatry, 136,* 1257–1262.

Blanchard, E. B. (1991). *Interview for irritable bowel syndrome.* Unpublished manuscript.

Blanchard, E. B., & Andrasik, F. (1985). *Management of chronic headaches: A psychological approach.* Elmsford, NY: Pergamon Press.

Blanchard, E. B., Martin, J. E., & Dubbert, P. M. (1988). *Non-drug treatments for essential hypertension.* New York: Pergamon Press.

Blanchard, E. B., O'Keefe, D. M., Neff, D., Jurish, S., & Andrasik, F. (1981). Interdisciplinary agreement in the diagnosis of headache types. *Journal of Behavioral Assessment, 3,* 5–9.

Bootzin, R. R., & Engle-Friedman, M. (1981). The assessment of insomnia. *Behavioral Assessment, 3,* 107–126.

Buss, A. H., & Durkee, A. (1957). An inventory for assessing different kinds of hostility. *Journal of Consulting Psychology, 21,* 243–248.

Diamond, S., & Dalessio, D. J. (1982). *The practicing physician's approach to headache,* (3rd ed.). Baltimore: Williams & Wilkins.

Ernst, F. A., Rupert, A. F., & Enwonwu, C. O. (1990). Manifest hostility may affect habituation of cardiovascular reactivity in blacks. *Behavioral Medicine, 16,* 119–124.

Ferguson, J. M., & Taylor, C. B. (Eds.). (1981). *The comprehensive handbook of behavioral medicine* (Vol. 2). Jamaica, NY: Spectrum Publications.

Ford, M. J. (1986). Invited review: The irritable bowel syndrome. *Journal of Psychosomatic Research, 30,* 399–410.

Ford, M. J., McMiller, P., Eastwood, J., & Eastwood, M. A. (1987). Life events, psychiatric illness and the irritable bowel syndrome. *Gut, 28,* 160–165.

Garrison, R. J., Kannel, W. B., Stokes, J., and Castelli, W. P. (1987). Incidence and precursors of hypertension in young adults: The Framington Offspring Study. *Preventive Medicine, 16,* 235–251.

Hollandsworth, J. G., Jr. (1986). *Physiology and behavior therapy.* New York: Plenum Press.

Horne, J. A., & Porter, J. M. (1976). Time of day effects with standardized exercise upon subsequent sleep. *Electroencephalography and Clinical Neurophysiology, 40,* 178–184.

Jenkins, C. D. (1978). A comparative review of the interview and questionnaire methods in the assessment of the coronary-prone behavior pattern. In T. M. Dembroski, S. M. Weiss, J. L. Shields, S. G. Haynes, & M. Feinleib (Eds.), *Coronary-prone behavior* (pp. 71–88). New York: Springer.

Jenkins, C., Rosenman, R., & Friedman, M. (1967). Development of an objective psychological test for the determination of the coronary-prone behavior pattern in employed men. *Journal of Chronic Diseases, 20,* 371–379.

Johnson, L. C., Burdick, J. A., & Smith, J. (1970). Sleep during alcohol intake and withdrawal in the chronic alcoholic. *Archives of General Psychiatry, 22,* 406–418.

Jorgensen, R. S., & Houston, B. K. (1988). Cardiovascular reactivity, hostility, and family history of hypertension. *Psychotherapy and Psychosomatics, 50,* 216–222.

Kales, A., & Kales, J. (1983). Sleep laboratory studies of hypnotic drugs: Efficacy and withdrawal effects. *Journal of Clinical Psychopharmacology, 3,* 140–150.

Kazdin, A. E. (1974). Self-monitoring and behavior change. In M. J. Mahoney & C. E. Thoreson (Eds.), *Self-control: Power to the person.* Monterey, CA: Brooks/Cole.

Kripke, D. F., Simons, R. N., Garfinkel, I., & Hammond, E. C. (1979). Short and long sleep and sleeping pills. *Archives of General Psychiatry, 36,* 103–116.

Lacks, P. (1987). *Behavioral treatment for persistent insomnia.* New York: Pergamon Press.

Latimer, P. R. (1981). Irritable bowel syndrome: A behavioral model. *Behavioral Research and Therapy, 19,* 475–483.

Manning, A. P., Thompson, W. G., Heaton, K. W., & Morris, A. F. (1978). Towards positive diagnosis of irritable bowel. *British Medical Journal, 2,* 653–654.

Mellinger, G. D., Balter, M. B., & Uhlenhuth, E. H. (1985). Insomnia and its treatment: Prevalence and correlates. *Archives of General Psychiatry, 42,* 225–232.

Novaco, R. W. (1975). *Anger control.* Lexington, MA: Lexington Books.

Parkes, J. D. (1985). *Sleep and its disorders.* London: W. B. Saunders.

Review Panel on Coronary-prone Behavior and Coronary Heart Disease (1981). Coronary-prone behavior and coronary heart disease: A critical review. *Circulation, 63,* 1199–1215.

Rosenman, R. H. (1978). The interview method of assessment of the coronary-prone behavior pattern. In T. M. Dombroski, S. M. Weiss, J. L. Shields, S. G. Haynes, & M. Feinleib (Eds.), *Coronary-prone behavior pattern* (pp. 55–69). New York: Springer.

Russo, D. C., & Budd, K. S. (1987). Limitations of operant practice in the study of disease. *Behavior Modification, 11,* 264–285.

Sandler, R. S., Drossman, D. A., Nathan, H. P., & McKee, D. C. (1984). Symptom complaints and health care seeking behaviour in subjects with bowel dysfunction. *Gastroenterology, 87,* 314–318.

Spielberger, C. D., Gorsuch, R. L., & Luschene, R. E. (1970). *STAI manual for the State–Trait Anxiety Inventory.* Palo Alto, CA: Consulting Psychology Press.

Spielberger, C. D., Johnson, E. H., Russell, S. F., Crane, R. J., Jacobs, G. A., & Worden, T. J. (1985). The experience and expression of anger: Construction and validation of an anger expression scale. In M. A. Chesney & R. H. Rosenman (Eds.), *Anger and hostility in cardiovascular and behavioral disorders* (pp. 5–30). New York: McGraw-Hill.

Suarez, E. C., & Williams, R. B. (1990). The relationships between dimensions of hostility and cardiovascular reactivity as a function of task characteristics. *Psychosomatic Medicine, 52,* 558–570.

Tunks, E., & Bellissimo, A. (1991). *Behavioral medicine: Concepts and procedures.* New York: Pergamon Press.

Turner, R. M., & Ascher, L. M. (1979). A within-subject analysis of stimulus control therapy with severe sleep onset insomnia. *Behaviour Research and Therapy, 17,* 107–112.

Waters, W. E. (1974). *Epidemiology of migraine.* Berkshire, UK: Boehringer Ingelheim, Bracknell.

Williamson, D. A. (1981). Behavioral treatment of migraine and muscle-contraction headaches: Outcome and theoretical explanations. In M. Hersen, R. M. Eisler, & P. M. Miller (Eds.), *Progress in behavioral modification* (Vol. 11, pp. 163–201). New York: Academic Press.

Williamson, D. A., Davis, C. J., & Kelley, M. L. (1989). Headaches. In T. H. Ollendick & M. Hersen (Eds.), *Handbook of child psychopathology* (2nd ed., pp. 317–326). New York: Plenum Press.

Williamson, D. A., Labbé, E. E., & Granberry, S. W. (1983). Somatic disorders. In M. Hersen (Ed.), *Outpatient behavior therapy: A clinical guide* (pp. 109–141). New York: Grune & Stratton.

Williamson, D. A., Ruggiero, L., & Davis, C. J. (1985). Headache. In M. Hersen & A. S. Bellack (Eds.), *Handbook of clinical behavior therapy with adults* (pp. 417–442). New York: Plenum Press.

III

Special Populations

12

Marital Dyads

GARY R. BIRCHLER AND LAUREN SCHWARTZ

DESCRIPTION OF THE PROBLEM

Since most clinicians are first taught to conduct diagnostic interviewing with individuals, the changes required for interviewing a marital dyad present a myriad of complications. First, while some categories of inquiry may be similar (e.g., presenting problems, developmental histories), the conceptual frameworks and methods used for dyadic interviews are highly variable and different from those used for individuals. In particular, the necessary emphasis placed on dyadic interactions and relationship factors can cause significant problems for dyadic interactions and relationship factors can cause significant problems for the inexperienced marital therapist. That is not to say that individual problems (e.g., depression, anxiety) are irrelevant in deciding the treatment of choice, but that even when they are present, there is a special requirement to understand how the marital relationship is affected by or contributes to the two individuals' problems.

Second, though this book is entitled *Diagnostic Interviewing*, there is as yet no standard diagnostic classification system for marital dyadic problems. Rather, using the interview method, this chapter will describe various aspects of the *clinical assessment* of married couples. Conceptualizing the clinical assessment of marital dyads as a prerequisite for treatment planning and intervention fits well with the basic intent of this book: the description of diagnostic interviewing procedures designed to enhance effective treatment.

The DSM-IV draft criteria (American Psychiatric Association, 1993) include several diagnostic categories that could pertain to marital dyads. The most likely diagnostic condition would be partner relational problem, which should be used when difficulties arise as a result of "interaction between spouses or partners characterized by negative communication (e.g., criticisms), distorted communication (e.g., unrealistic expectations) or non-communication (e.g., withdrawal) asso-

GARY R. BIRCHLER • Department of Veterans Affairs Medical Center, and University of California at San Diego School of Medicine, San Diego, California 92161.   LAUREN SCHWARTZ • Department of Rehabilitation Medicine, University of Washington, Seattle, Washington 98195.

Diagnostic Interviewing (Second Edition), edited by Michel Hersen and Samuel M. Turner. Plenum Press, New York, 1994.

ciated with clinically significant impairment in individual or family functioning or symptoms in one or both partners" (APA, 1993, p. U:4).

Typically, the individual symptoms suggested above take the form of an Adjustment Disorder, which is "the development of emotional or behavioral symptoms in response to an identifiable stressor(s) occurring within three months of the onset of the stressor(s)" (APA, 1993, p. S:1). For couples, the unnamed stressor might well be marital conflict. The DSM-IV draft further codifies adjustment disorders according to specific types of symptom expression, e.g., adjustment disorder with anxiety, with depressed mood, with disturbance of conduct, with mixed disturbance of emotions and conduct, with mixed anxiety and depressed mood, and unspecified other. Finally, certain marital dyads may also experience other DSM-IV-draft-identified problems related to abuse, e.g., physical abuse of adult or sexual abuse of adult. Within marriage, the former is exemplified by spouse beating, the latter by sexual coercion or rape (APA, 1993, p. U:5).

In practice, what is assessed and how it is assessed tend to be heavily influenced by the interviewer's theoretical orientation and the couple's presenting problems. For example, marital therapists who are more traditional and psychodynamically oriented may rely exclusively on the interview method for history-taking assessment information (e.g., Nadelson & Paolino, 1978).

In comparison, behaviorists, as well as strategic family therapists, may deemphasize history-taking and instead focus on here-and-now interactions. Moreover, so-called brief-treatment family therapists may use only a short problem-focused assessment interview and then proceed with strategic interventions within the first hour of contact (Segal, 1991). In contrast to psychodynamic, strategic family systems, and other approaches, many behaviorally oriented therapists engage the couple in a distinct *assessment* phase that is completed before formal treatment begins. Multiple methods, such as standardized paper-and-pencil measures and laboratory or home-based marital interaction observational systems, are used to gather diagnostic-type information that is used to develop specific treatment goals and strategies (e.g., Birchler, 1983; Bornstein & Bornstein, 1986; Haynes, Follingstad, & Sullivan, 1979; Jacobson & Margolin, 1979; Stuart, 1980; Weiss, 1980). Thus, in the behavioral approach, the clinical interview is a necessary but not sufficient tool for accomplishing a comprehensive assessment of the distressed marital dyad.

Third, even within the behavioral approach, there are some interesting questions concerning the role of the initial interviews with couples. For example, Haynes and Chavez (1983) state that clinical interviews are the "most frequently used, least investigated method of assessing marital distress" (p. 23). Bornstein and Bornstein (1986) note that "the initial interview may be the single most important session in all of conjoint marital therapy" (p. 34). Others have suggested that direct interviewing is readily available to all clinicians, is cost-effective, and constitutes the most common behavioral assessment instrument (Cormier & Cormier, 1985). However, Jacobson and Margolin (1979), offering an intriguing and contrasting perspective, state that "an initial interview is expendable as a means of obtaining assessment information" (p. 52) and assessment "is not the primary focus of an initial interview" (p. 53). These somewhat divergent viewpoints suggest that there may well be several important therapeutic objectives of the initial interviews. Nichols (1988) made the point that there are as many things therapists are looking for in the initial assessment phase as there are therapists.

To be sure, there is significant diversity in both basic theoretical and practical approaches to interviewing couples. However, in order to offer a coherent, and we hope, mainstream model of the interview assessment of marital dyads, the authors have relied primarily on the relevant literature produced over the past two decades by behaviorally oriented marital therapists who have described the interview process (e.g., Birchler, 1983; Bornstein & Bornstein, 1986; Haynes & Chavez, 1983; Jacobson & Margolin, 1979; Stuart, 1980; Weiss & Birchler, 1975). Also reviewed for this chapter, however, were the works of certain other well-known marital therapists or textbook authors who have incorporated systematic, behaviorally oriented assessment methods into their written descriptions of direct interviewing procedures (e.g., Cormier & Cormier, 1985; Glick & Kessler, 1980; Hof & Treat, 1989; Nichols, 1988).

Ideally, there will one day be a single standardized "diagnostic system" for marital dyads. Such a system would be designed to indicate the most appropriate method of treatment for a given couple (Jacobson, 1991). Today, such a system is far from reality, even though the field of marital therapy is increasingly embracing an integrationist perspective (e.g., Birchler & Spinks, 1980; Gurman, 1991; Segraves, 1982; Weiss, 1980, 1981). Nevertheless, given the practical challenge of being clinically competent in the practice of all types of approaches, most therapists end up learning well one or possibly two basic approaches. Since this focusing problem is particularly relevant for the therapist-in-training, this chapter will offer what the authors believe to be a basic, broadly endorsed, behaviorally oriented clinical interview format for assessing marital dyads.

In concluding these introductory comments, we should state that the following discussion pertains to marital couples seeking outpatient treatment for marital distress. While couples are occasionally seen on inpatient psychiatric units, in emergency settings, or via inpatient consultations from medical practitioners, most couples are seen as nonemergent outpatients in agency clinics or private offices. For purposes of this discussion, we will make the assumption that the necessary steps have been taken to arrange for both husband and wife to be seen at the initial contact.

PROCEDURES FOR GATHERING INFORMATION

Features of the Clinical Assessment Process

In his tour de force, *Helping Couples Change*, Stuart (1980) noted five essential features of a comprehensive assessment process. First, assessment should be *parsimonious*. That is, assessment procedures and sessions should not be dragged out interminably. Only information that is necessary to formulate and to implement a treatment plan need be gathered.

Second, marital relationships are so complex that a *multidimensional* assessment process is required. Several methods exist for gathering convergent and divergent information about marital satisfaction and interaction. Direct clinical interviewing is featured in this chapter. Other important methods include the administration of standardized paper-and-pencil inventories, direct observation of marital interaction in the clinic or at home, and home-based self and spouse observation (Birchler, 1983; Jacobson & Margolin, 1979; Margolin, Michelli, & Jacobson, 1988; Stuart, 1980; Weiss, 1980). Finally, consultation with former or concurrent therapists or other family members can often provide critical information.

Third, the information gathered should be *linked to specific treatment interventions*. Sometimes, in an effort to be comprehensive, therapists overwhelm clients with assessment procedures that become irrelevant to the actual treatment that is offered. Whether the method be history-taking, inventories, or observations of marital interaction, to the extent possible, the findings should be relevant to a differential diagnostic and specific treatment application.

Fourth, it should be noted that at intake, couples often present long-drawn-out, vague, tangential, and circumstantial descriptions of their experiences and concerns. One task for the therapist is to help partners be very *specific about their goals and perceptions of the problems*. Situational and functional analyses of complex marital interactions require a level of specificity that the therapist is invariably responsible for shaping. Only then can interventions be designed to resolve specific problems.

Finally, Stuart adds that the assessment process, per se, should have *value to the clients*. The goal would be that even if the couple decided to decline treatment, they would have profited from the experience in terms of a better understanding of how their marriage is functional and dysfunctional and what actions would be required to bring about certain improvements. A multidimensional assessment experience should provide couples with data and perspectives that they had not previously appreciated. Should the assessment process not be perceived as relevant to their needs, couples will tend to drop out of treatment or fail to gain maximum benefits from this rather elaborate process.

Objectives of the Initial Assessment Interviews

There is fairly good consensus among behavioral marital therapists concerning the strategic objectives of the initial clinical interviews (e.g., Birchler & Gershwin, 1990; Haynes & Chavez, 1983; Jacobson & Margolin, 1979; Stuart, 1980). In general, the overarching goals of the first several meetings with the couple are: (1) to screen clients for marital therapy, (2) to establish trust and rapport in a therapeutic relationship, (3) to gather diagnostic-type assessment information, and (4) to educate and orient clients to the assessment procedures and the therapeutic approach and to give feedback regarding the therapist's conceptualization of the marital discord and how this discord may be addressed in therapy.

Screening Clients for Marital Therapy

Frequently, the initial telephone contact provides the opportunity for the therapist to determine whether individual, marital, family, or even group therapy seems to be the treatment of choice. Otherwise, one possible outcome of a complete marriage-assessment process is the discovery that one or both spouses could benefit from individual therapy before, or sometimes concurrent with, couples therapy. Examples include ascertaining that one partner is using drugs, abusing alcohol, or engaging in an extramarital affair unbeknownst to the spouse. Occasionally, one partner may be psychotic, paranoid, brain-damaged, or sufficiently depressed or anxious to preclude conjoint therapy and require individual attention. Finally, it may be determined that one partner has decided to end the marriage but the couple is not interested in divorce therapy. Apart from these presentations, however, the majority of marital therapy intakes result in conjoint marital therapy as the treatment of choice.

Establishing a Therapeutic Relationship

Obviously, at the beginning of any therapeutic endeavor, one of the therapist's main objectives is to establish a sufficient degree of trust and rapport with the clients so that they will choose to participate openly in the assessment process and engage in therapy. Achieving such a rapprochement may be particularly important yet quite difficult in couples work, due to the highly sensitive and often threatening issues that arise in this arena (e.g., sexual dysfunction or possible termination of a long-term relationship). Moreover, such difficulty is underscored when the partners have different agendas for therapy or try to compete for the therapist's attention and allegiance (which are not uncommon occurrences). Additionally, couples often wait too long before they seek help for their problems. As a result, both partners frequently have strong feelings of resentment, hopelessness, and depression, and may selectively attend to and reciprocate their partner's negative behaviors (Birchler, Clopton, & Adams, 1984; Jacobson, Follette, & McDonald, 1982; Gottman, 1979). Consequently, it is important at the outset that the therapist attempt to neutralize or extinguish feelings of hopelessness and blame, generate positive expectations regarding the marriage and therapy, and establish himself or herself as a caring and competent therapist. Specific therapist behaviors that serve to facilitate reaching these objectives will be discussed in a later section.

Gathering Assessment Information

While some prominent clinicians suggest that assessment methods other than direct interviewing may be better suited for assessing marital problems (e.g., Jacobson & Margolin, 1979; Stuart, 1980), most marital therapists use a clinical interview as a primary tool for exploring and defining the problems that are impacting a couple. Certain aspects of the assessment interviews are designed to define existing problems related to the relationship (e.g., individual and collective perceptions of marital problems), to the individuals (e.g., background, psychiatric history, substance-abuse history, general coping style, current affective status, and overall health status), and to any external influences (e.g., familial, cultural, and socioeconomic factors). Many therapists also wish to delineate clients' strengths and resources in these same areas.

Educating and Orienting Clients to the Approach

A final major objective of the assessment interviews is to provide the couple with a reasonable understanding of the rationale and typical procedures of assessment and treatment. Anticipating for couples at each session what will happen next, indicating how and why certain information is to be gathered, and providing an appropriate rationale (including empirical data) for the approach are all important aspects of a successful marital-assessment process.

Interview Activities: Outline of the Information Exchanged

Introduction

In our practice, when the couple arrives for their first session, the first order of business is for them to read and sign a brief (two-page) description of the program. This document also includes an outline of the various conditions under which client confidentiality may be broken: (1) threats to harm self or others, (2) direct knowledge of child or elderly abuse, or (3) court orders in criminal proceedings. The clients also complete a one-page general biographical form. (Table 1 presents an outline of the interview assessment process)

Table 1.   Clinical Interview Assessment of Marital Dyads:
General Sequence and Content

Week 1:   Initial interview
1. Introductions and registration
2. Confidentiality[a]
3. Defining objectives of the session(s)
4. What brings you to the clinic?
5. Partners' goals and expectations
6. Analysis of presenting problems
7. Commitment to complete the evaluation (marital-relationship inventories handed out)
Week 2:   Second conjoint interview (inventories collected)
8. Communication sample of problem-solving abilities/style[b]
9. Relationship developmental history
10. Current status of relationship (continued)
a. Commitment: stability, steps toward divorce
b. Caring: support and understanding, sex and affection
c. Communication and problem-solving (see step 8)
d. Conflict resolution: anger management, compromise
Week 3:   Individual interviews with each partner
11. Assessment of individuals[a]
Week 4:   Third conjoint interview
12. Interactional summary of assessment findings and treatment contract

[a]The sequence may be altered, depending on clinic/practitioner policy.
[b]Optional but highly recommended assessment procedure.

Confidentiality

We suggest that the confidentiality issue be discussed at the beginning of the first assessment session. Some clinicians address this issue at the end of the first meeting or at the beginning of any individual assessment sessions. Others, unfortunately, do not discuss confidentiality at all. We highly recommend that this topic be covered very early in the assessment process because confidentiality in couples therapy is considerably more complicated than in individual therapy (cf. Karpel, 1980; Margolin, 1986). With the exception of the legal exceptions noted above, the ethical standards of the American Psychological Association (1981) and the American Association for Marriage and Family Therapy (1988) suggest that all information related to the therapist, in conjoint or individual meetings, be kept confidential—*strictly confidential*.

The practice of strict confidentiality in marital therapy can result in having to keep certain secrets, which some therapists believe to be contradictory to the ethical practice of marital therapy (Karpel, 1980; Margolin, 1986). For example, consider the situation in which the husband tells the therapist that he is having an affair and asks you not to tell his wife. However, the wife is working under the assumption that the therapist is helping to save the marriage as a mutual advocate. Keeping the husband's secret makes it difficult for the therapist to be a fair advocate for the wife and for the marital relationship. Maintaining this position implicitly condones the husband's affair.

An alternative policy with respect to confidentiality is to make clear to the couple at the outset that whatever *either* of them tells the therapist, alone or together, will be regarded as common knowledge that the therapist is free to share with both parties. Additionally, couples can be told that they may be encouraged to take responsibility for and to disclose their secrets during the conjoint sessions. In this instance, there is *no confidentiality* within the couple. There are no secrets. This position, too, is defensible, but not without its disadvantages. For example, the husband having the affair probably will not tell the therapist at all and undoubtedly the marital therapy could go on indefinitely, and most likely without success. To be conservative, beginning therapists should probably choose one of the two positions just discussed and accept the advantages and disadvantages.

There is, however, a third option: *limited confidentiality*, which offers yet another combination of advantages and disadvantages. The purpose of this option is to obtain as much critical information as possible without having to keep secrets incompatible with successful marital therapy. Couples are told that the therapist can be most helpful if he or she knows as much about the couple as possible. They are also told, however, that in instances in which information is provided on an individual basis (e.g., in paperwork, phone calls, or individual meetings), the therapist would like to have judicious discretion to use all information openly to promote the marital relationship. Should either partner specify that certain information be kept confidential, the therapist will honor this request and continue therapy, *on the condition that* the information held confidential neither poses an ethical problem nor compromises the mutually understood goals of marital therapy. Given the example of the classic and most frequent complication, the therapist learns from one partner that he or she is secretly having an affair and does not want the spouse to know. The therapist proposing to do marital therapy is in an ethical bind that can be resolved only by (1) the spouse being informed; (2) the affair being terminated, at least during therapy; or, as the last resort, (3) the therapist declining to offer marital therapy. In private, the partner having the affair is told that either one of the first two options must be exercised or the therapist must exercise the third option. In most cases, the partner is inclined to terminate the affair, at least temporarily, in order to continue with marital therapy. Obviously somewhat complex, the limited confidentiality option can provide the therapist with the most information and the fewest disadvantages. Very clear agreements, preferably written and signed, are required to exercise the limited confidentiality option successfully.

Defining the Objectives of the Session

Once the registration and confidentiality issues are addressed, the therapist outlines his or her agenda for the initial meeting. We usually indicate in conversational language that our goals are: (1) to learn what brings each of them to the session, (2) to learn what each person would like to gain from the process, (3) to better understand the basic problems and concerns about the marriage from each partner's perspective, and (4) to mutually decide at the end of the session whether to continue with the marital assessment process.

CRITICAL INFORMATION IN THE ASSESSMENT PROCESS

What Brings You to the Clinic?

This question begins an open-ended inquiry of both partners concerning who initiated the contact, the other's response to the suggestion, and why treatment is sought at this particular time. With these questions, an early attempt is made to assess the partners' relative levels of motivation for treatment, to ascertain who has more power compared to who is experiencing more emotional pain, and to determine whether there are significant precipitating events for seeking help at this time. In general, the strategy is (1) to reinforce the partners' motivational levels for assessment and treatment; (2) to respect the partner with the greatest power, while supporting the person in pain; and (3) to consider the treatment implications of any identifiable precipitants for seeking therapy.

Usually, when couples enter treatment, the power differentials of the relationship are being challenged. Quite often, the person most in pain has initiated contact and the person most powerful is less motivated for treatment. That is, the most satisfied partner comes to therapy relatively less desirous of significant changes in the relationship. Consequently, one early challenge for the therapist is to offer hope and support to the more distressed partner, while simultaneously assuring the most influential partner that important relationship gains can be made without significant personal losses. This task can be delicate, and the high rate of early dropout in therapy may be related in part to the failure in accomplishing this objective (Nichols, 1988).

The answer to another important question, "Why [seek treatment] now?," is sometimes difficult to discern, but any precipitants discovered can be instrumental for treatment planning. Typical precipitants include distressing marital or family life-cycle transitions, the breaking of a family rule (e.g., substance abuse, incest, violence, or infidelity), and threats of separation and divorce.

Partners' Goals and Expectations for Treatment

Before asking the partners for their perceptions of their problems, we like to ask them to express their positive expectations and goals for treatment. We believe that the extent to which partners respond with positive, specific, self- and relationship-oriented answers is directly related to a better prognosis for marital therapy. There is a significant difference between an answer such as, "I want Jane to stop nagging me and always picking fights about the time I spend with my friends," and one such as, "I enjoy and spend more time with my friends than Jane likes. We need to develop some fun activities for the two of us."

Unfortunately, in our experience, it is the unusual couple who can or will articulate such specific and constructive cognitions or behaviors. Partners rarely understand their issues from an interactional perspective or volunteer personal responsibility for change. Much more likely to be heard are vague, blame-framed references to *problems* identified by or blamed on their partners. It appears that couples have a need to tell the therapist about their complaints in terms of what they do not like about their partner or the relationship, rather than to make direct statements of what they want. Moreover, partners tend to adopt a defensive posture regarding their partner's dissatisfactions. They may spend much of their energy justifying their own past and present behaviors. Questions and answers concerning positive goals do not fit within their current paradigm. Therefore, on one hand, at this stage in the interviews, it is important for therapists to validate and normalize (if possible) each partner's complaints and behaviors.

On the other hand, given instances when partners do mention positive and specific goals, they should be reinforced strongly. In some cases, couples identify very general goals, such as, "Improve communication," "Stop fighting," "Improve our marriage," or "Become more trusting." However, whenever the opportunities present, we try to elicit, reinforce, and shape the expression of specific, constructive, and relationship-promoting goals. When the couple is unable or unwilling to discuss issues from a positive perspective, their problem-oriented responses serve as a natural lead-in to a discussion of the presenting problems.

Analysis of Presenting Problems

In the context of a contemporary multimethod assessment process, a number of self-report inventories complement the clinical interviews and serve to explicate most of the couple's problems. However, a discussion of such instruments is beyond the scope of this chapter, as they are presented elsewhere (cf. Birchler, 1983; Filsinger, 1983; Hersen & Bellack, 1988; Jacobson & Margolin, 1979; Margolin et al., 1988; Stuart, 1980). During the initial interview with a marital dyad, hearing the couple describe their problems in some detail is an important objective of all concerned. Couples come primed to tell their stories (i.e., *to make their complaints and to defend themselves*), and there is probably no appropriate way to avoid hearing them out. It is important to give partners "air time" to express their views, and in the process, significant information concerning the type and severity of their problems may be gleaned. Rather than survey in detail all the problems, we prefer to understand comprehensively a few of their major issues. Once an important problem is identified, we endeavor to help partners describe it in operational terms. Important aspects of most problems include: *onset, duration, past attempts at solutions* (including previous therapy experiences), *perceptions of responsibility*, and the variety of *antecedents* to and *consequences* of the problem. The following case excerpt will illustrate some of this inquiry process.

Bill and Mary, both in their early 40s, had been married for 15 years and had two children, aged 10 years and 18 months. Bill came alone to the mental health clinic seeking assistance in "trusting his wife," and the couple was referred for marital therapy evaluation. The couple arrived for the initial interview on time and were quite attentive and cooperative during the usual introductory paperwork and description of the goals for the first meeting.

The therapist asked what brought the couple to the clinic and their preliminary goals and expectations for treatment. Bill was concerned that he would do something wrong, or not do something right, that would lead his wife into having another affair or cause her to leave him again. Approximately 4 months previously, the couple had separated when Mary rather abruptly told Bill she wanted a divorce and wanted him to leave the house. Bill was shocked, but complied and set up his own apartment. Bill had suspected for a few weeks that Mary was "seeing someone else," but she denied doing so. Soon after the separation, Mary began a sexual relationship with Bill's best friend; she fully intended to divorce Bill. Within a few weeks, however, Mary not only lost her job, but that same day the boyfriend dumped her.

Interestingly, because of visiting the children and other practical reasons for keeping in contact, Bill and Mary began to support one another in their separate experiences of having been discarded by their significant other. Within 2 months of the separation, they were living together again trying to make a go of it. However, as one might imagine, significant damage had been done to the relationship because of the affair and the unilateral aspect of the separation. Currently, the two of them were having significant difficulty getting over the affair, and they were unable to address relationship factors that contributed to the marital difficulties in the first place.

Their generally stated goals for therapy were to put the separation and affair behind them, to improve communication, and to avoid relapsing into the situation that existed prior to the separation. We enter the dialogue about 25 minutes into the first session as the therapist is helping the couple to specify and analyze their problems:

THERAPIST: Bill, how can you best describe the major problem you are having right now in the relationship?

HUSBAND: For one thing, the affair seems to be on my mind a lot. I feel like I'm walking on eggshells. I don't know what to keep to myself and what to bring up to Mary.

WIFE: [Mary nods her head in acknowledgment.]

THERAPIST: How long have you felt this way?

HUSBAND: Mostly since we moved back in together. . . .

THERAPIST: About 2 months?

HUSBAND: Yes. If I bring up things about the affair, Mary gets mad. If I keep things to myself, she accuses me of withdrawing. I don't want to get back into the pattern we had before.

THERAPIST: What was that?

HUSBAND: I was overwhelmed by two jobs, financial problems, and our boy was an infant. I couldn't get out from under the problems, but I couldn't talk about them either.

WIFE: [Mary nods her head again.]

THERAPIST: Mary, how does Bill's experience compare with yours? Do you see things similarly?

WIFE: Bill calls me from work two or three times a day. He comes home for lunch several times a week. He never did that before. He tries to be nice, but I've told him he's smothering me. I need some space! Somehow we always end up arguing about the separation.

THERAPIST: And you've noticed this behavior how long?

WIFE: It started a few days after we got back together.

HUSBAND: [Bill looks somewhat perplexed.]

THERAPIST: What do you think Bill's behavior means?

WIFE: Well, he always wants to know what I'm doing. I can't talk to a man without him getting upset. I'm an outgoing person. My mom always said that I never met a stranger. I won't change that. He's got to trust me some time, doesn't he?

THERAPIST: Trust is clearly a critical issue for you both right now. Your difficulties certainly make sense, given what has happened. Tell me, over the past 2 months, what have you each tried to do to resolve this problem?

WIFE: I've told him to give me some space. I've got to be able to see my friends and family without Bill being there or questioning me. I'm tired of talking about the affair. I just want it behind me!

THERAPIST: Have your efforts worked?

WIFE: Not really. Sometimes he sulks or seems to try harder for a few days, but that only adds to the problem.

HUSBAND: [Bill looks earnestly concerned.]

THERAPIST: Bill?

HUSBAND: I just want to be with her—what's wrong with that? I can't believe she went out with Jack. I need to know what happened, but then talking about it really gets me upset and makes Mary mad.

THERAPIST: How have you tried to solve this problem?

HUSBAND: I try not to think about it, but I get afraid when Mary is at work or out in the evenings. Seems like it could happen again so easy. I try to pay more attention to her than before, but now she doesn't like it.

THERAPIST: Didn't you pay enough attention to Mary before the separation?

WIFE: He would hardly talk to us at all. We would have friends over, and Bill would tune out completely.

THERAPIST: When did you first notice Bill tuning out?

Wife: I think it started getting really bad after we moved to California—about 2 years ago.

Therapist: [Turning to Bill.] Do you remember this?

Husband: I don't remember spacing out with friends over. But I do know I was under a lot of stress after we moved out here.

Therapist: Were you able to share these feelings with Mary?

Husband: She had her own problems. We've had nine miscarriages, and she was having a difficult pregnancy with our son. I pretty much kept things to myself.

Therapist: Mary, if this was the case, was Bill's strategy helpful to you at the time?

Wife: No. I mean, I really felt alone. Bill was working all the time. We didn't even eat meals together. I didn't have anybody to talk to—except my family in Ohio, and then we argued about the phone bills.

Therapist: O.K., in view of the time, let me see if I can summarize my understanding of this problem *so far*. I want to thank you both for sharing your perspectives. It seems to me that your communication, both before and after the separation, has not worked as well as you would like, but both of you were well-intended. You alluded to some very important history, such as tremendous job stresses and major medical problems. We will need to learn more about these experiences later. However, to simplify, after you moved to California, pregnant and having to take on multiple jobs, the stresses increased for each of you. But somehow you had different styles of coping. Bill took the burdens on himself, and trying to protect you, Mary, perhaps he held too much inside. You felt isolated and alone and apparently couldn't ask for and get the support you needed from Bill either. Things got to the point where you two weren't connecting well at all and Mary bailed out.

At this point in time, whatever else has happened, the separation and affair have shocked your relationship. You now realize that something fundamental has to change in order to build a healthy, satisfactory marriage. But you're here because you're not sure what to do. And, a major complicating issue is the meaning and threat of the separation and affair itself. Given that the affair happened, your current reactions sound typical. However, it will take some time and considerable effort to rebuild trust—in both directions.

Bill, having once been burnt by isolating yourself, the insecurities caused by the affair have driven you to the other extreme: constantly attending to Mary, such that she feels smothered. Your protective vigilance is having the opposite effect of pushing her away. Mary, you are also caught in a dilemma. Once you were trusted implicitly and even had to find supportive social relationships *outside* the marriage. Now, essentially you don't feel trusted and are being asked to meet your social needs almost exclusively *within* the relationship. Also, at one time you desperately needed emotional contact with Bill; now, you sometimes find yourself resentful and put off by it.

How does this description sound so far?

Wife: I think that's pretty much what's happening now.

Husband: [Bill nods his head in agreement.]

Therapist: Well, as mixed up and confusing as this pattern may sound, as frustrating as it may be, I think we can understand what has happened, and I think we can get most of this straightened out. But right now, I would like to know if either of you would like to mention any other major problems currently affecting your relationship. Otherwise, I want to review briefly some other important areas of marital interaction.

In this example, we have learned, through discussion of the couple's identified major problem, that during some significant and very stressful transitions, the partner's divergent psychosocial coping mechanisms failed the relationship. Poor communication and unexpressed expectations led to a critical deficiency in support and understanding, which eventually affected at least the wife's essential level of caring and ultimately her basic commitment. Curiously, while we do not know what would have happened had the new boyfriend not dumped Mary, the affair has impacted on this marriage such that it will probably never again be the same. On the positive side, the couple demonstrated an amazing degree of friendly cooperation during the separation and an unusual cohesiveness during the initial interview. While a more detailed relationship and individual assessment is required, and their particular presenting problem generally is quite difficult to treat, it may be possible to help this couple save and improve this 15-year marriage.

This dialogue illustrates how a balance is kept in interviewing both husband and wife. Also, without resorting to a cookbook inquiry process, the therapist can gather information about the problem: onset, duration, past attempts at solution, partners' intentions and perceptions of responsibility, and at the very least global antecedents and consequences of the problem behavior. Finally, the problem is conceptualized and summarized in an interactional perspective that avoids blame, normalizes their affective reactions to the problem, and provides hope for improvement.

Much can be learned about this couple if a developmental and situational analysis is completed on two or three of the couple's high-priority problems. That is, a determination is made of what the problem is, when it started and how it developed over time, how each partner thinks and feels about the problem, what the antecedents and consequences of the problem are, and what attempts have been made to resolve (and sometimes to perpetuate) the problem.

Next, if not already discussed, in an attempt to probe for high-probability marital conflict, the couple is asked how they are doing in the following areas: sex and affection, finances and money management, vocational and leisure activities, general communication and conflict management, and various extramarital relationships (e.g., child-rearing, in-laws, affairs). Finally, it is usually a good idea to ask, "Is there anything else that you would like to tell me?" Sometimes an important surprise follows this question; someone has been waiting for permission to mention something important—something hitherto withheld.

In summary, the assessment information gathered thus far, including an in-depth analysis of the major problems, gives the therapist a reasonable understanding of the current status of the marriage, the nature and severity of the problems, and how the couple has experienced and responded to the problems. In most cases, our goal is to get this far by the end of the first 60- to 90-minute session. Depending on the therapist's and the couple's efficiency in communicating, sometimes gathering this much information from the point of introduction is too ambitious a goal. If so, the agenda is continued into the next session.

Nonetheless, whenever required by time constraints, the initial interview is concluded with (1) a brief summary of the proceedings, (2) therapist validation of the couple's decision to seek assistance, (3) a brief description of the remainder of the assessment process, and (4) an *explicit invitation* to the couple to commit to the remainder of the assessment process. To encourage this commitment, partners are assured that information-gathering *only* is the goal of the evaluation process, that no one will be blamed for the relationship's problems or asked to change during evaluation, and that after the final assessment meeting is concluded, both the therapist and each partner will have the opportunity to decide whether or not to commence therapy. Given these structured guidelines, virtually all couples decide at least to complete the evaluation process. Generally, the first session ends when the marital assessment inventories are explained briefly and handed to the couple for completion between sessions.

Relationship Assessment

The couple's reasons for seeking therapy, their goals and expectations for therapy, and an outline of the major presenting problems having been determined in the first session, the second session is devoted to further assessment of the functional and dysfunctional aspects of the marital relationship.

Communication Sample

Since one of our primary treatment emphases is on communication efficacy, we typically begin the second assessment session by obtaining a *communication sample*. Outside of behaviorally oriented programs, the directed problem-solving sample of marital conflict communication may be rare. However, it is easily obtained, and is an important and often unique piece of information that is not incompatible with most contemporary approaches to marital therapy (Birchler, 1979; Gurman & Jacobson, 1988). Basically, at the start of the session and it is to be hoped, before any other conflict-laden material is introduced, the couple is asked to provide a 10-minute sample of their communication. The therapist helps them to identify a current, relevant, unresolved, and moderately intense issue about which they disagree. Typical topics selected are management of finances, the lack of quality time together, or conflict involving a child, in-law, or other adult. The therapist may have to help identify an appropriate issue on the basis of problems discussed during the initial interview or obtained from a quick glance at the Marital Relationship Assessment Battery (Birchler, 1983), which usually has been completed and returned to the therapist at the beginning of this session.

Once a viable issue is identified, the couple is asked to spend about 10 minutes attempting to resolve the problem. The therapist acknowledges that they may not solve the problem in 10 minutes, but states that he or she is interested in observing how they go about attempting to resolve it. At this point, the therapist may leave the room and observe from behind a one-way mirror or on a video monitor, or may simply push back in his or her chair and ask the couple to proceed as though they were alone.

The observed communication sample may demonstrate any of a variety of deficits in performance or skill or both with respect to the partners' relative abilities to assert themselves, to maintain focus on the issue at hand, to listen to one another, to propose solutions to the problem, and generally to engage in constructive (vs. destructive) interaction. Following the communication sample, it is often helpful to ask the couple how similar the interaction was to what transpires at home and whether they indeed felt as though they came up with a solution during the discussion. If the observed interaction was not representative, the therapist should understand why not; on occasion, one might repeat the exercise to better approximate the couple's actual style of problem-solving.

A review of the technical literature on the analysis of marital problem-solving is beyond the scope of this chapter; suffice it to say that these abilities clearly discriminate between distressed and nondistressed couples (e.g., Birchler et al., 1984; Birchler, Weiss, & Vincent, 1975; Gottman, 1979; Jacobson et al., 1982; Vincent, Weiss, & Birchler, 1975). Summary and interpretation of the information obtained from this exercise ranges from the therapist making some personal notes for feedback and treatment planning to use of an in-session therapist rating scale (e.g., Basco, Birchler, Kalal, Talbott, & Slater, 1991; Floyd & Markman, 1984) to analysis using a sophisticated behavioral coding system [e.g., the Marital Interaction Coding System (Weiss & Summers, 1983)]. The communication sample provides a behavioral demonstration of how couples *actually perform* in the context of a marital conflict. It can validate or offer information to compare with the couple's self-report of their problem-solving and conflict-management styles.

Relationship Developmental History

Following collection of the communication sample, we then take a developmental history of the relationship. The goal of this inquiry is to focus on the initial positive attraction the partners felt for one another, while specifically addressing how and when the couple met, what attracted them to one another, courtship and dating experiences, and their decision to live together or to marry. Also, we assess initial expectations for marriage, early gender role and sexual adjustments, and similarities and differences in values. Finally, we like to review relationships to extended families, the cultural, social, and economic forces that impact the couple, and an assessment of marital and family life-cycle stages (cf. Birchler, 1992; Carter & McGoldrick, 1988).

Often, important information is gained during this developmental review. Information concerning early (and possibly continuing) stresses and problems is usually obtained. Partners describe experiences that have influenced their past and current levels of commitment, trust, caring, and patterns of communication and conflict resolution. Obviously, the number and severity of negative experiences can significantly impact on the prognosis and the challenge of marital therapy. Nevertheless, throughout this discussion, the therapist highlights the positive features of the couple's history and their current coping resources, while also empathizing with the partners' experiences of trauma and struggle. The findings from the relationship history contribute significantly to the therapist's emerging data base of factors that account for the present level of marital distress. Next in the interview sequence (see Table 1), it is appropriate to focus the assessment process on certain aspects of the two individuals who comprise the couple.

Assessment of Individuals

In the field of marital therapy over the past two decades, the importance ascribed to the assessment of each partner's personal history and development, their personality styles, and the existence of psychopathology has varied considerably. Traditionally, psychodynamic approaches have placed heavy emphasis on such factors as intrapsychic conflicts derived from one's family of origin, mate selection, and the interaction of partners' unconscious conflicts in the marital dyad (Meissner, 1978; Nadelson & Paolino, 1978). At the other extreme, both the family systems and the behavioral approaches have focused almost exclusively on here-and-now marital interaction [cf. Gurman (1978) for a detailed comparison of various treatment orientations].

Currently, in our assessment plan, we routinely devote at least one and occasionally two sessions to each individual, depending on the complexity of his or her past history or current ambivalence concerning goals for therapy. Individualized history-taking has seemed increasingly more appropriate over recent years, since (1) the number of cases in which there have been previous marriages and blended families has grown dramatically and (2) the likelihood of significant psychopathology in one or both partners has increased as the application of marital therapy has broadened to include identified patient populations (Jacobson & Gurman, 1988). In these situations, marital therapy is frequently more complicated and expectations for change quite variable. Accordingly, a better understanding is required of what past experiences and expectations each individual brings into the current relationship, especially any traumatic legacies from one's family of origin or previous relationships.

Obviously, one or even two hours of interview time provides only a brief review of the individual's history. At the outset of the individual assessment session, two goals are proposed to the client: (1) to give the individual an opportunity to talk about issues that may be difficult to discuss in the conjoint meetings and (2) to take a personal developmental history up to the time the present relationship was initiated. The objective of the personal history is to touch on the *important positive and negative highlights* of family childhood experiences, significant activities and relationships during school, and experiences related to previous meaningful intimate relationships.

Significant issues that may arise and should be noted during these individual sessions are histories of medical, mental, or substance-abuse problems, legal difficulties, or issues related to sexual fidelity or orientation. Indeed, we have found that information gathered during these individual sessions can be important in understanding individuals' past experiences that significantly influence their *current* behavioral patterns, cognitions, and affective perspectives. Recently, the MMPI has been added to our marital assessment battery. The MMPI has proven to be a relatively efficient tool in terms of facilitating our understanding of partners' personality dispositions. Most recently, the MMPI has been used to explore the utility of studying the potential interaction of partners' personality predispositions within the marriage. On occasion, MMPI interpretations have been used for strategic purposes during the feedback process to the couple. The use of the MMPI in this fashion has proved to be both interesting and extremely helpful, especially for certain couples in whom psychopathology is present. In sum, treatment planning may indeed be affected by individual partners' personal limitations and resources for change. These boundaries can best be illuminated by conducting individual assessment sessions.

INTERACTIONAL SUMMARY AND TREATMENT CONTRACT

The final conjoint assessment session has two objectives: (1) to summarize the findings of the multimethod assessment process and (2) to make the decision whether or not to enter marital therapy (i.e., the intervention phase). In providing feedback, an effective strategy is to describe to the couple the positive potential for change in their marital system, using the language and perspectives learned from and recently taught to them. In addition, any noteworthy limitations and challenges to the couple in reaching their goals are discussed.

First, the major analytical task is to conceptualize the problems and strengths in the marital dyad and then to attempt to summarize for the couple the multidimensional information obtained. Data come from the individual and conjoint clinical interviews, from the observed communication sample, and from the Marital Relationship Assessment Battery and the MMPI. Of passing note, much of the personal information gained throughout the assessment process about the individuals may or may not be related directly to the couple, particularly in a conjoint format. Disclosing such information depends on the couple's interest, on the therapist's strategic objectives in setting up the treatment contract, and, of course, on the quality of the information. That is, we try to ensure that any feedback is constructive for the individuals and for the relationship (i.e., in accord with the limited confidentiality agreement).

The comprehensive information accumulated throughout the assessment process can be organized into four requisite dimensions of marital intimacy—the 4 C's: Commitment, Caring, Communication, and Conflict resolution (Nichols, 1988). These dimensions are very similar to critical relationship processes and skills discussed by others (e.g., Olson, Fournier, & Druckman, 1987; Weiss & Birchler, 1975; Wynne, 1984). Adopting Nichols's labels, the 4 C's is an easy mnemonic for therapists and couples to remember; as such, it assists couples to understand and to categorize the comprehensive information summarized to them at this time.

The treatment plan is outlined for the couple with the goal of making improvements in these primary domains of relationship function. As appropriate, a certain rationale is presented to the couple regarding the requisites for a quality intimate relationship. First, from a biopsycho-social perspective, individuals must grow and develop to the point where each has whatever essential personal resources are required to establish and to maintain a healthy relationship. As therapists, we may oversimplify this basic concept as the *absence of disabling psychopathology*. Next, without *Commitment*, there will probably be insufficient trust and faith in the security and stability of the relationship to foster the development of long term intimacy. Commitment is largely a motivational variable, born of past and present interpersonal relationships. Of course, *Caring* behaviors are critical to a truly intimate relationship. Interestingly, caring behaviors derive from both motivational and instrumental (i.e., skill acquisition) determinants. Such behaviors encompass not only sex and affection but also the development of mutually rewarding activities, quality time together, and a real friendship experience offering interpersonal support and understanding. Beyond the basics of commitment and caring, a necessary vehicle for expressing these values, for building friendship, and for identifying and understanding important relationship issues is marital *Communication*. While the *will* to communicate is an important motivational variable, we believe that the presence or absence of the *skill* to communicate significantly helps or hinders most couples in their pursuit of an intimate relationship. Finally, since conflict is inevitable in marriage, couples must possess (or soon develop) *Conflict resolution* skills in order to manage anger and conflict such that they do not damage the other important aspects of their relationship. In sum, in our experience, couples find it easy to relate to the 4 C's as they try to comprehend what has gone wrong with their marriage and what aspects of the relationship require therapy.

Table 2 incorporates the variables discussed above and presents a therapist rating form that is being piloted in our clinic. We are gathering data on the probable difficulty level of, and perhaps the outcome prospects for, marital therapy with a given couple at varying levels of these dimensions. While as yet few empirical data have been collected, the information is presented here as a heuristic clinical tool to summarize levels of function/dysfunction in these areas. Our plan is to develop empirical weights for each level so that eventually the measure may be scalable. Our expectations are: (1) that couples who, at the end of the assessment phase, rate relatively lower across the five variables will prove to be more difficult to treat; and (2) that the therapeutic outcome prospects for such couples will also be relatively poorer.

Typically, the decision to commence (or not to commence) marital therapy is made at the end of the fifth session overall, which is the third and final conjoint meeting of the assessment phase. If the therapist, or one or both partners, decide that marital therapy *is not* indicated, the therapist carefully and sensitively discusses the reasons and goes on to make whatever referrals may be appropriate (e.g., individual psychotherapy, divorce mediation or therapy). If marital therapy *is* indicated, any number of content- and process-type problems identified during evaluation can be conceptualized according to the 4 C's and existing individual psychopathology. Therefore, the detailed interactional summary organized around the 4 C's has already formed the basis for the specific treatment goals. Issues relating to commitment, caring, communication, and conflict resolution are targeted for treatment in a planned sequence of interventions.

Unfortunately, for too many couples, the basic issue is either commitment to

TABLE 2.   Difficulty Level for Short-Term Marital Therapy: Therapist Rating Scale

Date: _____	Couple name: _____		Therapist: _____	
Significant individual psychopathology:	Mild–absent	Moderate	Major—one partner	Major—both partners
Couple commitment:	High	Fair	Low, mixed	Absent
Caring level:	High	Fair	Low	Absent
Communication:	Frequent, effective	Fair, intermittent	Poor, negative	Embittered, disrespectful
Conflict resolution:	Effective	Variable	Poor	Physical violence
Prognosis range:	Very good	Fair	Poor	Very poor

the relationship or basic caring for one another or both. In our experience, in the absence of fundamental levels of commitment and caring, interventions designed solely to increase communication and conflict-resolution skills are generally ineffective. In these cases, early interventions should focus on whether the partners can establish a basic sense of dyadic trust, security, and mutual attraction. For example, the therapist may assign simple exercises, in which the partners identify relatively nonconflictual independent or interdependent activities, and then encourage them to demonstrate follow-through regarding these behavioral agreements. Similarly, partners may be helped to develop independent and mutually rewarding activities that foster a feeling of enjoyment and togetherness. If these early interventions are successful in increasing the partners' levels of commitment and caring, then adding communication training and conflict-management skills to the therapeutic process can be an effective treatment.

On the other hand, in cases in which partners are committed and, even better, also experience a reasonable amount of caring for one another, then a program of communication, problem-solving, and conflict-resolution skills training can be initiated successfully at the outset of treatment. For a given couple, with these various goals outlined and endorsed, the treatment contract is confirmed and the formal intervention phase begins.

Do's AND DON'T's

Therapist Skills and Interview Behaviors (Do's)

Behaviorally oriented marital therapists are active participants in the therapeutic process. Efficiency, efficacy, and contemporary health care economics combine to mandate a briefer, more focused and directed therapeutic enterprise. Accordingly, there are a number of therapist skills and interview behaviors that are important in the clinical assessment process.

To enhance the prospects for gaining rapport and facilitating clients' positive expectations, the therapist, regardless of level of training, should be calm and exude confidence, competence, and enthusiasm. Throughout the assessment interviews, the therapist attempts to *sell* the couple on his or her capability as a therapist and on the efficacy of the chosen therapeutic approach.

For example, in an initial interview, the following dialogue is representative:

HUSBAND: [Looking skeptical] You look kind of young. Are you a student?

THERAPIST [Who is completing his predoctoral internship]: Not exactly. I have a master's degree in psychology, and I have been working with couples and families for over 2 years. This is my last year of training before I receive my doctoral degree.

HUSBAND: [Still testing] How long have you worked in this clinic?

THERAPIST: I've been here about 3 months. But as I said, I've been working with couples for about 2 years. In addition, I have constant access to two very experienced therapists who have been directing this couples program for many years. The approach developed here has been demonstrated to be very effective in helping couples who want to improve their marriages. We kind of use a team approach and you get the benefit of several experts consulting on your case.

The therapist maintains a supportive, information-seeking stance, probing for important personal information in a caring manner and using warm humor whenever appropriate. There are several other ways to facilitate this joining process. For example, emphasizing throughout the assessment process that you are all working as a team to evaluate the relationship and that ultimately they are the experts on their own relationship can minimize a couple's fear and defensiveness at this stage. Additionally, bringing in a cotherapist of the opposite gender can significantly facilitate joining with the couple and promote the concept of a team approach.

The therapist must also, however, maintain control of the interviews. Control techniques include effective interruptions, reframing problems as protective or coping mechanisms, summarizing and normalizing a partner's position, and directing who should talk and to whom at a given time. For example, during the second conjoint interview, the wife has shown a tendency to dominate the discussion with blaming-type comments. The therapist addresses John purposefully and probes for a positive theme:

THERAPIST: John, you said earlier that you were attracted to Linda because of her outgoing personality. She was cute, fun to be with, and was real interested in what you were doing. In your view, have those qualities changed?

HUSBAND: Not really. Linda still gets along well with people. Friends and family like to be around her. Except it seems like she and I don't have much fun any more.

WIFE: [Interrupting] We haven't got anything in common any more. Now that our kids have left home, John doesn't want to have much to do with them or me. He just goes to work and comes home and watches TV all night and all weekend. Then he gets mad when I want to go out or visit my family.

THERAPIST: [Interrupting] Linda, it sounds like you and John both agree that you still have lots of positive energy for socializing. You're the life of the party, but John hasn't been your date recently [smiling]. Initially, John was attracted to this, but now he says that the two of you don't have much fun any more. Would you like to spend more quality time with John?

WIFE: [Sarcastically] Yes, but not in front of the TV set!

THERAPIST: [Interrupting again] O.K. And John, would you like to spend more quality time with Linda?

HUSBAND: Sure, but I don't enjoy her family as much as she does.

THERAPIST: O.K., I understand. But I wonder if what has happened here isn't fairly typical. Your youngest child left home and moved out of town about a year ago, right?

WIFE: Yes.

THERAPIST: Unfortunately, many parents, in raising a family, inadvertently lose sight of the need to develop and maintain quality activities just for their own enjoyment. It's hard to make the couple relationship by itself a high priority. I suspect that both of you miss these fun activities and have gotten into the common rut of work, TV, and going your own way to socialize. Is that right?

HUSBAND: I guess so.

WIFE: Yes, we really haven't done much together since our daughter left home.

THERAPIST: Well, as I say, that's a typical development—and a problem we can certainly work on.

At all times, the therapist should model effective listening skills by paraphrasing, reflecting, validating feelings, and making empathic statements to support painful disclosures and to allay anxiety. Both partners have the right and the responsibility to participate in the assessment process; the therapist should take steps to involve them both in the description of their issues, experiences, thoughts, and feelings.

For example, in assessing a couple when the wife speaks only reluctantly:

HUSBAND: Ellen is never interested in having sex. I've given up asking.

THERAPIST: Ellen, Phil thinks you're not interested in having sex with him. What is your reaction to this?

WIFE: I don't know, I guess he's right." [Silence]

THERAPIST: Can you share your concerns? What is your sex life like with Phil?

WIFE: I guess it's not very good. When we do make love, Phil is in such a hurry. I just don't enjoy it very much.

THERAPIST: Is it painful? Do you feel you have enough time to get aroused? What would make it more enjoyable?

WIFE: Well, it's usually late at night when Phil is interested. I'm tired. I don't get wet like I used to and sometimes it hurts.

THERAPIST: Gee, no wonder you're less interested. I would think anyone who is tired, unaroused, and anticipating pain would be less enthusiastic about having sex. This is important information. Phil, were you aware of Ellen's experience?

HUSBAND: Not really. I know she's tired a lot, and by the time we get in bed it's 11:30 or 12:00. But I didn't know the other things. I just thought that if she was interested at all she'd probably want to get it over with and go to sleep.

THERAPIST: Well, without really clear communication, I can see how, for Ellen's sake, you might be in a hurry. Ironically, this strategy may have made the situation worse. What do you think, Ellen?

WIFE: I just wish we could be a little more romantic and not always get into these arguments about sex at midnight.

THERAPIST: You mean you think you would be more interested in sex if there were more romance, more energy available to enjoy sex, and more time to enjoy one another and to get aroused?

WIFE: Yes, that would sure help me.

HUSBAND: [Looks a little surprised, but attentive.]

THERAPIST: Yes, and if you were more comfortable and interested, I would think that the whole experience would be better for Phil, too, don't you think? [Looks at Phil.]

HUSBAND: That's right. I guess we got into some bad habits and haven't communicated about this very well.

THERAPIST: It's unfortunate how frequently this kind of pattern occurs in couples. But the good news is that improved communication, in a caring couple, can help to make significant improvements.

Obviously, the therapist keenly observes the couple and their communication patterns. At certain points during the assessment interviews, the partners are directed to talk with one another (e.g., the problem-solving communication sample). Verbal and nonverbal behaviors that suggest confusion or conflict for the couple are commented on and their meanings are explored. Using this technique, important relationship rules, roles, and expectations may be discovered.

For example, during the second assessment interview:

THERAPIST: Given what you've said, I'm very interested in why you moved from Arizona to California when you both had good jobs and Mike's big family lived nearby. I wonder if you two would review this decision together, while I watch and listen. But I may interrupt to ask questions, O.K.?

WIFE: [Looking at the therapist] I think Mike's family was part of the problem.

THERAPIST [Interpreting] Stacey, please discuss this with Mike.

WIFE: Your sister lived next door and I couldn't stand her telling me how to raise my kids when all four of hers were always in trouble.

HUSBAND: She didn't tell you how to raise your kids. You asked my mom about thumb-sucking, and Rose was just trying to help out.

WIFE: [Frowning and interrupting] Yes, I asked your mother, *not Rose*! It wasn't any of her business. How did she hear about it, anyway.

HUSBAND: [Acting defensively] Oh, you know my mom tells everybody everything. She doesn't know any better. Why do you have to be so sensitive?

WIFE: [Getting more angry] I'm not sensitive! I have a right to raise my kids without being criticized all the time!

THERAPIST: [Smiling] O.K.—thank you very much. Wow, there are a lot of strong feelings around this issue. [Addressing Stacey] I understand that the relationship between you and Mike's family was not on the best of terms. I wonder if you didn't feel a little outnumbered and maybe even that Mike didn't support you? [Looking at Mike] And Mike, I wonder if you felt caught in the middle on these issues—in a no-win position?

HUSBAND: I didn't like to take sides, but it was hard.

WIFE: Actually, I was a little jealous of Mike and his family and how close they were. Sometimes I didn't feel like I fit in.

THERAPIST: Well, it seems to me like this was a tough situation for both of you. Mike didn't want to criticize or anger his family, but in this situation you [looking at Stacey] apparently didn't feel the support you wanted. You know, it takes a lot of communication and good teamwork to establish the boundaries around a new family in the midst of one partner's extended family. I imagine things are easier in this regard now that you live in California.

WIFE: Yes, that part is a lot better.

It is important to allow an opportunity for each partner to tell his or her story. On one hand, while these descriptions are often blaming and defensive, if the therapist is too restrictive and disallows such ventilation of feelings (Stuart, 1980), the clients may not feel heard and may drop out of treatment. On the other hand, it is also important to limit the pervasive blame frame that couples bring to therapy by promulgating the *interactional view* whenever the opportunity allows. Accordingly, the couple's problems and strengths are described in interdependent relationship-oriented terminology. The relationship is conceptualized as an entity separate from and greater than the individuals. Individual growth potential is attributed to couples who can be genuinely collaborative with one another to improve the quality of their intimate relationship.

For example, near the beginning of an initial interview:

THERAPIST: Whose idea was it to seek marital therapy?

HUSBAND: [Looks toward the floor, silently]

WIFE: I've been trying to get Chuck to go to counseling for several years. Finally, I told him that either we get counseling or I'm leaving. I can't take it any more.

THERAPIST: So for you, Barbara, things finally got to the point where something just had to be done. What can't you take any more?

WIFE: Chuck's constant criticism and irritability. Nothing I do or the kids do is right. It seems like he hasn't been happy for years, and it's driving all of us crazy. Chuck's my husband, and I don't even know if I *like* him any more!

THERAPIST: I can hear that you're very frustrated and discouraged. It must feel lousy to wonder if you like your husband. I can understand that you are determined that things change. Chuck, how do you make sense of what Barbara is saying and feeling? What's your view?

HUSBAND: I've been busting my tail for over 20 years in the Marines. We've done very well as a family financially; we've only moved twice in the last 13 years. But I certainly don't get any respect at home. Barbara and the boys make a decision, and I have nothing to say about it. Of course this makes me irritable.

THERAPIST: Can you give me an example of a decision you've been left out of?

HUSBAND: Yeah! The damn car. Before the last cruise, I specifically told Barbara and Billie that three vehicles are enough to pay for, insurance and all. Then, against my wishes, they bought Billie a car anyway. I send the money home and they spend it however they please. I have no say in the matter—and naturally that ticks me off!

THERAPIST: So you feel kind of isolated and shut out or ganged up against when it comes to family decisions . . .

HUSBAND: [Interrupting] That's right!

THERAPIST: [Continuing] . . . and because of this situation, you feel disrespected and end up being irritable and critical, is that right?

HUSBAND: I guess so.

THERAPIST: So far, it sure sounds to me like each of you has lost your best teammate. Marriage works best as a partnership where both partners not only share the good and the bad, they consult one another on significant decisions, and they express positive and supportive attitudes toward each other and their children. I guess this process has broken down in your relationship, and you're here to try to fix it before the relationship comes to an end. Does that make sense so far?

HUSBAND AND WIFE: [Both look serious but nod their heads in assent.]

Finally, there are some therapist "Do's" in the event that so-called *resistance* behaviors are encountered during the assessment process (e.g., people are late for sessions, fail to complete agreed-on homework, present uncooperative attitudes). The basic strategy is first to try to ignore these behaviors in hope of extinguishing them. If such behaviors persist, the next step is to reframe them with a positive (i.e., functional) interpretation, such as: "You folks seem to have difficulty getting here on time. I wonder if your lateness isn't telling us something important about what is going on in the sessions?" Finally, if basic inquiry and reframing techniques are not effective, the next step is to confront them directly, for example: "We are not going to be able to help you if you are late consistently. Either we will have to resolve this problem, or perhaps now isn't the time to initiate this process." Detailed methods for identifying and dealing with various forms of resistance behaviors in marital therapy are beyond the scope of this chapter and are discussed elsewhere (e.g., Anderson & Stewart, 1983; Birchler, 1988; Jacobson, 1991; Spinks & Birchler, 1982.)

Therapist Don't's

Assuming that the therapist is knowledgeable and competent in basic interviewing skills (cf. Cormier & Cormier, 1985; see also Chapter 1), there are a number of additional situations to avoid in the assessment process with marital dyads. These pitfalls may be obvious, but they are nevertheless difficult to avoid, especially for beginning marital therapists. One should avoid the use of undefined jargon and pop psychology labels. Couples may be taught certain key phrases and concepts so as to understand the therapist's approach, but relatively more emphasis should be placed on understanding the couple's key phrases and relationship concepts.

The therapist should also avoid letting one partner dominate the session. There is a tendency for this to happen frequently. The idea is to control the dominance using assertive empathy and to involve both partners in the process of self-disclosure. In a similar vein, the couple should not be allowed to escalate their arguments and cross-complaints into an emotional exchange that is out of control. Indeed, some couples are all too practiced at escalating emotions to a highly destructive level at a moment's notice. However, beyond the most basic objective of baseline behavioral observation, escalating negative interactions should be controlled and avoided if possible. Usually, the therapist can cope with this problem by asking the partners to talk only to the therapist (i.e., not to engage each other). Using this technique, the therapist can summarize, rephrase, and validate partners' otherwise provocative negative statements. Also, the therapist may just have to interrupt and terminate escalating negative interactions, indicating that they are not productive and will be discouraged during the sessions.

Finally, during the assessment phase in particular, we believe that the therapist should neither actively take sides nor inadvertently be drawn into an alliance by sometimes desperate or manipulative partners. Maintaining a neutral stance in support of both individuals and the relationship is critical during assessment. This can be a very difficult task, and the case may require close supervision to accomplish it successfully.

Interestingly, the "Do's and Don't's" outlined above provide much of the substance of supervision of marital therapists in training. Indeed, even experienced therapists are not immune from occasional failure to manage these situations effectively. Therapists at all levels of training have rewarding successes and humiliating failures in their attempts to fully understand and to help marital dyads. Accumulated experience in marital therapy certainly helps, but in this field, one's learning process is never complete.

SUMMARY

This chapter has presented some basic interviewing strategies for assessing marital dyads in the context of a behaviorally oriented brief treatment approach. The outpatient assessment of marital dyads is carried out over several sessions, which include discussion and analysis of presenting problems, clients' goals and expectations for therapy, an *in vivo* sample of marital communication and problem-solving, and brief individual and relationship developmental histories. The basic outline of *what to cover* in assessing a marital dyad was complemented with suggestions of *how to cover* this extensive material. The content areas explored and the interview strategies used were designed to help the clinician understand the various presentations of marital dyads, to trace the development of relationship dysfunction, to determine the potential impact of the partners' individual issues, and to build a comprehensive data base for effective intervention planning. Important features of the clinical assessment process, strategic objectives of the interviews, the management of confidentiality issues, therapist "Do's and Don't's," and a basic scheme for presenting the multidimensional assessment results to the couple in preparation for the intervention stage were presented.

REFERENCES

American Association for Marriage and Family Therapy (1988). *AAMFT code of ethical principles for marriage and family therapists*. Washington, DC: Author.

American Psychiatric Association (1993). *Diagnostic and statistical manual of mental disorders*, 4th ed., draft criteria. Washington, DC: Author.

American Psychological Association (1981). Ethical principles of psychologists. *American Psychologist*, 36, 633–638.

Anderson, C. M., & Stewart, S. (1983). *Mastering resistance: A practical guide to family therapy*. New York: Guilford Press.

Basco, M. R., Birchler, G. R., Kalal, B., Talbott, R., & Slater, M. A. (1991). The clinician rating of adult communication (CRAC): A clinician's guide to the assessment of interpersonal communications skill. *Journal of Clinical Psychology, 47*, 368–380.

Birchler, G. R. (1979). Communication skills in married couples. In A. S. Bellack & M. Hersen (Eds.), *Research and practice in social skills training* (pp. 273–315). New York: Plenum Press.

Birchler, G. R. (1983). Marital dysfunction. In M. Hersen (Ed.), *Practice of outpatient behavioral therapy: A clinician's handbook* (pp. 229–269). New York: Grune & Stratton.

Birchler, G. R. (1988). Handling resistance to change. In I. R. H. Falloon (Ed.), *Handbook of behavioral family therapy* (pp. 128–155). New York: Guilford Press.

Birchler, G. R. (1992). Marriage. In V. B. Van Hasselt & M. Hersen (Eds.), *Handbook of social development: A lifespan perspective* (pp. 397–419). New York: Plenum Press.

Birchler, G. R., Clopton, P. L., & Adams, N. L. (1984). Marital conflict resolution: Factors influencing concordance between partner and trained coders. *American Journal of Family Therapy, 12*, 15–28.

Birchler, G. R., & Gershwin, M. (1990). Marital dysfunction. In M. E. Thase, B. A. Edelstein, & M. Hersen (Eds.), *Handbook of outpatient treatment of adults* (pp. 463–488). New York: Plenum Press.

Birchler, G. R., & Spinks, S. H. (1980). Behavioral-systems marital and family therapy: Integration and clinical application. *American Journal of Family Therapy, 8*, 6–28.

Birchler, G. R., Weiss, R. L., & Vincent, J. P. (1975). Multimethod analysis of social reinforcement exchange between maritally distressed and nondistressed spouse and stranger dyads. *Journal of Personality and Social Psychology, 31*, 349–360.

Bornstein, P. H., & Bornstein, M. T. (1986). *Marital therapy: A behavioral–communications approach.* New York: Pergamon Press.

Carter, B., & McGoldrick, M. (1988). *The changing family life cycle,* 2nd ed. New York: Gardner Press.

Cormier, W. H., & Cormier, L. S. (1985). *Interviewing strategies for helpers.* Monterey CA: Brooks/Cole.

Filsinger, E. E. (Ed.) (1983). *Marriage and family assessment.* Beverly Hills: Sage Publications.

Floyd, F. J., & Markman, H. J. (1984). Observational biases in spouse observation: Toward a cognitive–behavioral model of marriage. *Journal of Consulting and Clinical Psychology, 51,* 450–457.

Glick, I. D., & Kessler, D. R. (1980). *Marital and family therapy.* New York: Grune & Stratton.

Gottman, J. (1979). *Marital interaction: Experimental investigations.* New York: Academic Press.

Gurman, A. S. (1978). Contemporary marital therapies: A critique and comparative analysis of psychoanalytic, behavioral and systems theory approaches. In T. J. Paolino & B. S. McCrady (Eds.), *Marriage and marital therapy* (pp. 455–566). New York: Brunner/Mazel.

Gurman, A. S. (1991). Back to the future, ahead to the past: Is marital therapy going in circles? *Journal of Family Psychology, 4,* 402–406.

Gurman, A. S., & Jacobson, N. S. (1988). Marital therapy: From technique to theory, back again and beyond. In N. S. Jacobson & A. S. Gurman (Eds.), *Clinical handbook of marital therapy* (pp. 1–12). New York: Guilford Press.

Haynes, S. N., & Chavez, R. E. (1983). The interview in the assessment of marital distress. In E. E. Filsinger (Ed.), *Marriage and family assessment* (pp. 23–44). Beverly Hills: Sage Publications.

Haynes, S. N., Follingstad, D. R., & Sullivan, J. (1979). Assessment of marital satisfaction and interaction. *Journal of Consulting and Clinical Psychology, 47,* 789–791.

Hersen, M., & Bellack, A. S. (1988). *Dictionary of behavioral assessment techniques.* New York: Pergamon Press.

Hof, L., & Treat, S. R. (1989). Marital assessment: Providing a framework for dynamic therapy. In G. R. Weeks (Ed.), *Treating couples* (pp. 3–21). New York: Brunner/Mazel.

Jacobson, N. S. (1991). Toward enhancing the efficacy of marital therapy and marital therapy research. *Journal of Family Psychology, 4(4),* 373–393.

Jacobson, M. S., Follette, W. C., & McDonald, D. W. (1982). Reactivity of positive and negative behavior in distressed and nondistressed married couples. *Journal of Consulting and Clinical Psychology, 50,* 706–714.

Jacobson, N. S., & Gurman, A. S. (Eds.) (1988). *Clinical handbook of marital therapy.* New York: Guilford Press.

Jacobson, N. S., & Margolin, G. (1979). *Marital therapy: Strategies based on social learning and behavior exchange principles* New York: Brunner/Mazel.

Karpel, M. A. (1980). Family secrets. I. Conceptual and ethical issues in relational context, II. Ethical and practical considerations in therapeutic management. *Family Process, 19,* 295–306.

Margolin, G. (1986). Ethical issues in marital therapy. In N. S. Jacobson & A. S. Gurman (Eds.), *Clinical handbook of marital therapy* (pp. 621–638). New York: Guilford Press.

Margolin, G., Michelli, J., & Jacobson, N. S. (1988). Assessment of marital dysfunction. In A. S. Bellack & M. Hersen (Eds.), *Behavioral assessment: A practical handbook* (pp. 441–489). New York: Pergamon Press.

Meissner, W. W. (1978). The conceptualization of marriage and family dynamics from a psychoanalytic perspective. In T. J. Paolino & B. S. McGrady (Eds.), *Marriage and marital therapy* (pp. 25–88). New York: Brunner/Mazel.

Nadelson, C. C., & Paolino, T. J. (1978). Marital therapy from a psychoanalytic perspective. In T. J. Paolino & B . S. McCrady (Eds.), *Marriage and marital therapy* (pp. 89–164). New York: Brunner/Mazel.

Nichols, W. C. (1988). *Marital therapy.* New York: Guilford Press.

Olson, D. H., Fournier, D. G., & Druckman, J. M. (1987). *Counselor's manual for PREPARE/ENRICH,* revised ed. Minneapolis, MN: PREPARE/ENRICH.

Segal, L. (1991). Brief therapy: The MRI approach. In A. S. Gurman & D. P. Kniskern (Eds.), *Handbook of family therapy,* Vol. II (pp. 171–199). New York: Brunner/Mazel.

Segraves, R. T. (1982). *Marital therapy: A combined psychodynamic–behavioral approach.* New York: Plenum Press.

Spinks, S. H., & Birchler, G. R. (1982). Behavioral-systems marital therapy: Dealing with resistance. *Family Process, 21*, 169–185.

Stuart, R. B. (1980). *Helping couples change: A social learning approach to marital therapy.* New York: Guilford Press.

Vincent, J. P., Weiss, R. L., & Birchler, G. R. (1975). A behavioral analysis of problem solving in distressed and nondistressed married and stranger dyads. *Behavior Therapy, 6*, 475–487.

Weiss, R. L. (1980). Strategic behavioral marital therapy: Toward a model for assessment and intervention. In J. P. Vincent (Ed.), *Advances in family intervention, assessment and therapy* Vol. I (pp. 229–271). Greenwich, CN: JAI Press.

Weiss, R. L. (1981). The new kid on the block: Behavioral systems approach. In E. E. Filsinger & R. A. Lewis (Eds.), *Assessing marriage* (pp. 22–37). Beverly Hills: Sage Publications.

Weiss, R. L., & Birchler G. R. (1975). Areas of change questionnaire. Unpublished manuscript, University of Oregon, Eugene.

Weiss, R. L., & Summers, K. L. (1983). Marital interaction coding system—III. In E. E. Filsinger (ed.), *Marriage and family assessment* (pp. 85–116). Beverly Hills: Sage Publications.

Wynne, L. C. (1984). The epigenesis of relational systems: A model for understanding family development. *Family Process, 23*, 297–318.

13

Children

JEFFREY B. ALLEN AND ALAN M. GROSS

INTRODUCTION

The diagnostic interview with the child can be both difficult and rewarding for the behavioral assessor. The difficulty lies in the fact that children are complex and possess a communicative style very different from that of adults. While the child's interpersonal pattern is often complicated, it is also straightforward. To the clinician who is properly prepared for the situation, the interview provides access to the child's unique world and individual experiences. Such access allows for a more complete and accurate evaluation of the child's presenting difficulties. The challenge inherent in child assessment and diagnosis is undoubtedly linked to the multitude of developmental changes that occur during childhood.

When evaluating a child's functioning, a number of domains must be investigated, as even discrete childhood behavior problems can have numerous determinants. The social, developmental, intellectual, physical, educational, and affective realms need to be assessed, as all of these areas can influence the way the child functions in his or her environment. For example, childhood depression may manifest itself in symptoms of separation anxiety, enuresis, and conduct disorders (Kazdin, 1988). Unlike adult depressive symptom patterns, children show a much more diffuse and varied symptomatology throughout childhood. This age-related diversity is affected by the enormous developmental change that occurs during childhood. A thorough appreciation of the child's developmental status is necessary to comprehensively evaluate and treat even relatively focal behavioral problems.

Historically, behavioral assessment tended to focus on the direct observation and description of relatively specific target behaviors exhibited by the child. In the past, behavioral assessment was primarily concerned with obtaining frequency, rate, and duration measures describing the behaviors of interest and determining the consequences of these target behaviors (Mash & Terdal, 1988). While this approach was vital to the establishment of the empirical foundations of behavioral

JEFFREY B. ALLEN AND ALAN M. GROSS • University of Mississippi, University, Mississippi 38677.

Diagnostic Interviewing (Second Edition), edited by Michel Hersen and Samuel M. Turner. Plenum Press, New York, 1994.

assessment, it lacked the breadth of recent behavioral methods. Currently, there is a greater emphasis on evaluating the child as part of a larger network of interacting social systems (Patterson, 1982).

Just as the scope of behavioral assessment has evolved over the years, so too have the methods of evaluating the child. In general, current approaches include a greater variety of assessment tools and types of data (Evans, 1985; Kanfer, 1985). At present, there appears to be a growing appreciation for the value of interviewing teachers, completing behavioral checklists, and having the child self-monitor, as well as interviewing the parent and child. However, it is the clinical interview that guides and directs the implementation of these other strategies.

The purpose of this chapter is to discuss the major issues and components related to the diagnostic interviewing of children. The first part of the chapter is concerned with the general issue of classifying childhood behavioral problems. Next, the functions and components of the diagnostic interview are described. Following this material is a brief discussion of other assessment tools that may be used in conjunction with the interview. The chapter then addresses the importance of assessing the entire family system and attending to relevant development issues. Finally, a case study is provided to illustrate the proposed methodology for diagnostic interviewing of the child.

CLASSIFICATION

Classification is vital for the scientific development of any field. While this task is difficult for the general behavioral clinician, it is perhaps more difficult for the child behavioral assessor. Such difficulty arises primarily from the tremendous lack of information concerning etiology, familial patterns, and developmental aspects of childhood behavioral disorders. For this reason, most diagnostic categories have been generated on the basis of what clinicians agree they recognize from clinical descriptions as fitting what they see in their own practice (Rapoport & Ismond, 1989). The particular group of children seen by a given clinician may introduce a referral bias, which provides the therapist with an unrepresentative sample of a particular diagnostic population (Rapoport & Ismond, 1990). The paucity of long-term longitudinal studies with children only exacerbates this problem.

The chronology of revisions of the *Diagnostic and Statistical Manual of Mental Disorders* (DSM) reflects a steady increase in the number of specific diagnostic categories dedicated to child psychopathology. In the initial version of this classification system, DSM-I (American Psychiatric Association, 1952), childhood categories were largely absent. While the publication of DSM-II (American Psychiatric Association, 1968) provided some coverage of childhood diagnosis, there was ample dissatisfaction with the relative imprecision of the categories. Although there remain many issues related to the empirical robustness and clinical utility of DSM-III (American Psychiatric Association, 1980) and DSM-III-R (American Psychiatric Association, 1987) there is little question that the current offering is more refined and precise than earlier versions.

In general, DSM-IV (American Psychiatric Association, 1994) provides the same multiaxial diagnostic structure for childhood disorders as is used in adult classification. The classes of disorders that are relevant to childhood psychopathology can be subsumed under five major groups based on the primary area of disturbance. For heuristic purposes, these groupings include: intellectual, behavioral, emotional, physical, and developmental difficulties. The DSM-IV classification system requires that those disorders initially diagnosed in infancy, childhood, or adolescence be given Axis I status. Under DSM-IV criteria, both specific (e.g., reading, arithmetic) and pervasive developmental disorders will also be recorded along Axis I. As with adult difficulties, childhood disorders that do not warrant diagnosis as a mental disorder can be noted with a V-code (e.g., V62.30, academic problem). This designation reduces the social stigma attached to psychiatric labeling.

Accompanying the addition of new categories of childhood pathology is a decrease in interrater agreement. A larger number of diagnostic possibilities obviously leads to higher rates of clinical disagreement. This phenomenon is one rationale for the disconcerting findings by Mezzich, Mezzich, and Coffrian (1985) that clinicians making diagnoses from case vignettes showed no better agreement using DSM-III, despite clearer diagnostic criteria, than they did using DSM-II. While reliability issues still abound, there is also evidence that clinicians do agree regarding the broad category under which a particular behavioral problem should be classified. Apparently, disagreement within a broad category is much more common (Pendergast et al., 1988).

OBJECTIVES OF THE INTERVIEW

The diagnostic interview is often seen as a monolithic entity used to exhaustively evaluate the child. Perhaps a more realistic and appropriate objective would be to direct the course of the entire assessment process. That is, a function of the interview is to determine what other assessment methods need to be employed and how findings are to be interpreted. The more common objectives of the diagnostic interview include providing diagnostic information about the child's presenting problem, evaluating the child's larger environment (e.g., family, school, peers) in relation to his or her current difficulties, and evaluating the likelihood that the child will benefit from existing treatment options.

Generally, early diagnostic efforts tend to be aimed at screening and classifying the child's behavioral problems. This aspect of the interview involves the comprehensive evaluation of the child's social, intellectual, emotional, and physical development. Because of the complexity of children's psychological composition, a given presenting problem may be related to one of several diverse determinants. Thus, a child's depressive symptomatology may be viewed as an unchanging, chronic disease process when in reality it exists on a more transient basis governed by day-to-day events. For example, a child may be despondent one day because her father left for a business trip, while she may be despondent another day because of an argument with a friend.

A second objective of the interview is the complete assessment of the child's broader social environment. While the behavioral interview continues to be viewed as highly individualized and directed toward the child, it is not limited to assessment of the child. There is now consideration of a much wider range of variables, including such issues as family stress, the marital relationship, and the quality of parent–child interaction. These variables should also be subjected to assessment and possible intervention (Brody, Pillegrini, & Sigel, 1986; Pannaccione & Wahler, 1986).

Along with the evaluation of a broader set of variables comes the increased need for a greater variety of assessment methods than was characteristic of earlier approaches (Evans, 1985; Kanfer, 1985; Mash & Terdal, 1988). Direct observation, self-monitoring, formal testing, and the interviewing of parents or teachers may be incorporated with the behavioral interview of the child.

A third objective of the diagnostic interview involves the more pragmatic issue of treating a child's existing difficulties. While the initial interview with the child may be seen as a fact-finding session, the ultimate concern revolves around what can be done to assist the child in adapting more comfortably to his or her world. Evaluating the child's existing strengths and special competencies may not be immediately relevant to diagnostic decisions, but it is quite important in the development of treatment strategies. Assessing the motivation for treatment of the child and significant others can also aid in the selection of appropriate and effective intervention programs. Finally, the diagnostic interview can include the setting of realistic and specific treatment goals, which can be monitored throughout future involvement with the child. Thus, while treatment planning is not the primary objective of the diagnostic interview, it should be addressed so the child and significant others can be presented with useful prognostic information.

Although the goals of the diagnostic interview are similar regardless of the target population, there are a number of aspects of diagnostic interviewing with children that are very different from those of interviewing individuals with adult disorders. Unlike most adult patients who attend therapy after identifying themselves as having behavioral difficulties, a child usually sees the therapist because an adult (parent or teacher) has determined that a behavioral problem exists (Gross, 1985). Related to this issue is the reality that children also differ from adults in the amount of social control to which they are subject. A clear understanding of the specific controls and contingencies operating at the time of the assessment is vital to an accurate understanding of the child.

Behavioral assessment should also address the child's cognitive skills and intellectual functioning. Frequently, a child's behavioral symptomatology is related to learning difficulties, a circumstance that may necessitate a more formal evaluation of the child's intellectual or academic activities. Similarly, the clinician should be well-versed in developmental psychology in order to completely comprehend the nature and significance of the responses observed. Conduct at one age may not be predictive of later behavior. Reevaluation should be the norm in child diagnosis.

Perhaps the most unique aspect of the interview with a child concerns the relevance of parental and environmental variables to childhood behavior. Interviewers cannot simply assume that because a child is referred for evaluation, he or she exhibits behavior problems. Parents' perceptions of child behavior can be influenced by a variety of personal factors; therefore, the clinician must obtain multiple sources of information. Moreover, an assessment of parental adjustment and expectations about the behavior of children may be necessary before any determination of child deviance can be made.

DIAGNOSTIC INTERVIEW

Whether interviewing the parents, teachers, or child, the interviewer is attempting to gather considerable information. While a large part of the interview is directed toward the presenting problem, the focus of the interview should be much wider in scope. In addition to defining the problem behavior(s), the clinician should attempt to discover the associated antecedent and consequent stimuli, to assess the parents' mediational potential, to evaluate the youngster's strengths, and to identify possible rewarding and aversive contingencies to be employed in treatment. A developmental history should also be obtained. This information puts the child's behavior in perspective and contributes to determining the significance of the difficulty.

Interviewing the Parents

The initial meeting with the parent(s) can provide information about the child and the presenting problem, as well as information about the parents and the parent–child relationship. In the past, child assessment placed primary emphasis on gathering information directly relevant to the child or the parent–child relationship. At present, there is a greater appreciation for the importance of parental characteristics and personality traits that contribute to childhood functioning in both family and school environments (e.g., Forehand, Long, Brody, & Fauber, 1986). Furthermore, the affective status of the parents has also been linked to childhood behavior (e.g., Hammen et al., 1986). Moreover, there should be an attempt to focus on the child, the parent(s), sibling relationships, and the marriage, as well as the dynamics between these various systems (Mash & Terdal, 1988). Accordingly, an attempt should be made to determine how family difficulties as well as marital conflict are handled. Similarly, the parents' ability to cope with stressors outside the family should be evaluated. Questions such as "What do the two of you do to relax?" can be very helpful in assessing parental stress mediation.

The therapist begins the initial interview by gathering demographic information about the child (e.g., age, grade in school), then attempts to obtain a description of the problem. General questions from the interviewer, such as "What prompted you to come to the clinic at this time?" or "Can you tell me what problems you are having with your child?," can be used to initiate this process. Because the clinician is equally interested in gaining insight into what variables may be initiating and maintaining the child's behavior, specific questions regarding details of the response and situation in which it occurs should be asked: "Exactly what does she do?" "What do you do when he does that?" "Does it always occur at dinner time?" Additionally, information concerning frequency and duration of problem behaviors is collected.

Questions such as those suggested above serve to initiate the interview process, define the problem, and determine possible environmental stimuli related to its occurrence. Subsequent questions will be determined by the nature of the presenting complaint. Questions addressed to the parents and child presenting with attention-deficit disorder differ from those directed to the family of a depressed youth. The interviewer's questions are still intended to describe behaviors and identify associated stimuli. Familiarity with the essential and associated features of the various child syndromes is imperative for this process. Awareness of which behaviors typically covary with others determines the direction of the interview. For example, parents whose primary concern is their son's apparent inability to stay on task should be questioned about the occurrence of other behaviors known to covary with attention problems. This approach will help delineate the child's full range of responses in need of treatment, differentiate the disorder from similar childhood disorders, and yield useful data for determining the severity of the problem and the suitability of potential treatments.

Following this stage of data collection, the interviewer may begin to assess the child's behavioral assets. Asking the parents what behaviors they would like to see their child perform may yield this information (e.g., "What would you like to see him do in that situation?"). This line of questioning leads to the determination of appropriate alternative responses to teach the child. It also helps to assess parental expectation of child behaviors.

Parents should also be prompted for information about which stimuli serve as rewarding and aversive consequences for the child. This discussion can assist the therapist in determining possible contributors to the presenting problem and aid in the selection of an effective treatment plan. Asking parents about their child's likes and dislikes ("What does she do after school?" "Does he like TV?") is often an effective technique for gathering this information.

It is increasingly evident that behavioral assessment of the child should place greater emphasis on information reported by parents about themselves, such as self-reported perceptions and feelings (Patterson, 1982). While behavioral assessment traditionally focused on how parents reacted to the child's problem, clinicians currently place increasing value on parents' reports of their feelings, attitudes, and cognitions independently of the child's specific presenting problem (e.g., Sigel, 1985).

This increased focus on parental attitudes, values, and cognitions has generated a number of self-report measures intended for both research and clinical assessment of the parent. These instruments can assist the therapist in evaluating a number of parental dimensions, including general attitudes about children and child-rearing (Bristol, 1983), parenting self-esteem (Mash & Johnson, 1986), empathy (Chlopan, McBain, Carbonell, & Hagen, 1985), and satisfaction in areas concerned with spouse support (Guidubaldi & Cleminshaw, 1985). A thorough assessment of these parental variables provides a far broader understanding of the child's difficulties and gives the interviewer a more realistic appreciation for the parents' mediational capabilities. The success of any treatment intervention rests on the parents' ability and motivation to carry out the proposed intervention strategy.

One self-report scale that attempts to measure parents' attitudes concerning the relationship with their child is the Index of Parental Attitudes (IPA). The IPA is a

25-item scale designed to measure the extent, severity, and magnitude of parent–child relationship problems as seen and reported by a parent. Scores range from 0 to 100, with a cutoff score of 30; scores above 30 indicate the presence of a relationship problem with a child (Hudson, 1982). A second measure that tends to focus on the marital relationship is the Marital Comparison Level Index (MCLI) developed by Sabatelli (1984). This instrument has 32 Likert-type items used to assess spouses' perceptions of their marital relationship. Specifically, questions are intended to measure an individuals' perception of the degree to which his or her marital relationship is living up to his or her expectations. Items are scored by assigning values of 0 to 7 to each response and summing these scores. While a cutoff score is not employed with this index, higher scores indicate a more favorable evaluation of the marriage. Although these instruments may be initially implemented in diagnosis, their utilization may also assist in quantifying the progress of future interventions.

Interviewing Others

Other than parents, the child's teacher is perhaps the best source of information relevant to the youngster's behavior within a standard setting. On the basis of the child's interaction with many children at similar developmental stages, the teacher can also provide rough normative data concerning a number of variables. The teacher is a good reporter of the youth's social and peer-group functioning (Milich & Krelbiel, 1986). Teachers can also supply the clinician with a wealth of data related to the child's cognitive strengths and weaknesses.

Similar to the parent interview, teachers are asked to provide a description of the problem responses, the setting in which they occur, and possible controlling variables. Here again, interviewers should tailor their questions to evaluate hypotheses regarding potential behavioral syndromes.

Interviewing the teacher may lead to identification of areas of behavioral assets and deficits that are not easily obtained from parents. Social skills may be assessed by inquiring about the child's interactions with peers ("Does she have many friends?" "How does he interact with girls?" "With boys?" "Do the other children include him when they are selecting team players?"). Questions about academic performance may also delineate important areas for intervention. A good set of questions to ask in this area includes: "Does she do her homework?" "Are assignments completed on time?" "Relative to classmates, how would you evaluate his performance in math, reading, and other subjects?" "Does she have difficulty staying on task?"

Finally, the interview with the teacher should result in an assessment of the teacher's willingness to assist in further evaluation of intervention programs. Generally, teachers are very interested in the performance of their students. An interviewer who consults a child's teacher and shows sincere appreciation of the teacher's observations and comments is likely to elicit a cooperative response (Gross, 1985).

The clinician may also find it helpful to consider data derived from sources other than the parent or teacher. In many cases, valuable information can be gleaned from existing medical records or from the records of other professionals or social agencies with which the child and parent(s) have had contact (Johnson & Krelbiel, 1986). Consulting these sources often obviates some types of testing or provides a means for quantifying developmental change by comparing data obtained at two separate times.

Interviewing the Child

The structure and content of the initial interview with the child should be formulated in relation to the child's particular problem area, developmental status, and the nature of the referral question. While objectives vary, there is typically an attempt to glean information pertaining to the child's perceptions of himself or herself, the problem, and samples of how the child handles himself or herself in a social situation with an adult. The first meeting with the child should include a broad assessment of his or her views of the circumstances that brought him or her to the clinic, insight into his or her own difficulties, and understanding of the interview situation. In addition, the youngster's attitudes toward and perceptions of his or her parents, teachers, siblings, and peers should be explored (Hymel, 1986).

The interview with the child usually begins with the therapist asking why he or she thinks the interview is being conducted. Following the youngster's response, the therapist typically shares his or her own opinion about this issue with the child. The clinician's response should convey to the child that the entire family wants to make things more pleasant for everyone at home. The initial segment of the interaction should be nonthreatening to the child, as this is an important element in establishing rapport him or her. It is the therapist's responsibility to structure the interview so that anxiety and fears of negative evaluation are minimized and a sense of trust is instilled in the child. For this reason, the therapist should initially provide a structural framework for the interview. Providing the child with a brief agenda for the interview may be beneficial to this end.

In addition to providing descriptive data, interviewing the child and his or her parents also provides other very useful diagnostic information. This procedure affords the clinician the opportunity to directly observe how the parents and child behave during the interview. For example, observing the child's responses to questions may give an indication of the youngster's social-skills development. Moreover, the clinician can arrange the interview environment so as to allow firsthand observation of the target behaviors (e.g., attention deficit shown on a reading task, motor activity level, noncompliance). Observing the child and parents together may allow the interviewer to see how the parents respond to inappropriate child behavior. Despite the novelty of the interview situation and the possibility that the family is attempting to present itself at its best, or worst, the interview with the child and the family is the first direct observation provided to the therapist. The resultant information should be used to generate and evaluate diagnostic questions.

After the child is interviewed, the initial session is generally closed with a brief summary conference with the child's parents. During this time, the therapist presents his or her conceptualization of the problem(s) to the parents. Suggestions as to which problem area should be targeted immediately are also discussed. This summary provides parents with a framework in which to redefine and view the problem. When additional information is desired, this is also a good time for the therapist to give parents homework assignments (e.g., "Please write down each time you have a problem getting Jordan to finish eating. Also briefly describe the situation"). The closing moments of the interview can also be used to answer any questions the family has about the need for further assessment or the direction of future treatment.

Other Assessment Tools

While the diagnostic interview serves as the cornerstone of the child-assessment procedure, a number of other techniques and instruments provide valuable data as well. Structured and semistructured interviews, direct observation of the child, and formal psychological testing may also be incorporated into the diagnostic interview.

The structured or semistructured interview provides a prearranged format for discussing various topics and issues. The interviewer directs the conversation with the parents, and the opportunity to follow up on a related point is frequently a function of whether there is time remaining in the session after the predetermined questions have been addressed. A number of structured diagnostic interview scales have been developed. Although these scales have not enjoyed widespread use, there is growing evidence that such instruments will receive increasing attention due to their easy adaptability to computerized administration and scoring as well as the increasing administrative demand for assigning specific diagnostic labels to children (Stein, 1986). A number of these scales have recently been developed. Some commonly used instruments are the Diagnostic Interview Schedule for Children (DISC) (Costello, Edelbrock, Dulcan, Kalas, & Kleric, 1984), the Child Behavioral Checklist (Achenbach & Edelbrock, 1983), the Schedule for Affective Disorders and Schizophrenia for School-Age Children (Puig-Antich, Blau, Marx, Greenhill, & Chambers, 1978), and the Diagnostic Interview for Children and Adolescents (Herjanic & Reich, 1982).

The DISC contains 264 items and takes approximately 50–70 minutes to administer to each respondent (Costello et al., 1984). The scale is appropriate for children 6–7 years of age. The format of the DISC is highly structured and explicit. Furthermore, the structure of the interview is similar to a decision tree in that a "Yes" response may be followed with one series of questions and a "No" response may be followed with a different line of inquiry. Each item of the DISC is assigned a score of 0, 1, or 2, and these scores are summed to yield several symptom scores. Psychometric data on the DISC have been favorable, with interrater reliability scores ranging from 0.94 to 1.00 with an average correlation of 0.98 (Costello et al., 1984).

The DISC was developed with close attention to relevant DSM-III criteria. Furthermore, there are supplemental computer programs available for generating formal diagnostic statements. The highly structured format of the instrument also makes it a reliable device for measuring ongoing treatment effectiveness.

Although not a structured interview per se, the Child Behavioral Checklist (CBC) by Achenbach and Edelbrock (1983) represents extensive empirical and normative work. This scale contains 138 items and can be completed by a parent in approximately 20 minutes. This instrument is divided into two sections that assess the child's social competencies and behavioral difficulties in a number of areas (e.g., academic, interpersonal).

The CBC is appropriate for children aged 4–16 and has separate age/sex norms for three age groups: 4–5, 6–11, and 12–16. Factor analytical work generated a number of clinical syndromes such as Aggressive, Hyperactive, Depressed, and Anxious. Further analysis revealed two major groupings of scales in each age/sex group. One grouping was labeled Externalizing and referred to childhood difficulties related to being undercontrolled, angry, defiant, and aggressive. A second grouping was labeled Internalizing and resembled syndromes characterized by overcontrol, personality problems, shyness, and inhibition (Achenbach & Edelbrock, 1984).

It should be noted that the CBC is derived empirically from large clinical samples. Because of its empirical foundation, diagnostic categories represented by the CBC differ from those of DSM-III-R, which were not systematically derived. However, there are a number of similarities between the descriptive features of the two approaches (Achenbach & Edelbrock, 1989). Indeed, the CBC provides the clinician with an empirically based assessment device that can assist in relating an individual child's score to a normative population.

The Schedule for Affective Disorders and Schizophrenia for School-Age Children (K-SADS) was originally devised to assess depression as well as other diagnostic categories in children. This instrument has its origin in the Schizophrenic and Affective Disorders Schedule (SADS), which was constructed by Endicott and Spitzer (1978). Currently, two forms of the K-SADS are available. The Present Episode form (K-SADS-P) can be used as both a clinical and a research tool and focuses on existing psychopathology. The Epidemiological version (K-SADS-E) can be used in the diagnosis of both existing and previous episodes of psychopathology and behavioral disturbances.

The K-SADS is appropriate for children 6–17 years of age and is administered to the child's mother or primary caregiver. There are approximately 200 items on the K-SADS, yet the interview can usually be completed in an hour. During the initial, unstructured segment of the interview, the informant is generally asked to provide relatively detailed information concerning the child's presenting problems and symptoms. The second part of the instrument provides a more structured assessment of symptoms relevant to Axis I, DSM-III-R diagnosis. The final section of the K-SADS includes 7 observational items rated by the clinician.

The K-SADS-P is perhaps most helpful in monitoring behavioral change or treatment effects because it includes severity scales. These scales are generally scored on a 6- or 7-point range of severity and can later be used to discriminate relatively subtle behavior changes. Conversely, the K-SADS-E is entirely syndrome-based and can be quite helpful to the clinician interested in the child's long-standing psychiatric history. Psychometrically, both the K-SADS-P and the K-SADS-E have reflected good test–retest and interrater reliability (Chambers et al., 1985). Specifically, the interrater agreement concerning various symptoms and diagnostic syndromes has ranged between 0.65 and 0.96.

The Diagnostic Interview for Children and Adolescents (DICA) is a structural diagnostic interview designed for use in clinical and epidemiological research. The DICA is appropriate for children 6–17 years old and can be administered in approximately 60–90 minutes. The DICA and its companion instrument, the DICA-P, comprise three subsections. Part 1 contains 19 items dealing with baseline and demographic data. These questions are asked in a joint interview with the parent(s) and the child. Following Part 1, the parent(s) and child are separated and interviewed separately during Part 2. This section contains 247 questions grouped according to DSM-III symptom categories. Part 3 of the DICA allows the clinician to include observational data in the interview.

Although the DICA was developed on the basis of sound empirical work, data regarding reliability and validity need more extensive investigation. For example, parent–child agreement on Part 2 ranged from 0 to 0.87 using the Kappa Statistic (Herjanic & Reich, 1982). Inclusion of therapist observational ratings is a valuable addition to structured diagnostic assessment. Such ratings do indeed help to objectify follow-up assessment aimed at treatment evaluation.

Structured interviews have a number of appealing aspects. They increase the probability that interviewers cover the same material in a similar manner with all families. This method may be valuable in terms of providing a list of content areas that should be addressed during the diagnostic process. It is also conceivable that conducting very structured interviews helps the clinician develop a frame of reference from which to view child behavior problems. However, there may be times when the diagnostic situation demands more flexibility than is allowed with the structured or semistructured format. While there has been a recent surge in normative studies of these instruments, further work is needed to establish complete developmental norms. Finally, these scales were designed primarily to identify symptoms and generate diagnostic data; they may be less helpful in developing a treatment plan.

A second source of corroborative information is direct observation of the child. While early behavioral assessors placed an exceptionally strong emphasis on direct observation, there is now a much less exclusive focus on this procedure. This recent trend may be due to the increasing systems orientation in child and family assessment, as well as the current inclusion of cognitive and affective variables in the assessment process (Jacobson, 1985). In keeping with the interest in more molar behaviors exhibited by the child, there is at present more attention directed to "qualitative" aspects of the child's behavior (Mash & Terdal, 1988). Furthermore, there is increased interest in the way a target behavior is expressed. Recent work has indicated that nonverbal cues, such as facial expression, may provide information on family interaction styles that is overlooked with more simplistic coding strategies (Gottman & Levenson, 1986).

While many authors argue that the clinic is a highly artificial setting for observation, this view is in fact an oversimplification. Indeed, a well-implemented clinic observation procedure can provide very natural representative responses. Suitable scenarios that can be carried out in the clinic setting include free-play settings, role-play activities, and certain academic task situations. Observation of the child and parent in a free-play environment can provide a wealth of data in a relatively short period of time. This situation allows the observer to compare the overall style and quality of the parent–child interaction to that described by parents in the interview. This observation also generates data concerning the parents' social reinforcement and punishment styles.

Regardless of whether behavioral assessment is theoretically divergent from psychometric assessment, the use of developmental scales, intellectual tests, and achievement tests with children is quite common among behavioral therapists (Kaufman & Kaufman, 1983). Quantitative data from specific measures of intellectual, motor, perceptual, and social functioning can be clinically invaluable. A wealth of information also comes from observing the child as he or she deals with the test procedure. The astute clinician can also obtain data regarding the qualitative nature of a child's performance and reaction to the demands of testing. Specific information concerning how well the child attends to instructions, deals with distracting stimuli, and reacts to success or failure can also be gained during formal testing.

As information from formal testing is combined with interview and self-report data, diagnostic hypotheses may change dramatically. For example, a child initially referred by a teacher tentatively suggesting a diagnosis of mental retardation may be found to be in the "above average" range on formal IQ measures. Such new data may lead to further assessment, confirming an emotional rather than a cognitive origin for the child's poor classroom performance. Similarly, the discovery of deficient receptive language abilities may prevent the clinician from attributing the noncommunicative style of a youngster to depressive symptomatology. By allowing diagnostic hypotheses to unfold slowly and to be modified, reevaluated, or discarded, the therapist is able to construct a more complete and less biased clinical profile of the child.

Parental Characteristics

With considerable time having been spent on the structure and content of the interview process, it seems justifiable to discuss two issues that deserve further attention during the assessment process: developmental considerations and parental variables. While the inclusion of these topics may tend to extend the diagnostic interview, recent studies attest to the importance of these variables in the child's behavior.

Perhaps one of the most exciting new facets of behavioral child assessment is the recent focus on parental psychopathology in contributing to child behavioral disturbance. It is becoming increasingly obvious that the psychological constitution of parents can have a dramatic effect on the child. While parent–child interaction and parental responses to child behaviors have previously been the target of behavioral assessment, cognitive and affective variables exclusive to the parent have rarely been observed in child assessment. Specifically, parental characteristics of maternal depression and parental egocentrism have been implicated as having a role in childhood psychopathology.

Ferguson, Horwood, and Shannon (1984) investigated the relationship between maternal depression and child behavior problem in 1265 children. These investigators found that correlations between family life events and maternal reports of child-rearing problems were largely attributable to the mediating effects of maternal depression. It was suggested that the children of depressed mothers may respond to the mothers' depressive style by developing increasingly more behavioral problems. A second explanation suggests that depressed mothers perceive their children's behavior differently from nondepressed mothers. Regardless of the specific mechanism, however, maternal depression is a very important diagnostic clue.

Work by Hops et al. (1987) indicates that depressed mothers tend to display a more dysphoric affect with their children, as well as lower rates of happy affect. Furthermore, they are less rewarding in their interactions with their children. Although interview data alone may imply that a mother's affective state is contributing to a child's behavioral disorder, more formal measures may also be used. Asking parents to complete the Beck Depression Inventory (Beck, Ward, Mendelson, Mock, & Erbaugh, 1961) or the Self-Rating Depression Scale (Zung, 1965) may help quantify this influence.

A second major parental variable that should be considered in the assessment of child behavioral disturbance involves egocentrism. The work of Chandler, Piaget, and Koch (1978) suggested that egocentric thinking was common in the population of mothers with histories of serious psychiatric disorders. Furthermore, it was shown that children of such mothers were slower to relinquish their own egocentric thinking than were control children. This parental variable does not appear to be restricted to maternal influences. The Selfism Scale developed by Phares and Erskine (1984) appears to be well suited for the assessment of narcissism in parents.

Given the potential impact these parental variables can exert on the child, it may be worthwhile to spend some time discussing topics that can appear unrelated to the child's presenting problem. Points of inquiry may include asking the parents about their overall level of life stress and marital satisfaction.

Developmental Context

While the child may be referred to the clinic for a wide variety of difficulties, it is important to assess the nature and severity of the problem from a developmental context. Currently, there is more emphasis on the way the child's cognitive-developmental level influences how a particular behavior is perceived, interpreted, and labeled by adults. Bed-wetting, inability to read, and stranger anxiety are not considered problems in 2- and 3-year-olds, but are worthy of concern in 12-year-olds (Campbell, 1989). The specific developmental phase the child is in can also affect prognostic implications as well as treatment considerations. For example, it can be quite difficult to distinguish the characteristic emotional turmoil and lability of mood found in adolescence from significant depression disorder. This last point is paramount for the clinician as he or she begins to construct an intervention strategy and provides parents with feedback on potential outcomes.

The developmental context in which a particular behavior occurs is relevant to many aspects of the diagnostic process. First, as previously noted, the significance of a given behavior can be quite different depending on the age at which it occurs. Second, a complete appraisal of the child's cognitive development will assist the therapist in formulating realistic goals for treatment. The cognitive demands that can be placed on a 12-year-old in therapy are quite different from those applicable with most 8-year-olds. Finally, a comprehensive developmental assessment can aid the interviewer in identifying areas in which the child is relatively advanced in relation to his or her chronological age. These developmental strengths can then be used to a fuller extent in subsequent interventions with the child. For example, a highly verbal fifth-grader may use available communication abilities to enhance other social skills with peers.

An interviewer with a solid background in developmental psychology can tap into a wealth of data concerning the appropriateness of the child's development using primarily interview data. While a great deal of data can be generated by interviews with the child and significant others, more objective measures may also be employed. There are now available a number of developmental screening measures that can assist the clinician in evaluating the child's status in a number of developmental arenas. While many of the instruments available fail to meet crucial psychometric requirements, some are quite scientifically sound. Two such measures are the Minnesota Child Developmental Inventory (MCDI) (Ireton & Thwing, 1972) and the Vineland Adaptive Behavior Scales—Survey Form (Sparrow, Balla, & Cicchetti, 1984).

The MCDI is a standardized inventory useful in assessing the developmental status of children from age 6 months to 6.5 years. The MCDI contains 320 statements that describe the developmental behaviors appropriate for children of these ages. The inventory is administered in a written format that is completed by the child's mother or primary caregiver. Each of the 320 items is answered with a "Yes" or "No" response and can be scored by computer. The completed MCDI produces a profile that illustrates the child's unique constellation of strengths and weaknesses in eight developmental domains. Along with an overall developmental summary, the inventory contains scales that rate gross motor, fine motor, expressive language, comprehension, conceptual, situation comprehension, self-help, and personal–social development.

Results of the MCDI are interpreted in reference to age norms for each sex as developmentally delayed, borderline, or within normal limits. The relevant normative data are based on a sample of 796 white children aged 6 months to 6.5 years.

A second developmental instrument is the Vineland Adaptive Behavior Scales. The Vineland Scales are appropriate for children from birth to age 19. Administration of the scales requires a trained clinician and is based on interview data gathered from the child's primary caregiver. There are currently three forms of the Vineland, including the Survey form, which is used specifically for diagnostic and classification purposes. This scale consists of 26 items covering four domains of behavior (Communication, Daily Living Skills, Socialization, and Motor Skills). In addition to scores for the four domains, an Adaptive Behavior Composite and an optional Maladaptive Behavior Domain can be obtained.

The Vineland Scales represent an active effort to reduce the psychometric problems inherent in similar scales. The Survey form was normed on a randomly sampled group of parents or primary caregivers who responded with information on 3000 children between birth and 19 years of age. Along with matching 1980 census estimates concerning race, gender, and region of the country, the sample also included children with emotional disturbance and sensory impairment.

While neither of these instruments should be used in isolation, they can provide an objective measure of the child's developmental status that the clinician can include with more qualitative indicators. In this way, the therapist can compare the presenting problem to the child's development in other behavioral realms.

PRACTICAL CONSIDERATIONS

The approach described above provides a systematic method of diagnostic interviewing that is relatively successful. It emphasizes the importance of developing interview skills, as well as knowledge of the behavior patterns that characterize the various childhood disorders. Effective diagnostic interviewing also requires the ability to recognize and manage some of the common difficulties that may occur during the assessment process.

One major impedance obviously occurs when an attempt is made to interview a nonspeaking child. The child may be unable or unwilling to speak to the interviewer for a number of reasons. It is of initial importance to distinguish the child who is unable to speak from the youngster who has the verbal capabilities but refuses to talk. The latter category may include severely disturbed children, as well as those suffering from "elective mutism." Regardless of whether assessing communicative abilities is the explicit intent of the assessment, it is important to consider the effectiveness of the child's verbal skills. Such evaluation will establish the goals and limits of the interview with the child as well as dictate how much reliance will be placed on his or her nonverbal responses (Barker, 1990).

With children who have a pervasive language disorder, the interviewer should be careful to avoid talking down to the child. Instead, there should be an active attempt to use more facial expressions and body gestures when engaging these children. Furthermore, there should be a greater emphasis on nonverbal activities, such as drawing, playing, or acting out various scenarios relevant to the child's difficulties or current life situation.

With the child who refuses to speak, there is no simple solution for increasing participation in the interview. In many of these situations, the child also refuses to participate in nonverbal activities when asked by the therapist to do so. It is probably more appropriate to focus on the way the child reacts to the various stages of the interview process (Barker, 1990). In these situations, it is imperative to obtain a good history from parents, teachers, and other records (Barker, 1990).

Another problem encountered in diagnostic work with children is the failure of a child to clearly meet the criteria of one particular disorder. It is common for youngsters to display a variety of inappropriate behaviors that cut across a number of diagnostic categories. Moreover, developmental considerations may further hinder the assignment of a child to a particular category. In these cases, the best solution is to defer a diagnosis until more information can be obtained. The clinician and patient would best be served by using the diagnostic code that indicates that there are not enough data on which to make a diagnosis (DSM-IV 799.90) and then presenting descriptive information regarding the problem behaviors observed.

Although generally not a problem with young children, confidentiality can create difficulties for the clinician interviewing preadolescents and adolescents. Youngsters may be reluctant to discuss various aspects of behavior (e.g., sex, alcohol, suicide) for fear that this information will be presented to their parents. This reluctance results in an inaccurate representation of their responding as well as distrust between the child and therapist. There are no specific formulas for dealing with this dilemma, and to a degree the clinician must exercise his or her own judgment about revealing information to parents. However, one approach is to explain to the child and his or her parents that in most instances you will respect each individual's right to privacy, but information concerning behavior you feel may result in serious harm to the youngster (e.g., suicidal thoughts) will be passed on to the parents. Moreover, the youth should be forewarned when the clinician plans to share something with his or her parents (Gross, 1985).

Finally, starting the diagnostic interview can be problematic if the child reacts to the interviewer with fear and crying. Parents often fail to explain to their children why they are being taken to a therapist. Many parents simply inform their children that they are going to see a doctor. Some children also react negatively to the suggestion that they are to be left alone in the waiting room while their parents are interviewed. Having toys in the waiting room is frequently all that is required to entertain children while their parents are being interviewed. Spending a few moments engaged in an enjoyable activity in the waiting room with the child and his or her parents before taking the child into your office may also allay the child's apprehension. While these examples do not exhaust the difficulties that the therapist will encounter, they should serve to illustrate the value of solid preparation for the interview and the value of remaining calm and flexible during difficult situations.

While the consequences of classification have been presented, the stigma associated with labeling children deserves further consideration. When attaching a psychological tag to a child, the clinician should consider that any diagnosis may remain with the youth throughout childhood and into adulthood. Some critics would argue that labeling children creates a self-fulfilling prophecy in which the diagnosis negatively biases future evaluation of the child. Alternately, there is some support for the view that psychological explanations help temper social expectations and lead to greater acceptance and support. In general, it may be most helpful to avoid formally labeling the child and to focus on assessing and treating the cluster of behaviors that are evident.

CASE ILLUSTRATION

Having described a general diagnostic interviewing strategy for use with children, it seems appropriate to provide a case illustration of the application of these procedures. A clinical example of a diagnostic interview with Clovis, a 6-year-old Caucasian male diagnosed with an attention-deficit hyperactivity disorder (ADHD), is provided. Although only one diagnostic category is presented, it should serve to illustrate how diagnostic assessments with children involve the use of a general interview strategy and how the specifics of the interview process are shaped by the nature of the child's disorder and the clinician's familiarity with childhood diagnostic categories.

Attention-Deficit Hyperactivity Disorder (DSM-IV, codes 314.00, 314.01, and 314.09). The essential features of ADHD are developmentally inappropriate degrees of inattention, impulsivity, and hyperactivity. Children with the disorder generally display some disturbance in each of these areas, but to varying degrees (APA, 1987). The variability of these three symptom clusters has led to changes in the diagnostic criteria put forth in DSM-IV. Specifically, a diagnosis of Attention-Deficit Hyperactivity Disorder can be described as: predominantly inattentive type (314.00), predominantly hyperactive–impulsive type (314.01), or combined type (314.09). Associated aspects of the disorder include low self-esteem, mood lability, low frustration tolerance, temper outbursts, and motor–perceptual dysfunctions. Children usually begin to evidence the disorder by the age of 4, but may not be formally diagnosed until school-related difficulties arise. These youngsters usually demonstrate academic and social functioning impairment as a result of the disorder. Moreover, boys are 6–9 times more likely than girls to develop this problem.

Clovis was referred to the outpatient clinic through the school because of his general disruptiveness. His parents reported that he had difficulty staying on task and frequently behaved impulsively. At the initial interview, the therapist first met with Mr. and Mrs. B while Clovis remained in the waiting room. The therapist began the session by explaining the purpose of the first meeting and emphasizing how important it was that Mr. and Mrs. B describe Clovis's difficulties in detail.

THERAPIST: Let's start by having you describe what prompted you to come to the clinic.

MRS. B: Well, Clovis's teachers tell us that he needs almost constant supervision to prevent him from completely disrupting classroom activities. His second grade teacher says she is at the end of her rope.

THERAPIST: How long has this problem been described by his teachers?

MRS. B: Clovis went to a different school for kindergarten, but his teacher there also complained about the same things. He said that he was always jumping around or fiddling with something. He also commented that when he was misbehaving, he seemed to be uncontrollable and very difficult to discipline.

THERAPIST: How would you describe Clovis's behavior at home?

MR. B: He's just so hyper all the time.

THERAPIST: What do you mean when you say "hyper"? Can you be a little more specific?

MR. B: Sure, he just always seems to be on the go. It's like he has this motor inside him that always seems to be driving him.

THERAPIST: Could you give me an example of that?

MR. B: Yes, like the other day when I took him to the store. He couldn't stay with me for more than a few seconds at a time. Instead, he was climbing on lawn chairs and shopping carts. When he was staying with me, it seemed like he was constantly fidgeting or jumping around. So I know what the teachers are talking about when they say he can't sit still.

THERAPIST: When you were at the store, did Clovis ever seem to get settled?

MR. B: No, not at all. I even tried to tell him about some of the toys and games, but he doesn't ever seem to listen. I sometimes had trouble concentrating on schoolwork at his age, but I never was so consistently distractible just doing daily activities. Even when it seems to be something he likes, he just can't pay attention for any length of time.

THERAPIST: How about if you engage him in a game or play activity when it's just the two of you? Is his level of concentration better in that setting?

MRS. B: Not really. Yesterday, I was helping him build a house out of blocks, and he seemed to be interested in everything but the house.

MR. B: I've never seen him finish a game or project. If you send him off to do something, the smallest thing can turn him in a different direction.

THERAPIST: How is he around peers?

MRS. B: He is usually worse around the other children, because he leaves his own play activity and starts bothering them. I don't think he intentionally tries to hurt them; it's just that he is so active and physical that he doesn't know when to quit.

THERAPIST: Does he ever behave impulsively or unexpectedly?

MR. B: Oh yes, sometimes he scares me to death because he'll just run out into the street without looking for cars. And his teachers complain about him blurting out answers before they finish the question.

THERAPIST: So it doesn't seem like he thinks about the consequences of an act before doing it?

MRS. B: Right, it seems like he just jumps into something and thinks about it later. Like butting into other kids' games without considering how they might feel.

This first segment of the interview provides a description of Clovis's behavioral difficulties and suggests an attentional deficit. The interviewer then begins a line of questioning that assesses specific behaviors known to covary with the disorder, such as a high activity level, impulsivity, and distractibility. After determining the nature of Clovis's difficulty, the therapist now begins to explore environmental and situational variables that may be related to the problem. Then he inquires about desirable behaviors and potential rewards.

THERAPIST: You mentioned that Clovis is unable to complete tasks. How do you handle it when you want him to finish something?

MR. B: Well, most of the time we just stay on him until he does it. Homework seems to be the biggest problem right now. Nothing seems to work though. I've even spanked him a couple of times, and that didn't seem to faze him.

MRS. B: Yeah, I pretty much just have to sit next to him at the table to make sure he's doing what he's supposed to. Really, that's the only way to make sure he finishes his homework.

THERAPIST: What would you like to see Clovis do instead?

MR. B: I would like to see him be able to work on something until it's finished without having one of us over his shoulder.

MRS. B: I guess staying in his seat at school or when we're in public for a few minutes at a time is at the top of my list.

THERAPIST: What are some things Clovis really enjoys?

MRS. B: Well, he really loves any ball game. Baseball, football—throwing and catching.

THERAPIST: It sounds like you folks have had a lot to deal with lately. How do you feel like the two of you are holding up physically and emotionally?

MRS. B: Well, I know I've been pretty tired lately. If I'm not at school talking to one of Clovis's teachers I'm trying to keep him in line at home.

THERAPIST: Does it ever feel as though you just don't have the energy to deal with Clovis on some days?

MRS. B: Sometimes, but I always manage somehow.

THERAPIST: Have you noticed a change in your eating or sleeping habits recently?

MRS. B: No, not really. I think I'm pretty good at putting a rough day behind me and feeling refreshed the next morning

After gathering information relevant to diagnosis, situational variables, and potential rewarding stimuli, the therapist began to address the parents' ability to deal with the stress surrounding Clovis's current difficulties. After closing the interview with the parents, the therapist met with Clovis alone. This meeting provided an opportunity for the therapist to assess the child's insight into why he was brought to the clinic. It also allowed the therapist to observe the child directly.

THERAPIST: Do you know why you're here, Clovis?

CLOVIS: 'Cause Mom and Dad said so.

THERAPIST: Do you know why they wanted you to come here?

CLOVIS: 'Cause I don't do what they say?

THERAPIST: Well, they just want to see if all of you can do things without fighting, so that it's more fun at home. Would you like that?

CLOVIS: Yeah.

THERAPIST: What is the most fun thing you can think of doing, Clovis?

CLOVIS: Going to the zoo.

THERAPIST: What else do you like to do, Clovis?

CLOVIS: I like playing football.

THERAPIST: Well, we can play catch with that green ball over in the corner. Would you go get the ball for us, Clovis?

CLOVIS: Yeah, I'd like that.

On completing the interview with Clovis, the therapist met with Clovis's parents to summarize the information he had obtained and to clarify any questions or concerns they had. This time can also be used to set up future testing or observation sessions.

THERAPIST: Well, we have some good information to work with after today's meeting. You folks have done a fine job observing and describing Clovis's behavior, and it will be quite helpful in interviewing him. I would like to set up another appointment to assess Clovis's developmental progress a bit more formally. I'd also like to speak with his teacher about his current academic status.

MRS. B: We'll be glad to set up a second appointment and tell Mrs. Jones you'll be calling her. Is there anything we can help with?

THERAPIST: Yes, it also seems that some of the behaviors the two of you have been engaging in may be influencing Clovis's high activity level and impulsivity. Specifically, I would like the two of you to keep track of problem events and how you respond to them during the upcoming week.

MR. B: I think we can handle that.

THERAPIST: Here is a chart that will make the task a little easier for you. You write down what Clovis did, what you did, and the events surrounding the episode.

MRS. B: O.K., this makes a lot of sense to me.

THERAPIST: Again, you were both very helpful today with your descriptions and insights. Keep up the good work.

The information gathered during the initial interview indicated that Clovis was displaying a behavioral pattern consistent with the diagnosis of ADHD. After formal developmental testing and parental monitoring of the problem behavior, a treatment plan was formulated. Intervention consisted of medication obtained through a referral to a pediatric consultation as well as the introduction of behavioral management techniques at home and school. Working with Clovis's teacher and parents, a program was implemented that rewarded task-appropriate behavior and extinguished inappropriate behavior. A total of 22 sessions were required to effectively alter the behavior of Clovis and his family.

SUMMARY

It is clear that being a good diagnostician of childhood disorders involves more than interviewing skills and an understanding of the definitions of child psychopathology. Developmental considerations are of paramount importance in determining the significance of behavioral problems. Adult expectations can greatly affect the process of determining whether a youngster's responding is considered deviant. Moreover, diagnostic labels can influence adult reactions to children and their behavior.

The child clinician must be sensitive to a variety of factors that extend beyond identifying a cluster of target behaviors if the child is to benefit from the diagnostic process. Careful consideration of the variables that distinguish children from adults, while remembering that the goal of the diagnostic interview is to determine the child's problem such that an effective and efficient treatment program can be constructed, should allow the clinician to obtain maximum return on his or her investments in developing diagnostic interviewing skills.

ACKNOWLEDGMENT.   Preparation of this chapter was supported in part by National Institutes of Health Grant DE08641.

REFERENCES

Achenbach, T. M., & Edelbrock, C. (1983). *Manual for the Child Behavioral Checklist and Revised Child Behavioral Profile*. Burlington: Department of Psychology, University of Vermont.

Achenbach, T. M., & Edelbrock, C. (1984). Psychopathology of childhood. *Annual Review of Psychology, 35*, 227–256.

Achenbach, T. M., & Edelbrock, C. (1989). Diagnostic, taxonomic, and assessment issues. In T. H. Ollendick & M. Hersen (Eds.), *Handbook of child psychopathology* (pp. 53–73). New York: Plenum Press.

American Psychiatric Association (1952). *Diagnostic and statistical manual of mental disorders*, 1st ed. Washington, DC: Author.

American Psychiatric Association (1968). *Diagnostic and statistical manual of mental disorders*, 2nd ed. Washington, DC: Author.

American Psychiatric Association (1980). *Diagnostic and statistical manual of mental disorders*, 3rd ed. Washington, DC: Author.

American Psychiatric Association (1987). *Diagnostic and statistical manual of mental disorders*, 3rd ed., revised. Washington, DC: Author.

American Psychiatric Association (1994). *Diagnostic and statistical manual of mental disorders*, 4th ed. Washington, DC: Author.

Barker, P. (1990). *Clinical interviews with children and adolescents*. New York: W. W. Norton.

Beck, A. T., Ward, C. H., Mendelson, M., Mock, J., & Erbaugh, J. (1961). An inventory for measuring depression. *Archives of General Psychiatry, 4,* 53–63.

Bristol, M. M. (1983). The Belief Scale. In M. Bristol, A. Donovan, & A. Harding (Eds.), *The broader impact of intervention: A workshop on measuring stress and support.* Chapel Hill, NC: Frank Porter Graham Child Development Center.

Brody, G. H., Pillegrini, A. D., & Sigel, I. E. (1986). Marital quality and mother–child and father–child interactions with school-aged children. *Developmental Psychology, 22,* 291–296.

Campbell, S. B. (1989). Developmental perspectives. In T. H. Ollendick & M. Hersen (Eds.). *Handbook of child psychopathology* (pp. 5–28). New York: Plenum Press.

Chambers, W. J., Puig-Antich, J., Hirsch, M., Paez, P., Ambrosini, P. J., Tabrizi, M. A., & Davies, M. (1985). The assessment of affective disorders in children and adolescents by semi-structured interview: Test–retest reliability of the K-SADS-P. *Archives of General Psychiatry, 42,* 696–701.

Chandler, M. J., Piaget, K. F., & Koch, D. A. (1978). The child's demystification of psychological defense mechanisms: A structural and developmental analysis. *Developmental Psychology, 14,* 197–205.

Chlopan, B. E., McBain, M. L., Carbonell, J. L., & Hagen, R. L. (1985). Empathy: Review of available measures. *Journal of Personality and Social Psychology, 48,* 635–653.

Costello, A. J., Edelbrock, C., Dulcan, M. K., Kalas, R., & Klaric, S. (1984). *Report on the NIMH Diagnostic Interview Schedule for Children (DISC).* Washington, DC: National Institute of Mental Health.

Endicott, J., & Spitzer, R. L. (1978). A diagnostic interview: The SADS. *Archives of General Psychiatry, 35,* 837–853.

Evans, I. M. (1985). Building systems models as a strategy for target behavior selection in clinical assessment. *Behavioral Assessment, 7,* 21–32.

Fergusson, D. M., Horwood, L. J., & Shannon, F. T. (1984). Relationship of family life events, maternal depression, and child rearing problems. *Pediatrics, 7316,* 773–776.

Forehand, R., Long, N., Brody, G. H., & Fauber, R. (1986). Home predictors of young adolescents' school behavior and academic performance. *Child Development, 57,* 1528–1533.

Gottman, J. M., & Levensen, R. W. (1986). Assessing the role of emotion in marriage. *Behavioral Assessment, 8,* 31–48.

Gross, A. M. (1985). Children. In M. Hersen & S. M. Turner (Eds.), *Diagnostic interviewing* (pp. 309–335). New York: Plenum Press.

Guidubaldi, J., & Cleminshaw, H. K. (1985). The development of the Cleminshaw–Guidubaldi Parent Satisfaction Scale. *Journal of Clinical Psychology, 14,* 293–298.

Hammen, C. L., Gordon, D. S., Adrian, C., Burge, D., Jaenicke, C., & Hiroto, D. (1986, May). *Children of depressed mothers: Predictors of risk.* Paper presented at the annual meeting of the American Psychiatric Association, Washington, DC.

Herjanic, B., & Reich, W. (1982). Development of a structured psychiatric interview for children: Agreement between child and parent on individual symptoms. *Journal of Abnormal Child Psychology, 10,* 307–324.

Hops, H., Biglan, A., Sherman, L., Arthur, J., Friedman, L., & Osteen, V. (1987). Home observations of family interactions of depressed women. *Journal of Consulting and Clinical Psychology, 55,* 341–346.

Hudson, W. W. (1982). *The clinical measurement package: A field manual.* Chicago: Dorsey Press.

Hymel, S. (1986). *Computer assisted diagnosis for children and adolescents.* Unpublished manuscript. Toronto: Department of Psychiatry, University of Toronto.

Ireton, H. R., & Thwing, E. J. (1972). *Minnesota Child Development Inventory.* Minneapolis: Behavioral Science Systems.

Jacobson, N. S. (1985). The role of observational measures in behavior therapy outcome research. *Behavioral Assessment*, 7, 297–308.

Johnson, J. H., & Krelbiel, G. (1986). Issues in the assessment and treatment of socially rejected children. In R. J. Prinz (Ed.), *Advances in behavioral assessment of children and families* Vol. 2 (pp. 249–270). New York: Plenum Press.

Kanfer, F. H. (1985). Target selection for clinical change programs. *Behavioral Assessment*, 7, 7–20.

Kaufman, K. S., & Kaufman, N. L. (1983). *Kaufman Assessment Battery for Children*. Circle Pines, MN: American Guidance Services.

Kazdin, A. E. (1988). Childhood depression. In E. J. Mash & L. G. Terdal (Eds.), *Behavioral assessment of childhood disorders* (pp. 157–160). New York: Guilford Press.

Mash, E. J., & Johnson, C. (1986). *Norms for the Parenting Sense of Competence Scale*. Unpublished manuscript. Calgary: Department of Psychology, University of Calgary.

Mash, E. J., & Terdal, L. G. (1988). Behavioral assessment of child and family disturbance. In E. J. Mash & L. G. Terdal (Eds.), *Behavioral assessment of childhood disorders* (pp. 3–11). New York: Guilford Press.

Mezzich, A. C., Mezzich, J. E., & Coffrian, G. A. (1985). Reliability of DSM-III vs. DSM-II in child psychopathology. *Journal of the American Academy of Child Psychiatry*, 24, 273–280.

Milich, R., & Krelbiel, G. (1986). Issues in the assessment and treatment of socially rejected children. In R. J. Prinz (Ed.), *Advances in behavioral assessment of children and families* Vol. 2 (pp. 249–270). New York: Plenum Press.

Pannaccione, V. F., & Wahler, R. G. (1986). Child behavior, maternal depression and social coercion as factors in the quality of child care. *Journal of Abnormal Child Psychology*, 14, 263–278.

Patterson, G. R. (1982). *Coercive family process*. Eugene, OR: Castalia.

Pendergast, M., Taylor, E., Rapoport, J., Bartko, J., Donnelly, M., Zametkin, A., Ahearn, M. B., Dunn, G., & Wieselberg, H. M. (1988). The diagnosis of childhood hyperactivity: U.S.–U.K. cross-national study of DSM-III and ICD-9. *Journal of Child Psychology and Psychiatry*, 29, 284–300.

Phares, E. J., & Erskine, N. (1984). The measurement of selfism. *Educational and Psychological Measurement*, 44, 597–608.

Puig-Antich, J., Blau, S., Marx, N., Greenhill, L. L., & Chambers, W. (1978). Prepubertal major depressive disorders: A pilot study. *Journal of the American Academy of Child Psychiatry*, 17, 695–707.

Rapoport, J. L., & Ismond, D. R. (1989). *DSM-III-R training guide for diagnosis of childhood disorders*. New York: Brunner/Mazel.

Sabatelli, R. M. (1984). The Marital Comparison Level Index: A measure for assessing outcomes relative to expectations. *Journal of Marriage and Family*, 46, 651–662.

Sigel, I. (Ed.) (1985). *Parenting belief systems: The psychological consequences for children*. Hillsdale, NJ: Erlbaum.

Sparrow, S. S., Balla, D. A., & Cicchetti, D. V. (1984). *The Vineland Adaptive Behavior Scales: A revision of the Vineland Social Maturity Scale by Edgar A. Doll, Survey Form*. Circle Pines, MN: American Guidance Services.

Stein, S. J. (1986). *Computer assisted diagnosis for children and adolescents*. Unpublished manuscript, Department of Psychiatry, University of Toronto.

Zung, W. K. (1965). A self-rating depression scale. *Archives of General Psychiatry*, 12, 63–70.

14

Sexually and Physically Abused Children

Anthony P. Mannarino and Judith A. Cohen

Description of the Problem

There are at least two distinct roles that a mental health professional could be called upon to play when interviewing a child who has been abused sexually or physically or both. One would be that of a psychiatric/psychological interviewer whose major task is to determine the kinds of emotional and behavioral problems that exist because of the abuse. In this role, the interviewer would be assessing psychiatric symptomatology as reported by both the child and the parent(s) in order to generate a specific psychiatric diagnosis and a systematic plan for treatment. This professional role would be similar to that of other mental health professionals who routinely interview children who present with a variety of emotional and behavioral difficulties.

The second major role would be that of an investigative interviewer. In this capacity, the professional would be attempting to determine the likelihood that a child has been abused. Mental health professionals are increasingly being asked to take on this role in order to assist the child protective service system or juvenile court system in making an official abuse determination. For example, it would not be uncommon for a juvenile or family court judge to appoint a professional to independently interview a child so that additional information about an abuse allegation might be provided. This type of evaluation has increased dramatically over the past decade, particularly in response to the enormous rise in reports of sexual abuse.

This chapter will focus primarily on the role of the investigative interviewer. This is the role both professionals and laymen typically are referring to when the issue of interviewing abused children is raised. It is important to note that this role clearly falls within the general domain of forensic mental health. Accordingly,

Anthony P. Mannarino and Judith A. Cohen • Medical College of Pennsylvania, Allegheny General Hospital, Pittsburgh, Pennsylvania 15212.

Diagnostic Interviewing (Second Edition), edited by Michel Hersen and Samuel M. Turner. Plenum Press, New York, 1994.

whatever forensic standards and guidelines exist within each mental health profession regarding such issues as education, training, and relevant clinical experience are certainly applicable. Although the scope of this chapter does not permit a discussion of general forensic child mental health credentialing and guidelines, these matters are addressed elsewhere (Grisso, 1990; Schetky & Guyer, 1990).

SEXUAL VERSUS PHYSICAL ABUSE

As mentioned earlier, the need for investigative interviewing has increased sharply over the past decade in relation to the tremendous rise in reported cases of child sexual abuse. Since there is no medical evidence to substantiate sexual abuse in the majority of cases (Muram, 1989), there is often a reliance on verbal disclosures by the child to document that something inappropriate has occurred. These disclosures are frequently obtained during an investigative interview. Because such interviews are now widely conducted, guidelines have begun to emerge regarding interview protocols and practices, particularly for young children who may have been sexually abused (American Professional Society on the Abuse of Children, 1990).

This situation is in marked contrast to the situation with respect to alleged victims of physical abuse. Since the time Kempe and his associates coined the term *battered child syndrome* (Kempe, Silverman, Steele, & Droegemueller, 1962), documenting physical abuse has been based largely on medical evidence. In this regard, the presence of unexplained physical injuries that could not have resulted from an accident is the standard employed in most states to substantiate physical abuse. Although an alleged child victim may be interviewed, the physical evidence is paramount. Moreover, since many victims of physical abuse are very young (National Center on Child Abuse and Neglect, 1988), they are often not capable of providing verbal details about what may have occurred.

In light of this historical background, investigative interviewing has not played a major role in the area of child physical abuse. Moreover, physical abuse has commonly been perceived to be in the professional domain of the physician and not the mental health practitioner. In the last decade, there has been an increased emphasis on the emotional and behavioral difficulties that children experience as a result of physical abuse (Mask, Johnson, & Kovitz, 1983; Wolfe & Mosk, 1983). Accordingly, treatment programs to address these problems are being established. Within this context, children are interviewed about their psychiatric symptoms and also about such issues as their feelings about the abuse, the perpetrator, or both. Nonetheless, investigative interviewing to actually substantiate that physical abuse has occurred remains a relatively uncommon practice.

Since this chapter will largely focus on investigative interviewing, it will pertain primarily to sexually abused children. Any section that may be particularly relevant to physically abused children will be noted. (Also, although both boys and girls are sexually abused, the female pronoun will be used throughout for simplicity and because girls do have a higher incidence of sexual abuse than boys.)

Professional Issues

Prior to the discussion of specific interview procedures, several professional issues will be addressed. These are role definition and boundaries, interviewer biases, and confidentiality.

Role Definition and Boundaries

It is extremely important that the role boundaries of an investigative interviewer be defined prior to an evaluation. For example, the purpose of the interview(s), the limits of confidentiality, who will be informed of interview findings, and other matters must be clarified with all relevant parties. This process must also include attorneys if they represent any of the parties (e.g., child, nonabusive parent or other relative, alleged perpetrator). In some cases, a court order or other written document may specify the nature of the interviewer's role. In other instances, meeting with parents, other relevant parties, or both prior to interviewing the child may be sufficient. Regardless of how it is achieved, clarification of the interviewer's role can potentially help the professional avoid later confusion and misunderstanding. More important, it can reduce the probability that an abused child will be subjected to additional interviews by multiple investigators, which is a particularly traumatic outcome.

Interviewer Biases

Gathering information objectively is essential to the interview process, but may not be easily achieved in the emotion-laden area of child abuse and, in particular, child sexual abuse. Sexual abuse victims tend to elicit our sympathy and compassion. Moreover, many interviewers who have had extensive experience in treating abused children may believe that they rarely lie. Such beliefs may bias an interviewer toward the perspective that if a child alleges sexual abuse, it must necessarily be true.

In contrast, there has recently been tremendous concern about false allegations of sexual abuse, particularly in the context of child custody disputes (Gardner, 1987; Green, 1986). These concerns have intensified, in part, because of the media, which often sensationalize individual custody cases. Investigative interviewers who also conduct many custody evaluations may be inherently suspicious of any type of allegation, particularly if it is made by an angry parent. Such a bias may cause an interviewer to have serious doubts about the validity of a sexual abuse allegation, even prior to seeing the child.

These examples illustrate how our own subjective biases can reduce the objectivity of the interview process. Interviewers need to be aware of their biases and the impact of previous clinical experience so that they can proceed with interview protocols without unwarranted assumptions or compromised neutrality. Objectivity is a very important part of any type of assessment procedure, but it is even more critically required in the emotionally charged area of child sexual abuse.

Confidentiality

Mental health professionals can typically keep confidential the information provided to them during diagnostic interviewing and treatment. This ethical principle applies to children as well, except if there is potential danger to the child or another individual. In cases of investigative interviewing related to alleged child abuse, however, this principle no longer applies. In all 50 states, there are mandatory reporting requirements for mental health and other professionals if there is adequate suspicion of child abuse. Furthermore, in cases of alleged sexual abuse in which a professional is appointed by the court or hired by the local child protective services agency to interview a child, it is commonly assumed by all parties that the results of the interview will be shared with caseworkers, attorneys, and the court.

In light of these legal obligations and court-related concerns, it is essential that the interviewer inform an alleged abuse victim of the limits of confidentiality. This task may be a difficult one, particularly with very young children who have limited verbal understanding and perhaps some confusion about the purpose of the interview. Nonetheless, the interviewer should attempt to clarify confidentiality in a manner consistent with the child's developmental status. Such an open discussion may cause a child initially to feel reticent about talking of possible abuse, especially if there have been threats related to disclosure. However, directly addressing the issue of confidentiality will make it less likely that a child will subsequently feel betrayed when her disclosure of abuse is brought to the attention of a caseworker or the court. Particularly for sexual abuse victims, a sense of betrayal is an issue to which they are already acutely sensitive.

PROCEDURES FOR GATHERING INFORMATION

As mentioned previously, this section on specific data-gathering procedures will pertain primarily to sexually abused children.

General Issues

Number of Interviews

The manner in which an interviewer proceeds in obtaining information about possible sexual abuse depends, at least in part, on the child's age and developmental status. Although there may be pressure from the legal system to gather the relevant data in one interview, it may be impossible to do so. Particularly for younger children with limited verbal and cognitive skills, several interviews may be required. Moreover, it is critical to gain the child's trust and establish an atmosphere of warmth and encouragement. Achieving these goals may take many sessions. Accordingly, an interviewer needs to proceed slowly and cautiously. Raising the topic of sexual abuse before a child feels sufficiently comfortable may generate a great deal of anxiety and ultimately result in no disclosures.

Interviewing the Child without the Alleged Perpetrator

If a child has allegedly been sexually abused by a parent, it is certainly not appropriate for that parent to be present during any of the investigative interviews. In fact, the alleged perpetrator should not even accompany the child to the interviewer's office. In many sexual abuse cases, the victim has been threatened with some type of harm if there is any disclosure. Accordingly, the presence of the alleged perpetrator during an interview would be highly intimidating for the child.

In addition, many abuse victims maintain positive feelings toward the perpetrator, especially when the abuser is a parent. Often, children are afraid that the perpetrator will be punished or that the perpetrator will not be permitted any contact with her. These are significant reasons for a child not to provide information about sexual abuse. Obviously, then, the presence of the alleged perpetrator during the interview would only serve to reinforce these issues and make it extremely difficult for the child to be truthful.

Interviewing the Child without the Nonabusive Parent

In the majority of sexual abuse cases that are infrafamilial in nature, the child is brought to the examiner's office by the nonabusive parent. Nonetheless, every attempt should be made to interview the child alone. It may be difficult to do so with a young child who would experience much anxiety if asked to separate from her parent. Such anxiety can be alleviated by permitting the parent to remain in the office for 10–15 minutes so that the child can become more comfortable. Moreover, having a parent wait just outside the office or keeping the door ajar for a few minutes can be reassuring.

There are at least two reasons for interviewing a child in the absence of the nonabusive parent. First, if a parent is present, a child may feel compelled to say what she believes the parent wants to hear, although this may not necessarily reflect what actually occurred. For example, if a child knows that the parent does not believe that any abuse occurred, she may be highly reticent to make any disclosures in that parent's presence. Conversely, a child may feel obliged to agree with an angry parent who is alleging abuse by an ex-spouse, even if there has been no maltreatment. In either scenario, a child can be influenced about what is disclosed in order to obtain a parent's approval or, at least, avoid disapproval. Accordingly, the truth about the alleged abuse may not be revealed.

The second major reason for interviewing a child alone is related to legal issues. If charges are being pressed against the alleged perpetrator or if the case is being reviewed in juvenile or family court, the presence of a parent during the interview may be perceived as a contaminating factor. Although the interviewer may feel that a parent can help a child feel more relaxed and comfortable, the attorney representing the alleged perpetrator will no doubt suggest that the parent influenced the content of the child's statements. In a criminal proceeding, this could result in charges being dismissed; in family or juvenile court, the child might be forced to have unsupervised contact with an abusive parent because the allegations are seen as unfounded. Given the potential for such highly negative and potentially traumatic outcomes, the interviewer should make every attempt to interview a child alone so that findings will be more acceptable to the legal/judicial system.

Discussion of Normal Routines of Touching

When interviewing children in general, it is certainly appropriate to begin with warm-up questions related to school, activities, friends, and other familiar matters. Such a strategy is also helpful with children who have allegedly been sexually abused. However, instead of proceeding to questions about inappropriate touching, it is useful for the interviewer first to elicit information about normal routines of touching. Doing so will help the child to feel comfortable talking about different kinds of touching experiences. Routines such as those that occur during bathtime (e.g., "Who helps wash you?" "Who washes your hair?") and the child's perception or experience during routine medical examinations should be explored. In addition, questions can be asked about normal displays of affection between parents and the child and how she feels about being kissed, hugged, and otherwise shown affection. Very young children sometimes inadvertently provide information about inappropriate touching in response to these routine questions.

During this segment of the interview, it is very important that the child's terms for various parts of the body, including the private parts, be determined. In this regard, it is quite likely that a child will use idiosyncratic descriptions to identify the private parts, such as "pee-pee," "stick," "peachy," "bum," and the like. Occasionally, children will utilize adult terminology (e.g., "penis," "vagina"), especially if they have participated in prevention programs or treatment related to sexual abuse. However, age-appropriate terms are more typically used, particularly by young children. In either case, without knowledge of the child's terminology, it may be extremely difficult for the interviewer to interpret statements that the child makes later in the session about possible sexual abuse.

Essential Data to be Gathered

Questioning a child about inappropriate touching or possible involvement in sexual activities is a very difficult and sensitive part of the interview process. In this regard, it cannot be overemphasized how critical it is that the child supply the information about any alleged abuse. Leading questions are almost always inappropriate, although an inexperienced interviewer may not realize that a specific question is leading. (Leading questions will be discussed more extensively in the "Do's and Don't's" section.)

Details about the Abuse

In addition to obtaining information about the identity of the alleged perpetrator and the specific nature of the sexual acts perpetrated against a child, other details need to be explored. These details would include the number of abusive episodes, where the abuse occurred, the whereabouts of the child's primary caretaker (if different from that of the abuser) when the abuse occurred, and the child's feelings about the incident(s). Moreover, the following issues should be addressed: threats or promise of rewards made by the perpetrator, reasons for delaying disclosure if there has been a delay, and whether the alleged perpetrator told the child to keep the abuse a secret. It is also important to ascertain the child's feelings with respect to who is responsible for the abuse, whether she has felt emotional support since the disclosure, and what she believes the consequences are for the alleged perpetrator and herself, now that the abuse has been disclosed.

Children will vary, of course, in the amount of information that they can provide, depending on their age, level of trust, and other factors. Moreover, disclosure may occur gradually, with more and more details being given over time. Nonetheless, even children as young as 3 years old can provide some basic details about what may have occurred. This information is critical in helping the interviewer eventually determine the likelihood that a child has been sexually abused.

Interviewer's Reaction to Disclosures

The interviewer's reaction to the information provided by the child can be a critical determinant as to how much additional information is disclosed. An interviewer who is judgmental of the alleged perpetrator or who reacts strongly to horrible details may make the child feel scared, guilty, embarrassed, or responsible for what happened. Any of these feelings will inevitably result in the child's being reluctant to talk further about any alleged abuse. It is essential, therefore, that the interviewer be calm and nonjudgmental when details are being provided.

It may take extensive experience in interviewing sexually abused children to achieve this type of emotional reaction. Professionals are as human and prone to strong and judgmental responses to the disclosure of sexual abuse as are lay members of society. Being aware of one's own feelings about sexual abuse and monitoring one's emotional reactivity to this issue can help the professional respond to the information provided by alleged victims in an encouraging but objective, neutral, and nonjudgmental manner.

Use of Anatomically Correct Dolls

Anatomically correct (AC) dolls were originally designed as a diagnostic tool to assist interviewers in assessing young children or older children with limited verbal skills. It was hoped that children who could not use words to describe any alleged sexual abuse could demonstrate with the dolls what was perpetrated against them. Unfortunately, as reviewed by White and Santilli (1988), a great controversy has evolved over the appropriate use of AC dolls in interviewing alleged abuse victims.

One of the greatest concerns about the utilization of AC dolls has been that they are suggestive to young children and that this suggestiveness could result in their simulating explicit sexual play with the dolls even in the absence of previous sexual abuse. However, recent empirical studies have failed to support such a contention. For example, Sivan, Schor, Koeppel, and Noble (1988) found no demonstrations of simulated sexual intercourse in their sample of 144 3- to 8-year-old non-sexually abused children observed in free play with AC dolls. Similarly, Everson and Boat (1990) reported that only 6% of their non-sexually abused 2- to 5-year-old subjects demonstrated behavior clearly suggestive of sexual intercourse during a doll interview. Thus, there is little empirical support for the notion that AC dolls elicit representational explicit sexual behavior in "normal" nonabused children.

In light of these recent findings, professionals can perhaps feel more comfortable in using AC dolls during play interviews. Nonetheless, scientific data about their diagnostic utility remains limited, and interviewers should continue to utilize them cautiously. There are some ways, though, in which their use may facilitate the interview process. For example, an interviewer could present a set of AC dolls to a child in order to help identify the terms that she uses for the private parts of the body. Moreover, an alleged victim could be asked to use the dolls to demonstrate the sexual activities that she was forced to engage in. The interviewer could then determine whether such demonstration corroborates the verbal statements made by the child earlier in the interview. Consistency between demonstration with AC dolls and any verbal statements would support a child's credibility in most cases.

It is worth adding that at present, the diagnostic usefulness of AC dolls in the *absence* of verbal allegations by the child is unknown. Therefore, an interviewer's conclusions based only on a child's play interaction with the dolls would certainly be highly speculative in nature. Moreover, such clinical findings would be severely challenged in most legal jurisdictions.

CASE ILLUSTRATIONS

The two cases discussed below illustrate some of the data-gathering procedures described in the previous section. In both cases, the names have been changed to protect the identity of the victims.

Case 1

This case involved a 4-year-old boy named Joey who was allegedly sexually abused by his father during visits. The parents were divorced, and the father had partial custody of Joey every other weekend. The mother had become suspicious of possible sexual abuse because of Joey's use of precocious sexual terms and excessive masturbation immediately after visits with the father. When she had asked her son about possible inappropriate touching, he responded that "Daddy" had been touching him "down there." Prior to this child's being interviewed, the attorneys for both parents agreed that an evaluation could be performed by a court-appointed professional. The following dialogue demonstrates questions about normal routines of touching and general questions about inappropriate touching.

During the first interview with Joey, which lasted 45 minutes, there were a series of warm-up questions about preschool, play interests, and other mundane matters. Normal routines of touching were then discussed.

INTERVIEWER: Joey, do you ever go to the doctor?

JOEY: Yes.

INTERVIEWER: What does the doctor do?

JOEY: He looks at my ears.

INTERVIEWER: Oh? Does he do anything else?

JOEY: He listens to my heart. And sometimes he touches my tummy.

INTERVIEWER: I see. You know, it's okay for a doctor to touch children in these kinds of ways. He's just trying to help you. Another kind of touching is when you take a bath and somebody helps to wash you. Do you like taking a bath?

JOEY: Sometimes. But I hate cold water.

INTERVIEWER: Me, too! Does anyone help you while you're in the tub?

JOEY: Mommy and sometimes Daddy.

INTERVIEWER: What do they do?

JOEY: They wash my hair. Sometimes the water gets in my eyes. Yuk!

INTERVIEWER: That does feel bad. Who washes the rest of you?

JOEY: I do.

The interviewer then asked Joey about washing the private parts of his body. In the context of this discussion, he indicated that his word for penis was "pee-pee" and his word for the anal area was "bum." Later in the interview, after some play activities, other types of touching were discussed.

INTERVIEWER: Joey, we've been talking about different kinds of touching today. Like going to the doctor or at bathtime. Another kind of touching is when someone hugs or kisses you and you feel good inside. Does that ever happen to you?

JOEY: Yes. My mommy hugs me. I hug her back.

INTERVIEWER: Anyone else?

JOEY: My grandma.

INTERVIEWER: That's nice. Those are good kinds of touching. They make us feel happy inside.

The interactions discussed above helped Joey to become comfortable talking about different kinds of appropriate touching. The interviewer observed that questions of this type did not upset him in any way. The interviewer also learned the terms Joey used to identify the private parts of the body. Additional play time was then provided. This is important, especially for a young child with a relatively limited attention span. Questions were subsequently asked about inappropriate kinds of touching:

INTERVIEWER: Joey, you've told me about touching which makes you feel good inside. Other kinds of touching make us feel sad or unhappy inside. Has that ever happened to you?

JOEY: Yeah, Billy hit me with a car. So I punched him.

INTERVIEWER: You must have been really mad! Is Billy your friend?

JOEY: Yes.

INTERVIEWER: Well, sometimes even friends fight. Has there ever been another time that you felt sad or unhappy about a kind of touching?

JOEY: Yeah, with my Daddy.

INTERVIEWER: I see. Can you tell me what happened?

JOEY: He touched my pee-pee.

INTERVIEWER: Oh. How did he do that?

JOEY: [Rubbing his genital area] Like this.

INTERVIEWER: Did anything else happen?

JOEY: I sucked his pee-pee. Stuff came out. I drank it until it was all gone.

This disclosure made Joey quite anxious. Accordingly, the interviewer decided to discontinue this line of questioning until the second interview. At that time, additional details were gathered.

Space does not permit a discussion of the second interview, but it was important to convey to this child that he had not done anything wrong and that he was brave for having talked about what had happened to him. This type of encouragement is totally acceptable and particularly significant for young children. It is important to emphasize, though, that children should receive words of encouragement and positive feedback no matter what is disclosed, even if there is a denial of abuse or if there are inconsistencies in their statements.

Case 2

This second case involved a 9-year-old girl named Jennifer who was allegedly sexually abused by her father over several years. This was an intact family with two younger siblings. Jennifer had initially disclosed the abuse to her mother, who did not believe her. She subsequently told her maternal grandmother, who called the local child welfare authority. Jennifer and her siblings were then placed in temporary foster care because her father would not leave the home. Soon afterward, a local juvenile court judge ordered an evaluation to assess Jennifer's credibility regarding the abuse allegations.

The excerpts that follow illustrate procedures for alleviating a child's anxiety, gathering details in a nonleading manner, and obtaining information about a child's feelings about the alleged perpetrator and abuse.

Jennifer knew that she was going to be questioned about the alleged sexual abuse. Despite warm-up questions, she remained quite anxious.

INTERVIEWER: You seem to be kind of nervous.

JENNIFER: [Shaking head affirmatively] I am.

INTERVIEWER: Do you know why you're here?

JENNIFER: Yes. But I don't want to talk. Can you ask my caseworker what happened? She knows.

INTERVIEWER: It's really hard to talk about these kinds of things, isn't it? Most children do feel nervous or afraid. It's okay if you feel this way.

JENNIFER: I just can't talk about it. It's too embarrassing. Please ask my caseworker.

INTERVIEWER: Did you know that I talk to lots of children about different types of touching experiences? It is scary, but after a while, kids usually feel okay.

This exchange did seem to help Jennifer to become more comfortable. After a brief discussion of different kinds of touching, questions were asked about inappropriate touching:

INTERVIEWER: Have you ever been touched in a way that made you feel upset or uncomfortable?

JENNIFER: Yes.

INTERVIEWER: Can you tell me about it?

JENNIFER: You know that's why I'm here. Please ask my caseworker.

INTERVIEWER: I could, but it's important that I hear from you, too. Can you tell me about what happened?

JENNIFER: Well, it was my father. I'm too shy to talk about it.

INTERVIEWER: You're doing fine! Go ahead with what you were going to say.

JENNIFER: [After a few seconds] My father, he touched me.

INTERVIEWER: I see. Can you tell me more?

JENNIFER: He touched me on my bottom. He put his pee-pee in my bottom.

INTERVIEWER: Did anything else happen?

JENNIFER: He made me touch it with my mouth.

INTERVIEWER: Touch what?

JENNIFER: His pee-pee.

INTERVIEWER: Where did this happen?

JENNIFER: In the bathroom or the cellar.

INTERVIEWER: Of a house?

JENNIFER: Yes, our house.

INTERVIEWER: Was anyone else there when he would do these things to you?

JENNIFER: No, we were always alone.

INTERVIEWER: I'm not sure how often this happened.

JENNIFER: Lots of times.

INTERVIEWER: Can you tell me how often that means?

JENNIFER: Every week. Sometimes more.

Jennifer did a good job providing details about the alleged abuse. Encouragement was offered as well as positive feedback that she was trying very hard to remember what happened despite her embarrassment and anxiety. General questions were used so that Jennifer could provide the information about what had occurred. This is important, even if questions have to be repeated or if the interviewer appears to the child to be a bit "dumb" or "slow." Again, leading questions should be avoided, whenever possible.

After more information about details was gathered, questions were asked about Jennifer's feelings about what had happened:

INTERVIEWER: How did you feel when your father did these things to you?

JENNIFER: I felt bad.

INTERVIEWER: How did you feel about him?

JENNIFER: Mad. How could a father do this stuff? I told my mother, but she didn't believe me. She said he was just putting medicine on me, but you don't put medicine on with a pee-pee!

INTERVIEWER: Does she believe you now?

JENNIFER: I think so.

INTERVIEWER: How do you feel toward your father now?

JENNIFER: I love him. But I'm still mad. He has to go to some kind of doctor to get healed. That's what Mommy said.

INTERVIEWER: How do you feel about being away from home?

JENNIFER: Sad. Maybe it's my fault. Maybe I shouldn't have said anything. He could get into trouble.

INTERVIEWER: What kind?

JENNIFER: Go to jail.

INTERVIEWER: How would you feel about that?

JENNIFER: A little happy and a little sad. He did some nice things with me, too.

This excerpt illustrates the kinds of feelings that are commonly found in sexually abused children, such as their sense of betrayal, their ambivalence toward the perpetrator, and their feelings of responsibility for the abuse. Questioning a child about her feelings is important not only for investigative purposes, but also for clinical reasons. Resolving these kinds of feelings is typically a critical component of treatment for most child victims.

INFORMATION CRITICAL TO MAKING A DIAGNOSIS

General Concerns

Although interviewing a child with regard to possible sexual abuse is a critical part of the diagnostic process, other assessment procedures are also necessary. In this regard, a medical examination is typically suggested despite the absence of physical findings in the large majority of cases (Muram, 1989). Nonetheless, a physician can rule out sexually transmitted diseases and also provide assurance to the child and parents that she is not "damaged." In addition, interviewing the nonabusive parent to obtain background information and history, interviewing the alleged abusive parent when allegations arise during custody disputes (Benedek & Schetky, 1987), and gathering data from collateral sources are important diagnostic procedures.

In drawing conclusions regarding the likelihood that a child has been abused, interview findings must be evaluated in the context of other sources of data. Nonetheless, there are a number of criteria that can be used in examining interview results that do relate to a child's credibility. (For a parallel discussion, please see Myers et al., 1989.) It must be strongly emphasized, though, that the presence or absence of any of these factors does not confirm or disconfirm abuse and that there are many exceptions to the broad guidelines suggested below.

Convincing Details

It bears repeating that children will vary widely in the amount of information that they can provide about alleged abuse depending on such factors as their chronological age, developmental level, anxiety, and level of trust. Also, disclosure often occurs gradually, with more details discussed over time. Nonetheless, children who can provide convincing details are likely to be perceived as more credible than those who give only minimal information such as "Daddy touched my pee-pee." Generally, it has been our clinical experience that even preschool children can specify where the abuse occurred, whether anyone else was present, and some details about the exact nature of the inappropriate touching.

Age-Appropriate Terminology

As noted previously, it is common for abuse victims to use their own terminology to describe the private parts of the body and what sexual acts they were forced to engage in. Accordingly, interviewers can expect to hear such words as "pee-pee," "stick," and "peachy" to describe the private parts and statements such as "Daddy put his thing in my bum" or "He made me rub it" to describe the actual sexual experience. Of course, some children will use adult terms, especially if they have been in therapy related to possible abuse, have participated in sexual abuse prevention programs, or have parents who taught them the more sophisticated terminology. Generally, though, most actual abuse victims will use words and descriptions that are consistent with their age and overall developmental status.

Consistency

It is inevitable that alleged child sexual abuse victims will not be totally consistent from one interview to the next or across interviewers with regard to the information that they provide. Again, age, developmental level, and other factors will be important influences. In addition, inconsistencies can result because different questions are asked by different interviewers. The gradual disclosure of more details over time may also result in apparent inconsistencies. Nonetheless, if a child's statements are generally consistent, this factor would support her credibility.

Affect Consistent with Allegations

In our clinical experience, when a child has truly been sexually abused, her affect is usually consistent with the allegations. Thus, embarrassment, anxiety, shame, and fear are commonly found when a victim is providing information about the abuse. However, there are numerous exceptions to this general guideline. Children who have been interviewed several times or have been in therapy related to the abuse may present details in a relatively straightforward manner without significant distress. Also, children who have received much emotional support from parents after disclosure may feel reasonably comfortable in talking about what occurred. Accordingly, this factor has to be carefully considered. The absence of anxiety or other signs of emotional distress when discussing the allegations does not necessarily diminish a child's credibility.

Other Factors

There are other factors that merit some attention. The interviewer must try to assess whether a child has been coached or influenced with regard to the information that she provides. Particularly with young children, it is useful to ask directly whether anyone has told them what to say. Again, however, caution must be exercised. Sometimes, even in legitimate abuse cases, a parent instructs the child, "Tell the doctor the truth" or "Just say what happened." Also, it is important to evaluate whether an alleged victim has any motivation to make a false allegation.

Older children or adolescents who have more advanced sexual knowledge and possible sexual experience are more capable of fabricating abuse. They may do so out of anger, a desire to seek retaliation for perceived rejection, or to gain attention.

Again, it cannot be emphasized enough that the criteria presented above are very broad guidelines and that many children who have actually been abused may meet some criteria but not others. Determining whether a child has been sexually abused is a very serious and complex task, which requires the integration of interview findings with data from other assessment procedures and from sources other than the child. Unfortunately, in some cases, the information gathered may be inconsistent or conflictual and leave the interviewer feeling very uncertain about the probability of abuse. In these situations, it is strongly recommended that the interviewer not hesitate to express this uncertainty in any written report that is prepared.

DO'S AND DON'T'S

Leading Questions

Interview procedures for abused children have come under attack in recent years because of a concern that leading questions are frequently used. Particularly with regard to sexually abused children, there have been reported cases in which evaluations have been judicially challenged because of the perception that leading questions contaminated the findings (White, 1990). This issue becomes an even greater concern when investigators are not adequately trained in interviewing abused children. It can hardly be overemphasized that although an inexperienced interviewer may understand that leading questions are inappropriate, he or she may not be aware that a particular question is leading.

It is essential that during the interview process, the child provide the information about any alleged abuse to which she has been subjected. Leading questions are not acceptable, except in emergency situations in which a child's safety would be clearly endangered if she remained in a potentially abusive environment. To illustrate, asking a child, "Did Daddy touch your pee-pee?," particularly if it is an initial question, is leading in at least three ways. Specifically, this type of question incorporates the assumptions that the child has been touched inappropriately, that the father is the perpetrator, and that genital fondling was the type of sexual activity that occurred. It is worth adding that young children have a propensity to respond affirmatively to yes/no type questions, particularly in an attempt to gain the interviewer's approval. Leading questions can therefore result in a child's being guided or influenced to provide a specific response that may or may not reflect the reality of what actually happened.

The following dialogue illustrates how leading questions can contaminate interview findings:

INTERVIEWER: Do you know why you're here today?

CHILD: [Nods affirmatively.]

INTERVIEWER: Good. Can you tell me how your Daddy touched you?

CHILD: He touched me in a yukky way.
INTERVIEWER: Did he touch your pee-pee?
CHILD: Yes.
INTERVIEWER: Did he put his pee-pee inside of your pee-pee?
CHILD: I think so.

In contrast, the following dialogue illustrates more appropriate general questions in which the child supplies the information about what happened:

INTERVIEWER: Has there ever been a time that you were touched in a way that made you feel upset or bad?
CHILD: Yes.
INTERVIEWER: Can you tell me about that?
CHILD: My daddy touched my pee-pee.
INTERVIEWER: I don't quite understand. Can you tell me more about what happened?
CHILD: He touched my pee-pee with his pee-pee.
INTERVIEWER: How did he do that?
CHILD: He put it inside me.

As noted earlier, an interview replete with leading questions may be challenged in court and possibly be rejected. This outcome may result in the judge's ordering a new evaluation, which is inherently more stressful for the child. Furthermore, the court proceedings in such a case may become even more prolonged. It is therefore critical to avoid leading questions not only to ensure that valid, reliable information is obtained but also to increase the likelihood that one's findings are perceived as objective within the legal system.

Interviewer Response to Child's Statements

In a previous section of this chapter, there was brief discussion of how the interviewer's reactions to a child's disclosures may affect the remainder of the interview process. This issue will be more fully elucidated here. Many children who have been sexually abused have kept the abuse a secret for a considerable time. Disclosure of what occurred is typically very upsetting and is frequently accompanied by anxiety, shame, or embarrassment. An interviewer who responds negatively to a child's presentation of details will likely make her feel even more uncomfortable. Further disclosures would then be improbable. This type of inappropriate emotional reaction is illustrated below.

INTERVIEWER: Can you tell me more about what happened?
CHILD: He made me put it in my mouth. He made me lick it.
INTERVIEWER: How horrible!
CHILD: [No response, appearing sad.]
INTERVIEWER: It was disgusting what he did. No wonder you have a hard time talking about it.

In a similar vein, being judgmental of the alleged perpetrator will likely result in an exacerbation of a child's fear that her disclosures may cause something bad to happen to him. Again, this will have a dampening effect on the likelihood of additional statements.

INTERVIEWER: How do you feel about what your daddy did to you?
CHILD: Bad. I'm very angry at him.
INTERVIEWER: You should be! He's a wicked man. How would you feel if he goes to jail?
CHILD: Half and half. Happy but a little sad, too.
INTERVIEWER: I understand, but he deserves to go for what he did.

More appropriately, the interviewer needs to respond to a child's disclosures in a relatively benign and straightforward but supportive manner. Responding in such a manner will lessen her anxiety and not make her feel that she has done anything wrong or that she is bad. Furthermore, a neutral perspective should be maintained toward the alleged perpetrator, with a focus on the child's feelings, not the interviewer's. In this regard, it may take many interviews with abused children for a professional to learn to achieve this type of constructive emotional response.

In addition to the aforementioned issues, this chapter has focused on several other interviewing features that can have a serious effect on the outcome of the interview process. These issues include the manner in which the question of confidentiality is addressed with the child, whether the child can be interviewed alone, and what reasonable conclusions can be drawn on the sole basis of child's interaction with anatomically correct dolls. (Please see the appropriate sections for further discussion of these issues.) It cannot be emphasized too strongly that professionals who interview allegedly abused children face a difficult and complex task. It is essential to proceed cautiously, as the stakes are too high to do otherwise. Using biased interview procedures lacking in objectivity or deriving conclusions that are not supported by the data may potentially result in greater stress for a chid who has already been subjected to a traumatic life event.

SUMMARY

This chapter has focused on investigative interviewing with physically and sexually abused children, although most of the discussion has been geared toward the latter group. General professional issues have been addressed, including role definition and boundaries, interviewer biases, and confidentiality. In addition, case illustrations have been presented to highlight specific interviewing techniques and to demonstrate how certain procedures are inappropriate in these types of cases.

It has been emphasized throughout the chapter that determining that a child has been abused is a difficult and complex task. Although broad guidelines were suggested in order to make such a determination, cases do vary tremendously, and many abused children will not meet one or more of these criteria. Interviewers must therefore proceed cautiously and draw conclusions based on an integration of interview findings with data from other assessment procedures and from sources other than the child.

References

American Professional Society on the Abuse of Children (1990). *Guidelines for psychosocial evaluation of suspected sexual abuse in young children*. Chicago: Author.

Benedek, E. P., & Schetky, D. H. (1987). Problems in validating allegations of sexual abuse. Part 2. Clinical evaluation. *Journal of the American Academy of Child and Adolescent Psychiatry, 26*, 916–921.

Everson, M. D., & Boat, B. W. (1990). Sexualized doll play among young children: Implications for the use of anatomical dolls in sexual abuse evaluations. *Journal of the American Academy of Child and Adolescent Psychiatry, 29*, 736–742.

Gardner, R. A. (1987). *The parental alienation syndrome and the differentiation between fabricated and genuine child sex abuse*. Cresskill, NJ: Creative Therapeutics.

Green, A. (1986). True and false allegations of sexual abuse in child custody disputes. *Journal of the American Academy of Child and Adolescent Psychiatry, 25*, 449–456.

Grisso, T. (1990). Evolving guidelines for divorce/custody evaluations. *Family and Conciliation Courts Review, 28*, 35–41.

Kempe, C., Silverman, F., Steele, B., & Droegemueller, W. (1962). The battered child syndrome. *Journal of American Medical Association, 181*, 17–24.

Mask, E., Johnson, C., & Kovitz, K. (1983). A comparison of the mother–child interactions of physically abused and non-abused children during play and task situations. *Journal of Clinical Child Psychology, 12*, 337–346.

Muram, D. (1989). Child sexual abuse: Relationship between sexual acts and genital findings. *Child Abuse and Neglect, 13*, 211–216.

Myers, J. E., Bays, J., Becker, J., Berliner, L., Corwin, D. L., & Saywitz, K. J. (1989). Expert testimony in child sexual abuse litigation. *Nebraska Law Review, 68*, 1–145.

National Center on Child Abuse and Neglect (1988). *Study findings: Study of national incidence and prevalence of child abuse and neglect*. Washington, DC: U.S. Department of Health and Human Services.

Schetky, D. H., & Guyer, M. J. (1990). Civil litigation and the child psychiatrist. *Journal of the American Academy of Child and Adolescent Psychiatry, 29*, 963–968.

Sivan, A. B., Schor, D. P., Koeppel, G. K., & Noble, L. D. (1988). Interaction of normal children with anatomical dolls. *Child Abuse and Neglect, 12*, 295–304.

White, S. (1990). The contamination of children's interviews. *The Child, Youth, and Family Services Quarterly, 13*, 6–18.

White, S., & Santilli, G. (1988). A review of clinical practices and research data on anatomical dolls. *Journal of Interpersonal Violence, 3*, 430–442.

Wolfe, D., & Mosk, M. (1983). Behavioral comparisons of children from abusive and distressed families. *Journal of Consulting and Clinical Psychology, 51*, 702–708.

15

Neurologically Impaired Patients

THOMAS J. BOLL

INTRODUCTION

In clinical psychology practice, despite its varying degrees of reliability and validity, the interview is an appropriate and, in many instances, excellent technique and procedure for obtaining information about the patient that is necessary and may be sufficient for a diagnosis. Furthermore, the clinical psychology interview is not only capable of allowing the clinician to make yes/no decisions with regard to diagnostic possibilities and probabilities, but is also adequate for obtaining information that allows sufficient descriptive information that a comprehensive evaluation can be said to have been accomplished along with whatever diagnostic or other formal classificatory activities are required.

In many instances, of course, interviewing is supplemented in a variety of ways. History may be provided from outside sources, and that material certainly should be reviewed. Such material includes medical, behavioral, academic, occupational, social, and previous psychological data and experiences. Supplementation is also provided by direct psychological examination through testing. This testing can provide objective data in a number of areas that cannot be precisely assessed, such as level of intellectual functioning, quality of verbalization under various sorts of structured and standardized types of provocation, and willingness to admit to subjective difficulties and complaints as opposed to willingness to provide them in a somewhat more extemporaneous fashion such as occurs in an interview. Although interviews may be more or less structured, psychological testing is always structured and therefore represents useful contrast, just as outside information and information from significant others provides useful contrast as well as the information itself when this information is compared to the direct commentary and revelations of the patient. All this is covered extremely well in the other chapters of this volume and is stated here in very brief form only to note the contrast between the interviewing that may take place in areas outside neuropsychology and the way neuropsychologists use the interview format.

THOMAS J. BOLL • University of Alabama at Birmingham, Birmingham, Alabama 35294.

Diagnostic Interviewing (Second Edition), edited by Michel Hersen and Samuel M. Turner. Plenum Press, New York, 1994.

The interview in clinical neuropsychology may be qualitatively different from the interview in all other areas of clinical psychology. One of the interesting differences between neuropsychological and other formats of practice is that an interview may be conducted both before and after the formal examination process. Doing so is neither necessary nor required, but can, under the correct circumstances, provide very useful information. These interviews can be collapsed into one, and if only one should be conducted, it is probably most useful to conduct it after rather than before the formal and standard neuropsychological examination.

One reason for recommending a posttesting interview is that usually the information that is typically of most importance to have prior to testing can be obtained by technical personnel who will be conducting the formal aspects of the examination, e.g., testing. Obviously, if the neuropsychologist himself or herself is conducting the examination, the information will also be obtained and can be utilized with or without the inclusion of a formal period of interview. Additional information typically obtained prior to testing, such as historical and documentary evidence from a variety of sources, can also be obtained by personnel other than the neuropsychologist. Many of the documents forwarded with the patient or obtainable in the medical chart are well-preserved and can be utilized at any time prior to coming to final conclusion and writing a report. Information can also be obtained from a patient questionnaire to be filled out by the patient or significant others with or without the examiner's help. While this information may indeed need to be supplemented, questioned about, and discussed, these activities need not occur prior to the more formal aspects of the examination.

One purpose of the initial interview is to put the patient at ease and indicate to him or her what the procedures for the day will be. This too can be done by well-trained personnel in the neuropsychologist's office, as these procedures are easily described and understood and can be communicated not only to the patient but also to significant others accompanying the patient so that they will have an idea of what is to be expected.

Finally, information about impediments to testing is typically seen as an important aspect of preexamination interview data-gathering. Issues such as physical impediments to either the sensory system (e.g., blindness, deafness) or the motor systems (e.g., paralysis or tremulousness) certainly can and must be observed and commented on by the examining person whether or not the neuropsychologist has made similar commentary. Difficulties in cooperation or frank unwillingness to cooperate are also identifiable and should be part of the behavioral note. Issues of undue anxiety, depression, or claims of emotional distress can certainly be noted as can unusual verbalization, motor activities, threats, aggressiveness, and lack of appreciation for the nature of the tasks as expressed by multiple, often irrelevant complaints about having to be subjected to the examination in the first place. Behavioral manifestations that may or may not interfere with the examination should also be noted.

Observable symptoms in the area of general mental status may become a focus of attention, and this focus may persist throughout the entire examination process. Such symptoms include issues of capacity to speak, general historical knowledge, and ability to delineate one's symptom picture and complaint profile. Thoughts, perceptions, and general verbalization skill should be noted. It is important to identify issues such as attentional capacity, apparent insight, and ability to maintain appropriate interpersonal style during what is often a relatively lengthy and sometimes fatiguing and even provoking examination process.

LANGUAGE

Language functioning of both a receptive and an expressive nature should be evaluated. Initially, the speech pattern may be the first observable sign of a disorder in the language mechanism. Such issues as articulation deficit may or may not signal central nervous system impairment. Word-finding difficulty, paraphasia, unusual patterns of speech, and obvious difficulties in comprehension are more likely to indicate a central nervous system origin. In some patients, linguistic deficits may significantly compromise their ability to undertake a number of formal neuropsychological activities, and the examination may therefore have to be organized in such a way as not to place the patient in double and triple jeopardy with regard to the objective test results. A patient who has a mild speech disorder or has some slight dysnomia is quite likely to be able to take the vast majority of neuropsychological procedures well. On the other hand, a patient with relatively global and severe dysphasic deficits may well wind up doing poorly on a wide range of apparently different tests for the same underlying reason, thereby giving the misimpression of a more global cognitive deficit when, in fact, it is the global nature of the language system dysfunction that is being expressed.

MOTOR AND SENSORY SYSTEM

The *motor and sensory system* is subject to direct interview and observational examination as well as direct and formal neuropsychological examination. Tremor, ataxia, athetosis, unsteadiness, clumsiness, and marked alteration in tone are findings that should have correlates, not only in the history and presenting complaints but also in the formal examination itself, and therefore are important to identify. Motor mannerisms that may reflect tics or unusual habit patterns rather than motor impairments should also be identified, as should such deviations from normative behavior as hyperactivity and marked motoric slowness.

DISRUPTIONS IN THE COGNITIVE APPARATUS

Disruptions in the cognitive apparatus—such as confusion, disorientation, severe impairments in various aspects of the memory system, and apraxia, both observed and complained of, as well as impairments in judgment, insight, planning, perception of current and past functional capacity, appreciation of current and future deficits in performance of a wide range of routine activities, and disruptions in the attentional mechanism as these are identified by the patient, reported by significant others, and/or noted in written historical information—should, once again, find correlates in the direct examination and appear in a fashion entirely proportional, one with the other. If there is no such proportionality, it may be that the patient has picked certain aspects of the examination in which to manifest these symptoms, either intentionally or otherwise. Certain types of circumstances, such as work stress or pain, are more prone to drive specific symptoms to expression, thus providing information that may be very helpful in a variety of postexamination management circumstances.

AMNESIA

Reports during interview of *significant amnesia* such as total loss of historical information and incapacity to recount many aspects of one's personal history, in the absence of severe dementia, are unlikely to be correlated with neurological disorder. The origin for this symptomatology is most likely to be found in motivations for exaggeration or, in the rare instance, hysterical amnesia. Patients who cannot recount the simplest aspects of their present and past life circumstances are either severely neurologically impaired in a fashion easily subject to documentation and appreciation from a variety of examination modalities or fall into the category of patients whose current life circumstances are likely to provide the sustaining motivation for this apparent symptom picture. Emotionally based or hysterical amnesia, relatable to a general or specific life event or set of stressors, is a diagnostic consideration. Patients who show no confusion throughout the event, but who develop and report amnesia at some later time, are likely to be demonstrating an emotional and nonneurological syndrome. Patients without obvious neurological disorder or emotional etiology for their amnesia, but who are involved in litigation, while possibly quite righteous with regard to a number of complaints, may have very specific motivation for self-identifying symptoms.

This is not to say that specific tests of malingering need always be given, but rather that careful correlation of history, current situations, objective examination, and direct observational information needs to be made in order to determine which aspects of any patient's complaint pattern are documentably relatable to the primary and possibly the secondary aspects of his or her injury or illness and which may exist and be sustained on the basis of more self-serving motivations.

DEFICIT AWARENESS

Although some patients will overidentify deficits, some patients with well-documented neurological disorders will actually misrecognize or actively deny functionally impairing conditions. Family members may also have very imperfect appreciation of or misunderstand the nature of the patients' deficits. Just as some patients without neurological disorder are prone to overcomplain, patients with general neuropsychological and neurologically based deficits may feel that they can accomplish many tasks that are beyond their capacity and may become quite resentful about any imposed restrictions. Family members may misidentify a patient's apraxia as arthritis or other medical difficulties. In some cases, the onset is so gradual that all involved accommodate to the patient's increasing disability. The patient's restriction in activities may be viewed as due to depression or other personality change rather than as an increasing neurological incapacity to manage usual and routine activities that were once enjoyed.

Neurologically impaired patients may insist on being allowed to return to work or school, to drive, and to utilize various equipment despite the very clear danger involved in performing such activities. Many patients with neurological disorder are not only highly motivated to return to full functioning and desperate to prove their competence, but also genuinely lacking in awareness that certain incapacities have caused them to be less able to manage or to sustain a previously performed activity. It may be only when the results of that activity are demonstrated to be entirely unacceptable that the patient can recognize that something has gone wrong and even then may resist the obvious interpretation. Excuses may be made, such as not having one's glasses or having had a poor night's sleep or not having been given a fair chance. These excuses are not made out of a contrary attitude, but out of a genuine, neurologically based, incapacity to perceive and appreciate the nature of the relationship between one's actions and their consequence and outcome.

DEVELOPMENTAL BACKGROUND

Observation of background information and life pattern of social activities, occupation, and educational accomplishment can be aided by data from IQ and academic achievement portions of the neuropsychological examination. Such scores may represent an underestimate of a patient's premorbid functioning. Nevertheless, many neurological conditions, particularly conditions that are generalized, relatively mild, and without neuropathological correlate, exert substantially less effect on a patient's stored fund of knowledge and general information than on other intellectual processes. This aspect of patient functioning is best assessed by such tests as the Wechsler Adult Intelligence Scale and the Wide Range Achievement Test. Scores on such tests are reasonable estimates of that level below which patients did not function prior to their suspected central nervous system event. Selected use of subtests, however, has not been found to be warranted. Many persons without neurological disorder have a relatively variable capacity to perform on the several subtests of the Wechsler Scale. Within the normative population, a 6-point subscale disparity between high and low score is routine. There is no reason to believe, therefore, that the highest or lowest or any other particular score is specifically reflective of premorbid achievement or premorbid preexisting deficits. Rather, the overall level of functioning, particularly in the context of other historical information such as occupational and educational attainment, provides at least a floor below which one need not go in interpreting other measures more sensitive to the effects of subtle central nervous system impairments.

Measures of IQ performance that fall distinctly out of line with hypothesized premorbid functioning should lead to interview questioning about the actual nature of educational attainment, rather than a blanket acceptance that all high school diplomas have been earned with equal merit and by overcoming equal academic challenge. A surprisingly low IQ may call into question the actual nature of the patient's occupational attainments and lead to a more in-depth description of the nature his or her actual duties that can be very revealing, both positively and negatively, as to the patient's lifelong capacities and achievements.

Even particular patterns of intellectual functioning such as significant Verbal–Performance discrepancies may be relatable to lifelong patterns of learning impairment or lifelong patterns of nonimpaired specific proclivities. The patient who never read much, but who has always been a mechanical marvel, who now, following a mild head injury, is uncertain whether he should return to work may well be revealing essentially no change in an IQ pattern in which the Performance IQ is 15–20 points higher than the Verbal IQ. Except for relatively severe, generalized brain injury or highly lateralized brain conditions, this pattern of Verbal–Performance disparity is less likely to be relatable to a neurological event than to other factors independent of and preceding the neurological disorder. This knowledge is critical in making judgments about the patient's capacity to resume occupational tasks and to appreciate the nature of the actual damage done by the injury as well as to recognize areas of functioning that have not been damaged or for which damage has been relatively insignificant to the person's functional capacity.

As an example of the necessity for this knowledge, a patient who had sustained two very minor head injuries, for which overnight hospitalization and observation was the only treatment in each instance, was referred with complaints of total occupational and significant generalized functional disability involving all aspects of his day-to-day performance. His measured IQ was found to be at the top of the range of mild mental deficiency. This was inconsistent with a bachelor's degree from a well-respected university and ownership of a business of substantial size and considerable success for the last 20 years. The patient was now claiming total inability to manage business and routine household financial activities. He demonstrated deficits not only on tests of short-term memory, which correlated well with the patient's subjective complaints of daily memory difficulty, but on tests of background skills as measured by the Wechsler Scale as well.

The dramatic nature of the difficulties experienced by the patient, which far exceeded expectation on the basis of his injury, suggested that considerable additional information would need to be acquired during the interview. The patient was queried about a variety of other neurological background factors without evidence of additional damage, diseases, or dysfunction. He described a set of symptoms, corroborated by his wife, that suggested significant depressive illness. Psychiatric evaluation again revealed a patient who initially appeared sufficiently impaired to warrant hospitalization. When, despite treatment, his symptoms persisted, a discussion of the advisability of ECT was initiated. Shortly after this discussion, the patient appeared to begin to benefit from pharmacological intervention and participated increasingly actively in a number of ward-based treatment programs to the extent that his clinical manifestations of depression were almost absent and his subjective report of well-being was incompletely but significantly improved.

Because of this improvement, it was deemed appropriate to reexamine the patient to determine whether, in fact, his difficulties had been due to his depression. If indeed this was the case, it would be anticipated that the depressed neuropsychological functioning would be greatly improved.

On reexamination, the patient, despite his protestations of improved functioning, performed equally poorly on every neuropsychological measure from tests of most subtle and sensitive attention and memory mechanisms to measures of background skill and abilities such as intelligence and academic competence. These findings were now even more incongruent and out of proportion to his reported injury and current reported circumstance. Because of the suspicious nature of his results, or at least because of the entire absence of any explanation that was scientifically acceptable, the patient was given a blood test to determine his antidepressant drug level. It was determined that the patient, despite repeated complaints regarding appropriate side effects, had no identifiable level of medication in his system whatever.

The results of the neuropsychological examinations and their lack of correlation with minor head injury along with the negative medicine screen were reported to his attorney when it was learned, rather late in the game, that indeed a legal matter was in process. Unlike most circumstances involving a minor head injury, however, in this case the patient was not suing for damages secondary to real or imagined injuries. Rather, in this case, the patient was being sued. The suit had nothing to do with the head injury, however. Indeed, the patient was being sued for embezzlement, and in the process of a more thorough investigation, it turned out that the head injury and claimed disability served two purposes. The first purpose was to allow the patient to draw on an extravagant and recently acquired disability policy that provided him with a significant income. The second purpose was to provide evidence of mitigating circumstances with regard to his responsibility for actions that took place after the head injury occurred.

When the attorney found out that the patient was not neuropsychologically impaired in a fashion consistent with minor head injury and that he was not medically or psychiatrically impaired in a fashion consistent with depressive illness, the patient was confronted with a choice. The choice was to drop the claim for head injury and depression as mitigating circumstances and as a claim for disability payments or to enter the hospital with pharmacological intervention being carefully monitored. The patient, realizing that actually taking the prescribed dosage of medication without an underlying depression would lead to a very impaired condition that would be obvious to everyone, and very different from that which he had claimed he had experienced following his pretended utilization of the antidepression medication, then capitulated and no further claims based on injury or injury-related difficulties were entered.

This case documents the value not only of good information-gathering with regard to ancillary services (e.g., medical, legal), but also the value of the posttesting interview as a qualitative and clinically honed data-gathering instrument available to bring together all sources of information in the most focused and efficient fashion. As the examination is largely technical in nature and as the background information is, in fact, gathered in a fashion that tends to summarize material already available, it is these parts of the overall evaluation process that should be done in the broadest and most thorough fashion, and it is the interview that should be accomplished in the most specific, clinically relevant, and informed manner, utilizing all available information to bring to final conclusion the results of all aspects of the neuropsychological consultation.

It is always appropriate, but certainly not always necessary, to obtain information from significant others. Significant others may not be readily available, and the patient may choose not to have significant others participate in the examination. It is often the case that information from significant others would not provide sufficient additional information to warrant the extra time and expense required on either person's part. Many neurological disorders are well documented. The referral information or the patient's report or both can be sufficient for all necessary considerations. The neuropsychologist's judgment represents the major factor in determining what areas of information will be gathered as well as the order in which and the sources from which that information will be obtained.

THE TIMING AND PURPOSE OF INTERVIEWING AND OBSERVATION

The claim is often made, but fortunately not frequently carried out, that one of the purposes of the initial interview is to determine the nature of the problem that the patient is manifesting so that tests can be selected that specifically fit those deficits. If this process were indeed carried out, it would represent a relatively serious mistake and an initial error that would likely fatally flaw the neuropsychological examination from then on. This rationale for how to proceed is flawed in several ways. The first flaw is found in the suggestion that one can, through interview, correctly identify the nature of a patient's problem with sufficient clarity that psychological testing can in fact be specifically directed to all relevant aspects of the patient's functioning. While specific issues such as dysphasia or paralysis or severe memory difficulties or generalized dementia can certainly be identified, these deficits are often not the reason that a neuropsychologist is consulted. If a patient has obvious deficits, it may not be necessary for the neuropsychologist to provide additional information. If it is, it still may be the case that the patient has other deficits not so obvious or masked by these more obvious impairments. In like fashion, it may well be the case that the patient's deficits are very subtle, not known even to the patient for a variety of reasons and poorly appreciated by significant others. In many instances, in fact, patients are unaware of their own deficits, specifically deny their deficits, or fail to appreciate that the deficits they have are present because their life activities do not call on functioning in those areas.

Therefore, unless the examiner feels that his or her interview is equivalent to a comprehensive neuropsychological examination, the likelihood of missing these areas of potential interest and therefore not examining for them is very high. That is one reason that almost all neuropsychologists, whatever their claimed theoretical affiliation, utilize some standard procedures to provide a reasonably comprehensive coverage of known and agreed-on areas of neuropsychological functioning as well as, of course, tailoring their examination in the appropriate fashion to deal with issues that are of critical importance while not unduly wasting the patient's time chasing irrelevancies.

A second flaw in the rationale for highly selective test administration following interview is the assumption that it is areas of deficit alone that are to be pursued. It is very interesting and important to know where the patient has deficiencies and what these deficiencies are. The neuropsychologist must measure them sufficiently well to appreciate their impact on day-to-day functioning. Such an assessment cannot be made, however, without an understanding of those areas in which the patient functions in an intact fashion. This intact functioning provides a very important contrast against which the impaired performance can be judged. It also provides very important information with regard to how the patient may be compensating or areas in which the patient may be able to function even in the presence of those deficits. It also provides an aspect of information about the patient's capability to participate in various rehabilitational activities, educational procedures, and vocational pursuits. A strictly "deficit-search" approach espoused by some extreme advocates of individual test tailoring would be counterproductive because such a search would do nothing more than document the very reason for the referral: Something is wrong with the patient. The lack of comprehensiveness as well as the lack of evenhandedness in this approach would leave the neuropsychologist, and the patient and referring source, roughly where they were before the referral was made.

In like fashion, one who mindlessly sticks to the same group of tests independent of the patient's characteristics would be performing equally unacceptably in neuropsychological terms. An elderly patient would not receive a children's battery. A person who is severely demented would not have the same tests as one who is being evaluated for very subtle impairments. Someone who is quadriplegic would not benefit from attempts to go through a rather extensive motor and sensory examination, and a patient with various sensory difficulties such as vision and hearing would need to have the examination tailored, as would a patient who is functionally illiterate. It also is the case that certain conditions such as traumatic brain injury, brain tumors, strokes, and degenerative disease have been studied rather thoroughly. Many aspects of these conditions are well understood with regard to their most usual and most expected types of neurocognitive impairments. For that reason, patients with these presenting historical conditions can be given an examination that relies on the best scientific information available in attempting to appreciate the nature of the patient's relative strengths and weaknesses, particularly as these strengths and weaknesses may have been contributed to specifically by that condition. Even here, however, the examination must be sufficiently general and respectful of the neurological generalities of all brain disorders so as to provide information as to whether or not other conditions may be significantly affecting the results for better or for worse. Such conditions as malingering, symptom exaggeration, emotional disturbance, other neurological disorders, and lifelong handicaps and impairments must be taken into account. Issues of proportionality of disorder to dysfunction can be assessed only through an examination that provides opportunity for unexpected as well as expected outcomes.

In neuropsychology, as in other areas, the interview is more than simply a conversation. It also is an opportunity for behavioral observation. The behavioral observation as well as the conversation need not be limited to the interaction between the doctor and patient, but may involve significant others as well. While the involvement of others may be much more important in some areas and less important or not necessary at all in others, information should be obtained with an eye toward the patient's actual past, current, and future situation, and this situation may differ considerably depending on the patient's age and neuropsychological as well as psychosituational circumstance. As an example, a child obviously has rather different needs for a caretaker than does an elderly adult who is beginning to show the initial signs of senility. Also, the environment is prepared differentially to provide those sorts of caretaking duties, and the patient's own ability to accept being cared for may differ importantly in those situations.

Likewise, a person with very good motor skills and independence behaviors who has sustained significant loss in higher mental functions will require and accept caretaking activities differently from one who has sustained devastating damage to the motor system but whose higher mental processes are entirely intact. To an even more subtle degree, someone who has sustained serious injuries to the brain resulting in significant impairments to problem-solving, learning, memory, and attentional processes is very different from one whose brain damage has produced what is frequently referred to as a frontal lobe deficit in which memory and past store of information may be quite intact and yet the capacity to utilize this ability to any productive end may be severely damaged.

Someone whose actual cognitive and motor systems are reasonably intact but whose emotional disruption secondary to organic damage is severe represents yet another kind of caretaking challenge. The nature of the challenge must be seen to interact with the patient's age and stage of physical, mental, and social independence now and at the time of the injury. For example, the patient may have been quite normally dependent prior to an accident that occurred in early childhood. Now that the patient is nearing his or her 25th birthday, the level of acceptability of this dependence and the capacity of the environment to provide dependent care may have changed considerably. Therefore, what may have been the questions of anxious parents about a 6-year-old with regard to distant, future concerns are now the concerns of more elderly parents who recognize the permanence as well as the immediacy of their child's problem and their own increasingly limited capacity to substantially improve their child's ability to live independently. Now that neurological stability (lack of likelihood of significant additional recovery) has been repeatedly documented, long-term care of an appropriate practical and affordable nature must be sought. Issues of vocational options and concerns about long-term financial issues must be tended to, and in such circumstances, as in situations in which a patient is seriously mentally ill, the interviewer may in fact spend more time with caregivers, both professional and family, than with the patient himself or herself in what could be formally described as an interview situation. Even relatively brief interviewing and behavioral observation in such circumstances may be entirely sufficient, along with an adequate neuropsychological examination, to document the nature of the patient's condition, and the questions that need to be addressed must be handled in the context of significant others.

Yet another difference between the traditional mental health and the neuropsychological interview situation is the objectively verifiable nature of the patient's disorder. The mental health arena often deals with hypothetical constructs and agreed-on diagnostic criteria for events for which no criteria of a biological nature can be obtained. In neuropsychology, things are often substantially different. If a patient has a brain tumor or has had a stroke or a significant traumatic brain injury, these conditions are quite readily identifiable. One can obtain information with regard to a variety of the aspects of these conditions, such as size, location, time of onset, and past, current, and future medical course. Other conditions, such as multiple sclerosis, degenerative diseases, and infections, to name a few, can also be documented as to their presence and neurological extent. Therefore, issues of proportionality play a significant role in the neuropsychological interview. It is possible to determine whether the patient demonstrates neuropsychological deficits in performing various tasks. It is also possible to determine whether these performances as measured objectively fit the patient's subjective complaints.

Furthermore, and perhaps more important, it is possible to determine whether the patient's subjective complaints and neuropsychological results actually fit the biological entity about which the patient is complaining. For example, if a patient has been found to have a meningioma overlying the convexity in the orbital frontal area, but not only complains of severe memory deficits but also points out that these memory deficits include a total inability to recall his or her past life, the likelihood that this complaint relates to the meningioma must be seen as exceedingly small. In like fashion, if the patient had sustained a very mild head injury with less than 20–30 minutes of unconsciousness with a Glasgow Coma Scale of 15 in the emergency room and essentially normal radiological findings, the presence of total incapacity to find one's way in life, which is actually worsening as time goes on, would be entirely nonproportional. It may well be that the patient is experiencing a secondary emotional reaction or is engaging in an active process of symptom enhancement. On the other hand, if a patient has sustained multiple cerebral contusions and has been unconscious for several weeks and has had significant motor and sensory deficits as well as marked neurological confusion that has resolved in a predictable fashion over a period of many months, the presence of substantial neurocognitive deficits would be entirely expected and likely to be directly connected to that injury.

The proportionality issue in the neuropsychological situation is thus quite different from that in the mental health situation, in which a specific trauma, be it developmental or represented in a one-time event, cannot, with the same degree of precision, be predicted to produce relatively similar outcome across patients. Therefore, the role of objective neuropsychological tests in validating the information from interview rather than simply supplementing it is quite specific to the neuropsychological enterprise. The role of medical historical information in validating as well as supplementing the neuropsychological information obtained from testing and interviewing is also a part of the overall evaluative activity. If any of these sources differ significantly from the others, explanations must be obtained. Issues such as emotional disruption or intentional production of symptoms will have to be considered and thus represent yet another area for the neuropsychological interview and general evaluation process to pursue.

Qualitative and quantitative aspects of the actual examination are not mutually exclusive. The patient may provide quantitative data on an objective personality examination of psychological distress and depression. These conditions may be noted qualitatively in behaviors observed throughout the examination. During the interview, affect and mood may be noted to be areas of difficulty. The interview may reveal a variety of reports by significant others consistent with these observations. The referral may indicate poor occupational performance in motor-based tasks. The patient may demonstrate impairment when asked to perform such tasks. This finding, in conjunction with description by family members of the patient's inability to perform certain simple tasks, may lead to a diagnosis of apraxia, which could, in the hands of a less skillful clinician, be misidentified as clumsiness secondary to arthritis or even another neurologically based motor difficulty that would suggest a different disorder altogether. Qualitative evaluation of neuropsychological data and qualitative appreciation of the nuances of patient complaints and historical information are every bit as important as signs and cues obtained from direct, one-to-one observation.

Just as one must not be slavishly adherent to the use of a particular set of tests, one must not be slavishly adherent to the use of one particular point in time during which observations and information can be obtained. Rather, the entire context of the neuropsychological evaluation is grist for the neuropsychologist's interpretive mill. Only the neuropsychologist can determine whether more or less information in any one of those areas is required in order to make a confident diagnosis, useful description, and appropriate recommendations to meet the patient's clinical need. To say that more information could always be obtained is to state a trivial truth. The question is not whether or not more information could be obtained but whether or not more information is needed to provide the patient a competent evaluation and clinically useful service.

Obtaining all possible information simply because one can is just as professionally indefensible as not obtaining information that has specific clinical relevance. Knowing what information to seek is part of the neuropsychologist's task, as is knowing when that task has been completed. There may still be issues in the patient's life to be resolved. Such issues, however, may be better resolved by other professionals such as attorneys, vocational rehabilitation specialists, radiologists, orthopedists, or specialists in other disciplines. So, too, the specifics of an educational curriculum may be better laid out by a trained educator than by a pediatric neuropsychologist, even though the neuropsychologist may be able to describe, in helpful and critical terms, the parameters of the child's neurocognitive operations as these will interact with any formal didactic enterprise. The same holds true in the vocational area. While the specifics of one job vs. another may not be the neuropsychologist's purview, the patient's general capacities to manage a variety of cognitive, motor, sensory, and affective challenges may provide critical guides for the vocational expert in determining which set of jobs to choose.

This information should serve as a lead into the interview process in neuropsychology. However, it must be recognized that the overall evaluative context is largely indivisible with regard to final conclusions, and that parts of the interview and behavioral observation may occur at various times—before, during, or after the formal examination itself. Finally, the interview may be conducted at least in part by people other than the interpreting neuropsychologist. With this in mind, the following outline for neuropsychological interview and behavioral observation is offered.

One mechanism for structuring an interview is a formal questionnaire format or rating scale, such as that proposed by Levin et al. (1987). The neurobehavioral rating scale proposed by Levin and associates provides information in 27 areas, including attention, somatic concern, anxiety, emotional withdrawal, guilt feelings, memory problems, decrease in motivation, suspiciousness, fatigue, motor retardation, hallucinatory activity, planning, and mood, as well as comprehension and speech deficits. This rating procedure casts patients on a 7-point rating scale and is typically filled out by an interviewer either in direct contact with the patient or with information provided by significant others where appropriate. Another semistructured interview developed in the Neuropsychology Laboratory at the University of Alabama at Birmingham is designed to aid the clinician in systematically covering areas of potential relevance to the patient's functioning.

Patients referred to a neuropsychologist are at least suspected of having a neurological disorder. This, of course, is not the case for patients in general clinical psychology, the majority of whom do not have and have never been suspected of having a neurological disorder. While all clinicians must be sensitive to the manifestation of physical conditions including pharmacological side effects, the issue is particularly relevant at all times in neuropsychology because of the very nature of the enterprise. For this reason, the diagnostic interview should include systematic questioning in a number of neurological areas as well as systematic questioning of areas that are not particularly associated with neurology but that will provide information about other aspects of medical functioning that may produce symptoms similar to those that result from various sorts of neurological insult and injury (see the Appendix for this interview format).

Initial aspects of the clinical neuropsychological interview involve nothing more or less than meeting the patient, observing his or her physical and social demeanor as introductions are made, and observing the context in which he or she presents (e.g., hospital or outpatient waiting room, well or shabbily dressed, clean or unkempt, with or without significant others, able to move in an appropriate fashion) and appearance of good or poor health in general terms or specific characteristics such as paralysis, obesity, blindness, language, or coordination impairments, as well as psychological problems such as anxiety, depression, confusion, or disorientation that may or may not result from purely neurological disorders.

After initial observations have been made and the patient has been escorted to and comfortably seated in the office or examining room, questions about the patient's perceived reason for neuropsychological referral are addressed. Most commonly, it is my practice to ask patients why they have been referred before I tell them. This gives me a sense of their own comprehension of the circumstances, the level of curiosity they are able to manifest, and the level of initial comfort with the environment, as well as, in many instances, the adequacy with which the referral has been handled by the referring parties. Patients may need reassurance at least as much as they need additional information. Information concerning congruity between the patient's perceptions and those of significant others, if it is available, many also be a help in understanding whether or not the patient has been given information and whether it has been either understood, ignored, forgotten, or never adequately comprehended. Following this discussion, an explanation of the rationale of the referral source, to the extent that it adds to or deviates from the patient's understanding, is provided.

Additionally, explanation of the nature of the examination is given so that the patient will have an opportunity to relax and recognize that no painful or invasive procedures are to be part of this examination and to allow the patient to make arrangements, if they have not already been made, for the duration of the examination, be it one hour or several hours, with regard to such issues as transportation, lunch, and arrangements for getting off work or out of school. Having this conversation in the presence of significant others often relieves the patient, who then understands that this is indeed what has been agreed on. If the patient is unaccompanied or for other reasons significant others are not available, the patient is still provided ample opportunity to ask questions and to have uncertainties addressed prior to engaging in a set of procedures that are not, in any way, routine or familiar with regard to the patient's past experience in most instances.

The interview also provides an opportunity to observe any impediments to the examination. Patients with visual difficulties may not have brought corrective devices, and this lack may in itself require rescheduling or calling the patient's room and having glasses brought over. Difficulty with hearing may alter the presentation of tape-recorded tests. Specific motor impairments may limit the nature of the examination in those areas. Likewise, significant emotional disruption may suggest a higher level of reassurance and encouragement for this patient than would be required for another patient who seems more comfortable with the overall examination procedures.

It is important to obtain the greatest possible level of cooperation from the patient, and doing so often entails increasing the patient's comfort level so that anxiety, distress, and hesitance do not unusually interfere with the ability to take the test. If it is perceived that sources of interference do exist, this interference must be taken into account with regard to any interpretive comments that are made. Obviously, there are many reasons for poor performance on neuropsychological tests besides neurological damage. It is important that the neuropsychologist recognize this possibility and make every effort to remove extraneous causes of poor performance and to understand the nature of those nonneurological causes that cannot be removed so that appropriate interpretations can be made.

Perhaps this is an appropriate time to caution against the "see-a-score-cite-a-lesion" school of neuropsychology that seems to believe that all bad performances on neuropsychological tests are due to neurological causes. Obviously, one of the major purposes for the posttest interview, behavioral observation, history-taking, and symptom-evaluation portion of the neuropsychological evaluation is, as mentioned earlier in this chapter, to determine the proportionality between the patient's alleged neurologically based symptoms and any documented neurological disease or disorder. It is the case that very mild and radiologically invisible neurological changes can produce subtle neurocognitive deficits, particularly on a temporary and resolving basis. These deficits may not be at all apparent in the interview portion of the evaluation due to their subtle nature and their interference with areas not easily assessed outside formal measurement. It is not true, however, that entirely invisible changes in brain function can produce severe neuropsychological impairment without any corroborative information whatsoever with regard to the patient's medical and neurological condition. Patients who have severe neuropsychological deficits are most likely to have recognizable neuropathological correlates, while patients with mild and transient neuropsychological deficits may have neuropathological difficulties that are not readily available to external identification and therefore clinical correlation.

Deviations from this rule of proportionality must be made with the greatest caution and only in the context of available scientific information. In the presence of deviations from proportionality, all efforts must be made to determine other possible causes of neuropsychological deficits such as emotional dysfunction, general premorbid adjustment, secondary gain, symptom enhancement, premorbid nonneurological–medical difficulties, and other coexisting conditions that affect the patient's performance on a nonneurological basis. Failure to take these factors into account is likely to leave the impression that all patients who do poorly on neuropsychological tests have some form of neurological disorder, even in the absence of adequate and independent criterion information. It may, in fact, foster an impression that in some instances such criterion information is not necessary. Nothing could be further from the truth. Criterion information is always necessary, and where it is lacking, neuropsychology is placed at a disadvantage. That neuropsychology may represent the frontier and become the criteria in newly discovered disorders of relatively mild neuropsychological and neurological significance is part of our scientific heritage. It is the case, however, that this process occurs in instances of mild or transient disorders, on one hand, or disorders that are discovered in their very earliest phases that do go on to subsequent neuropathological recognition, on the other. Failing one of these possibilities, the greatest likelihood is that problems other than neurological problems are responsible for the patient's difficulties both subjectively and on objective neuropsychological examination.

The interview is particularly useful in sorting out this type of diagnostic dilemma. For this reason, once again, the value of the posttesting interview is demonstrated. Once information from history, observations, and formal examination is available, the examiner's ability to focus questioning in areas of perceived uncertainty is enhanced greatly. Prior to the formal examination and evaluation of a variety of other materials, the field of inquiry is relatively wide open with respect to possibilities for difficulties and proposed solutions. Once substantial data have been gathered, the number of alternatives has, in most instances, been significantly limited, and the examiner's ability to focus the interview on issues of remaining uncertainty has been greatly improved.

AREAS OF MORE FOCUSED INVESTIGATION THROUGH INTERVIEW AND TESTING

Memory

Memory functioning seems to be the core of concern for many patients referred for neuropsychological evaluation. The reason is in part that memory is a word much more commonly used than intelligence when one thinks of mental failings and difficulties. It is very uncommon for a patient to complain of changes in intelligence or intellectual functioning or cognition. It is common for people, patient and family, to complain of memory difficulties. These difficulties may be associated with age, illness, injury, or physical or mental stress, as well as the exigencies of day-to-day activity. The appearance of memory difficulty may not signal the presence of a neurological etiology, or a treatable neurological disorder or neuropsychological disability.

Memory and learning affect day-to-day performance ability. Complex memory functions can be subdivided usefully and easily assessed and can be discussed without undue technical complexity. Memory can be divided along a timeline beginning with immediate memory, such as is often seen in tests such as Digit Span and in daily life is frequently referred to as "phone number memory." At the other end of the spectrum is distant or historical or personal memory. This later memory involves the content of knowledge that we have accumulated over the years and is least likely to be disrupted by mild or generalized neurological disorders. Memory of accomplishments of an educational and occupational nature, as well as information about personal life, including children, family, marriages and divorces, residences, and other such data, is quite resilient to other than severe neurological disruptions.

The intermediate forms of memory are those wherein most difficulties lie with regard to day-to-day complaints. These memories are also most likely to be disrupted by mild as well as severe neurological insult and illness. Short-term memory refers to a time span ranging from several minutes to several hours. Long-term covers a time span from an hour to several days. Short-term and long-term memory serve as the core of daily or functional memory around which our acquisition of knowledge, maintenance of trains of thought, and ability to sustain ongoing pursuit of various occupational and academic activities occurs. Patients with these kinds of difficulties very commonly complain of being disrupted in the middle of activities, losing track of what it is they are doing, becoming lost, forgetting directions, instructions, and occurrences, and having to be constantly reminded by notes and other mnemonic devices in order to be able to manage even relatively simple and routine activities.

Patients with such deficits are most commonly at a severe disadvantage in any sort of educational situation. In occupational circumstances, their disadvantage is going to vary significantly depending on the intellectual nature of their work as well as their familiarity with it. Patients who perform relatively routine and nonintellectual work may be able, even with a relatively notable memory problem and especially under appropriately supported circumstances, to manage at least reasonably adequately. On the other hand, patients who have jobs with highly intellectual demands or who are in positions in which new learning is required are at maximum disadvantage. Unfortunately, it is also the case that memory is rarely damaged in total isolation, and therefore other aspects of cognitive processing, important for performance of academic and occupational tasks, are not available in fullest extent to support the patient's requirements to manage day-to-day activities. Therefore, what may be presented as simple memory problems may turn out to be deficits in a number of areas, not the least of which are attention and concentration as well as other aspects of problem-solving and mental speed. For this reason, the latter areas must also be inquired about as well as directly examined.

With regard to the modalities and material of memory, it is possible to assess memory using tactile, auditory, and visual materials. The modalities of memory, including language and spatial functions, can be assessed as well, and the interaction of these materials and modalities with various temporal distances of memory can give a reasonably complete picture of those aspects of mnemonic functioning that are likely to create problems in a patient's day-to-day activities. The data from such an examination can then serve as a guide to those areas of day-to-day activity to be discussed in the interview tailored to the patient's individual circumstance.

While there is no specific trick to *interviewing about memory*, or about anything else for that matter, there are specific aspects of memory dysfunction relatable to the commonly occurring mild brain injury that can be very helpful in determining whether or not there is any likelihood at all that brain injury has occurred. It can also be helpful in determining proportionality that can be utilized in assessing the nature of the patient's claimed difficulties and his or her performance on formal examination procedures. Three aspects of amnesic difficulties are commonly associated with mild and, of course, more severe brain injury. The first is amnesia for the *event*. Patients who remember their accidents in detail have not had a traumatic brain injury, with the following exception: Patients can sustain focal, penetrating brain lesions without loss of consciousness or amnesia. These lesions, however, are never lacking for documentation.

The second type of amnesia is *retrograde*, which refers to that point of time prior to the accident that is forgotten. When interviewing a patient 1 month after a severe head injury, days of lost time may be part of the patient's recital of difficulties. The patient may not remember the party or getting ready for the party or the day of the party or even going to work the day before the party. On being interviewed 3 or 4 months later, however, the patient may well remember the day before the party, getting ready for the party, and even driving to the party, but still have no memory of the party itself, much less of driving away and being involved in an accident 5 miles away. The patient may recover additional memories that involve activities much closer to the accident. Many patients will attempt to stimulate their memory by actively thinking about it or engaging others in conversation. Others think that various sorts of medication or even hypnosis might be helpful in causing them to recover their lost memory. This likely will not be the case. Other patients are concerned that they will remember the accident and that the memory will be very traumatic, and they begin to worry about being saddled with the memory of a frightening set of experiences with which they may not be able to cope. This, too, does not occur, and patients can be reassured that the amnesic period may continue to shrink toward the accident, but memory of the accident itself will never return.

The third area of amnesia is that period of time following the accident for which the patient has no memory. This is referred to as *posttraumatic* amnesia. Posttraumatic amnesia, unlike retrograde amnesia, is fixed, and the patient will therefore be able to give a relatively consistent account at 1 month, 3 months, and even 3 years of that first set of memories after which memory was reasonably consistently present and before which the patient has no recollection. Some early, postaccident, event such as an ambulance ride or painful emergency medical procedure may be followed by an additional period of amnesia for events in the hospital. These early memories are called *islands* and typically occur in the first third of the overall posttraumatic amnesic period. Whatever the length of the posttraumatic amnesic period, the patient can be reassured that this period is stable and that nothing can be or need be done to reestablish memory of lost events. The presence of a permanent posttraumatic amnesic period does not in any way imply that the patient has a continuing significant memory problem or memory disorder. Rather, it implies that the patient has lost a period of time in his or her life, but this is not necessarily incompatible with normal current functioning of the overall memory mechanism. Nevertheless, there is a reasonable correlation between length of posttraumatic amnesia on one hand and severity of residual sequelae on the other.

Many patients feel that the accident itself has been productive of significant emotional pathology. There are many ways in which patients can gain this impression, and interviewing is an ideal format to determine the patient's sense of emotional distress as it is associated with various aspects of their injury or illness. If a patient is amnesic for the event and a period of time surrounding the event, the likelihood that the event will be psychologically traumatic approaches zero. One can hardly be traumatized by something about which one has no recollection. On the other hand, if one can recount in graphic detail the fear, the pain and surrounding noise and commotion of an injury, this memory may be a source of significant posttraumatic disruption even though it may be the case that no neurological injury has occurred. This differential is best handled in the interview format. There are no psychometric tests for these types of amnesias, and tests of emotional dysfunction can produce results suggesting significant psychological distress without in any way revealing the cause for that distress.

Personality

With regard to personality changes, the most common complaint and description of a patient by significant others is that the patient has a totally different personality. Personality, when described by significant others, often refers to a combination of psychological features that involve intellect and capacity to function, rather than those things that psychologists perceive as the formal aspects of personality structure. Nevertheless, various aspects of personality, such as aggressiveness, empathy, industriousness, stability, and interpersonal warmth and sensitivity, may have changed significantly. In like fashion, other difficulties such as anxiety and depression as well as lethargy and disinhibition are reported. Many patients who perceive themselves as having lost capacity are depressed, and this depression may actually outlast the neurological consequences of the injury or illness. Many patients who attempt to return to full functioning too rapidly, while they are still experiencing various cognitive disruptions, find that their return to work or school is very unsuccessful. An unsuccessful return to work or school can result in a very frightening failure, loss of a job, or damaged school record and may result in a career change or an alteration in future academic plans that could have been avoided if the patient had simply returned to work or school at a later time or in a more gradual and supported fashion. Fear, anxiety, and depression resulting from these very negative experiences following illness can become the major source of difficulty and even disability and may be the major issue that requires treatment following neurological disorder.

Patients with neurological impairment are often easily upset and irritable and able to tolerate only a much reduced level of social and environmental stimuli.

Patients may become confused, disrupted, disorganized, and uncomfortable even in familiar surroundings such as church and shopping malls because of the degree of commotion. In like fashion, because of this tendency to be easily disrupted by children running around the house or commotion at the dinner table, patients with a neurological disorder may spend more time alone and in secluded environments. This retreat may be perceived as depression, when in fact it is a very appropriate self-protective mechanism to dampen and control the amount of stimuli that the patient perceives as highly irritating. It is far better to have a patient in a protected environment than to expose him or her to overstimulation that results in irritable and aggressive outbursts that can be perceived as far more unacceptable by significant others. More important, however, it is critical that significant others understand the nature of these personality changes. It is only through adequate interviewing of the patient and significant others that information about these changes can be communicated.

Because the validity of personality tests as these tests relate to the specific neurological correlates of personality functioning is poorly understood, the utilization of formal personality-testing devices should be seen as ancillary. There is no evidence that any personality profile or code type on any of the popular personality measures is specific to neurological pathology. That is not to say that changes in personality style and the presence of personality dysfunction itself are not validly represented, but rather that the relationship between that personality style and specific brain disorder has not been sufficiently established. Therefore, many patients with neurological disorder may well express substantial distress on a variety of personality measures that may reflect either the direct consequences of the disorder, preexisting difficulties that may or may not have been exacerbated, or the secondary consequences of the neurological disorder as it has had a negative impact on the patient's life. For these reasons, it is imperative that interview information accompany psychometric measures of personality evaluation. Personality change may be primarily irritability and lethargy following initial neurological insult, or anxiety and depression secondary to loss, or a more permanent organic personality disorder directly relatable to neurological disease. The personality change may relate to a reaction to other medical conditions and to dysfunction secondary to nonneurological injuries or deficits, e.g., pain, not related to central nervous system damage.

Another category of personality change is that falling under the general term of *frontal lobe syndrome*. Patients with frontal lobe disorder very frequently experience two types of difficulties. The first type is with initiation and suppression. Patients frequently fail to appropriately initiate actions in a variety of areas, thereby appearing lazy, disinterested, unmotivated, and disorganized, and may, because of this failure, experience difficulties in performing job-, school-, and home-related duties. Patients may also have a difficult time suppressing behaviors once they have been initiated. A second type of difficulty may leave patients unresponsive to subtle and even obvious cues suggesting needed behavioral modifications. Interpersonal style may be described as clumsy, boring, aggressive, insensitive, or immature. Such behavior requires considerable understanding and structure for the patient to cope with social expectations and achieve appropriate levels of occupational productivity.

Such a disorder, while on occasion temporary, is not infrequently permanent and requires a significant, long-term, alteration, not only in the patients' work- or school-related environment but also in family relationships. Increasing degrees of responsibility for various aspects of the patient's social and occupational activities may fall to significant others. This shifting of responsibility may substantially alter the personal relationship that existed prior to the neurological event. Issues of whether or not the patient can take adequate responsibility for financial activities, child-rearing, and other adult behaviors must be decided for the patient. Significant others may find this situation unacceptable in their lives and be forced, in their own mind, to terminate their relationship with the patient. This rupture, obviously and in turn, produces its own difficulties. Whereas a patient might be reasonably productive under a highly structured, supportive, and encouraging environment, this same patient may become thoroughly disorganized and dysfunctional in a situation without such structure and support.

With regard to the role of the clinical interview, it is frequently these patients who are the least aware of or least able to describe adequately the nature of the difficulties they are experiencing. In fact, such patients often grossly overvalue their own participation in a wide variety of activities and underestimate the nature of the difficulties they are experiencing. They may set goals that greatly exceed their capacity. In these circumstances, an overall understanding of the patient may not be adequately achieved through direct contact. While it may not be necessary to interview a significant other to determine that the patient has a severe frontal lobe deficit, it may be critical to discuss this situation with the family in order to determine how much help, if any, can be obtained and what the limits of these helping circumstances are.

Executive Functions

Neuropsychological tasks associated with damage to the frontal lobe and associated structures often are conceptualized under the rubric of *executive functions*. These functions include not only the aforementioned personality-related features of an individual's neuropsychological style but also some more cognitive features. Such features as the capacity to plan, to organize, to anticipate future consequences, to focus and sustain attention, to be vigilant even under disruptive circumstances, and to change set and maintain sufficient cognitive flexibility, or alternate between two thoughts that are going on simultaneously, often are associated with anterior brain impairment. Once again, as with personality functioning, a number of formal examination procedures have been developed that claim to measure frontal lobe deficits. While they seem, at least on face-valid grounds, to measure the functions mentioned above, there has yet to be an adequate demonstration that any specific test or set of tests is indeed sensitive to damage to the frontal lobe in any exclusive or specific way. Because no specific test battery or individual test has been found to be particularly sensitive to this area of the brain, the interview plays an important role in assessing the validity of the complaints, the nature of the complaints, and the patient's abilities to describe and even manifest these complaints in a fashion consistent with the historical, medical, and psychometric data that are being simultaneously accumulated.

SUMMARY

The interview is in fact the beginning of treatment as well as part of the evaluation. Information can be provided to help the family and the patient understand that the patient's behavior is an expected and, in many instances, temporary part of his or her overall condition. During the interview, with the benefit of medical and neuropsychological examination data, it is appropriate and helpful to begin the process of modifying the environment and initiating the remedial coping strategies. This process provides immediate relief and can also aid in the evaluation of the patient's and family's ability to comprehend and comply with treatment efforts.

The interview in neuropsychology, while different in many respects, plays an important role in many evaluations. It also plays a role in the initiation of treatment whether or not this is done by the neuropsychologist or by a colleague in a related field or specialty. The uniqueness of the postexamination interview technique in neuropsychological practice has been discussed by others (e.g., Swiercinsky, 1989) and is recommended as a useful way to maximize efficiency, specificity, and completeness of the patient's evaluative service.

APPENDIX: STRUCTURED CLINICAL INTERVIEW FORMAT

The clinical interview is a fundamental instrument for gathering information. In addition, it serves the function of facilitating rapport and building trust between the interviewer and the patient/family. Conducting an interview is a dynamic process requiring professional judgment and skill.

A clinical interview is *not* a checklist; it is *not* another form to fill out, file, and forget. For this reason, many of the questions intentionally are left as open-ended inquiries. Some areas of exploration have been listed as topics, with the expectation that the interviewer will supply the actual question most appropriate for that client. For example, "coping style" can be investigated by the question, "How do you typically handle stress?" A more concrete client may need examples from his own history, e.g., "How do you feel and what do you do when you . . . ?" The interviewer understands the essential concerns and considerations for the particular client and is therefore able to shape questions and probe appropriately during the interview. The terminology is amended according to the comprehension and comfort level of the individual client and the family.

This approach is intended to afford the interviewer a great deal of flexibility in conducting the session. In the experience of the interviewer, a particular type of injury, psychosocial background, premorbid personality, or regional characteristic might require a variety of individualized adjustments. Questions regarding sensitive topics such as finances, religion, and sexual behavior may need modification. Each professional will employ his or her own unique style of interaction, suitable to the client/family and to the interviewer's own personality.

The same structured format assures standardization of coverage and therefore allows use in research undertakings while maintaining sufficient flexibility for clinical application.

CLINICAL INTERVIEW

Name _____   Medical Record # _____

Address _____   SSN _____

_____   Date of birth ___ Age ___ Sex ___

Home phone _____   Height ____ Weight ____ Race ____

Work phone _____   Insurance company _____

Date _____ Interviewer _____   Insurance policy # _____

In an emergency, contact (name) _____ at (phone) _____

Persons present during interview: _____

Are you currently: single married separated divorced widowed? (circle one)
   For how many years? _____

Have you been previously married? If yes, list previous spouses, number of
years married to each spouse, and children resulting from each marriage.

_____

Who lives with you in your home? _____

_____

FAMILY (names, ages, residence, health, education, occupation)

Spouse: _____

Children: _____

_____

_____

Father: _____

Mother: _____

Brothers: _____

Sisters: _____

FAMILY RELATIONSHIPS (Describe how you get along) _____

_____

Where were you born and raised? _____

_____

EDUCATION

How far did you get in school? (highest grade completed) _____

What kind of student were you? (usual grade in school) _____

Were you ever held back or required to repeat a grade? If so, state which grades and explain the circumstances. _____

Have you ever had homebound instruction or tutoring? If so, state the subject matter and explain the circumstances. _____

Have you ever been placed in any special education class? If so, describe.

_____

Advanced training or higher education? (Specify school, major, etc.) _____

MILITARY SERVICE

Highest rank attained: _____

Type of discharge: _____

OCCUPATIONAL HISTORY: Trace a consistent history from school to present; include the job title, type of work, years employed, reason for change:

Previous: _____

_____

_____

Present: _____

Particular problems in school/at work: _____

DISABILITY STATUS _____

To what extent do you consider yourself disabled? _____

PRESENT FINANCIAL SITUATION

How are you managing financially? (income, bills, savings) _____

_____

Do you have insurance? (medical, life) _____

Do you have a will? A living will? _____

To what extent do you feel that your personal affairs are in order? _____

_____

PRESENTING PROBLEM

Give a brief history of your condition. _____

_____

What brings you here today? (name of referral source; expectations)

_____

Do you notice anything that makes your condition better or worse?

_____

Have you ever had surgery associated with this condition? If so, specify procedures and dates. _____

Date of the accident or event that brings you here; please describe.

_____

Major complaint(s): _____

_____

What medications do you take? _____

_____

Describe how you manage your medication schedule. _____

_____

Have you experienced any medication side effects? (depression, sexual function) _____

_____

MEDICAL HISTORY

Primary physician: _____

Last medical examination: _____

Accidents; head injuries: _____

Serious illnesses; neurological disorders: _____

Surgeries; other medical procedures: _____

Other hospital admissions: _____

Other medical problems: _____

SYMPTOM CHECKLIST

Have you ever experienced any of the following symptoms? If yes, describe the symptom or illness, when it started, and how long it lasted.

Loss of consciousness	Yes	No	_____
Weight changes	Yes	No	_____
Pain (describe/area)	Yes	No	_____
Shakiness	Yes	No	_____

Muscle jerks or twitches	Yes	No	_____
Unusual odors or tastes	Yes	No	_____
Blurred or double vision	Yes	No	_____
Ringing in ears	Yes	No	_____
Bowel or bladder change	Yes	No	_____
Change in speech	Yes	No	_____
Change in sleep pattern	Yes	No	_____
Change in energy level	Yes	No	_____
Change in stamina	Yes	No	_____
Change in motivation	Yes	No	_____
Change in sexual interest	Yes	No	_____
Frequent headaches	Yes	No	_____
Dizziness	Yes	No	_____
Allergies	Yes	No	_____
Asthma	Yes	No	_____
Seizures	Yes	No	_____
Toxic exposure	Yes	No	_____
Meningitis or encephalitis	Yes	No	_____
Diabetes	Yes	No	_____
Rheumatic or scarlet fever	Yes	No	_____
Glasses/contacts	Yes	No	_____
Hearing aid	Yes	No	_____

Other physical problems: _____

_____

PHYSICAL

Do you notice, or do others tell you that they notice, changes in your physical appearance (including dress, grooming, gait, posture, mannerisms)? If so, please describe. _____

_____

What physical limitations, if any, have you noticed? _____

_____

Have you noticed any increased difficulty in performing your normal activities? If so, please describe. _____

In what specific ways do you anticipate that this experience may affect your life-style? _____

_____

Describe a typical day. Tell me what you do from the time you wake up in the morning until the time you fall asleep in bed at night. _____

_____

_____

_____

EMOTIONAL

Do you notice, or do others tell you that they notice, changes in mood, personality? _____

_____

Have you ever had psychological or neuropsychological testing? If yes, please describe areas of concern and assessment results. _____

_____

To what extent have you experienced emotional distress? Describe periods during which you have felt depressed or anxious. _____

_____

_____

Have you ever received psychological treatment (counseling) or psychiatric intervention (medication)? If yes, please describe the nature of the psychological problem. _____

_____

The treatment or intervention. _____

_____

Have you ever experienced hallucinations? If so, please describe the experience and the circumstances. _____

Have you ever (If yes, please explain):

considered suicide? _____

attempted suicide? _____

been abused, physically or sexually? _____

harmed yourself or anyone else? _____

Does anyone in your family have a history of psychiatric disturbance or trouble with their nerves? If yes, please describe. _____

HEALTH HABITS

Exercise habits: _____

Dietary habits: _____

Substances (specific information about age begun, amount, historial usage, current usage, or date discontinued):

tobacco: _____

alcohol: _____

drug history: _____

LEGAL

Are you currently involved in any type of legal proceedings? _____

Do you have a valid driver's license?	Yes	No
Have you ever been convicted of a DUI?	Yes	No
Have you ever been convicted of a crime?	Yes	No

If so, please explain. _____

COGNITIVE

Do you notice, or do others tell you that they notice, changes in thinking ability, memory? _____

Who runs the errands, pays the bills, and balances the checkbook? Could you perform these tasks? _____

_____

PSYCHOSOCIAL

Whom would you go to for advice or assistance? _____

_____

Describe your spiritual life. _____

_____

Describe your social support network and any group memberships. _____

_____

Describe your friendships and the quality of relationships. _____

_____

What do you do for fun? (hobbies, interests) _____

What community resources are available in your area? _____

How do you solve problems? (problem-solving, decision-making) _____

How do you handle stress? (coping strategies, defense mechanisms)

How would you describe yourself? _____

Is there anything not addressed in this interview you would like to add?

Interviewer's observations/comments: _____

CHART REVIEW

REFERENCES

Levin, H. S., High, W. M., Goetag, K. E., Sisson, R. A., Overall, J. E., Rhodes, H. M., Eisenberg, H. M., Kalisky, Z., & Gary, H. E. (1987). The Neurobehavioral Rating Scale: Assessment of the behavioral sequelae of head injury by a clinician. *Journal of Neurology, Neurosurgery and Psychiatry, 50,* 183–193.

Swiercinsky, D. (1989). *Manual for the adult neuropsychological examination.* Springfield, IL: Charles C. Thomas.

16

Older Adults

ROGER L. PATTERSON AND LARRY W. DUPREE

INTRODUCTION

Interviewing older adults is often associated with some type of assessment of the individuals or their situations or both. Frequently encountered objectives usually include the determination of one or more of the following: (1) cognitive functioning, (2) emotional status, (3) need for resources, and (4) ability to utilize objects, materials, and resources in order to function successfully in required activities of daily living (ADLs). This chapter will present a type of interview involving an assessment that both simplifies and improves on this process. The method to be explained and illustrated uses the Behavioral Interview (BI) techniques developed by Pascal and Jenkins (1961) combined with a focus on problems that are widely recognized to be prevalent in elderly populations. Their interview method achieves its usefulness by seeking to determine the way an older adult *interacts* with his or her personal social and material environment so as to maintain (or fail to maintain) a desirable level of functioning. In contrast, most other approaches have sought to measure resource availability and abilities of the individual as separate entities. The authors seek to make the case that discovering the unique way the particular person interacts with his or her own environment can provide much more direct information regarding strengths and deficits in the person–environment system.

Before the BI techniques as used with older adults are presented in more detail, some more general interviewing and assessment issues will be considered. First to be presented are general issues relating to identifying and investigating problems of older adults. Next will be a discussion of some psychodiagnostic problems frequently encountered in elderly populations. The last section will expand on the rationale and technique of the use of the BI techniques with older adults, including an illustrative example.

ROGER L. PATTERSON • Department of Veterans Affairs, William V. Chappell, Jr. Outpatient Clinic, Daytona Beach, Florida 32117-5115. LARRY W. DUPREE • Florida Mental Health Institute, University of South Florida, Tampa, Florida 33612.

Diagnostic Interviewing (Second Edition), edited by Michel Hersen and Samuel M. Turner. Plenum Press, New York, 1994.

PROBLEMS IN IDENTIFYING AND INVESTIGATING BEHAVIORAL PROBLEMS OF OLDER ADULTS

Influence of Ageism

There are many reasons for the mental health of older adults to be passed over. The attribution of most unwanted changes or behavior in late life to normal aging by older adults, by their families and friends, as well as by practitioners, is well under way. Also, numerous studies have described the influence of both cultural and professional ageism on case-finding, assessment, and treatment of elderly individuals, as well as on the underutilization of mental health services. In our culture, ageism reflects a personal revulsion to, and distaste for, growing old, and a fear of powerlessness, "uselessness," and death. Even older adults participate in aging stereotypes, along with other family members and members of their community/culture. Thus, stereotypic beliefs act as barriers to asking for or considering mental health care (Bernstein, 1990; Butler, 1969, 1980; Butler & Lewis, 1977; Dupree, O'Sullivan, & Patterson, 1982).

In the mental health field, ageism has become professionalized. Many mental health specialists share their culture's negative attitudes toward elderly people. Professional ageism includes a belief that aging means inevitable decline, pessimism about the likelihood and speed of change, and the belief that it is futile to invest effort in a person with limited life expectancy (Butler & Lewis, 1977). Of course, such beliefs may not be verbalized, but the resulting behavior manifested by professionals correlates highly with such views. Professional ageism impacts program funding, case-finding ("marketing"), assessment, treatment recommendations, and outcome. In the words of Dupree et al. (1982), ". . . Views associated with professional ageism (particularly those noting that mental illness in old age is inevitable, untreatable, disabling, and irreversible) become a self-fulfilling prophecy, leading to a lack of prevention and treatment which in turn tends to confirm the original belief" (p. 10).

Researchers have documented over the last 10–15 years how social work, medical, and mental health professionals have been influenced by ageism (Gatz & Pearson, 1988; Kimmel, 1988; Meeks, 1990; Palmore, 1990; Schaie, 1988). This influence among professionals in various mental health settings is manifested by a lessened desire or ability to attract, retain, assess, and treat older adults with mental health problems.

Conceptualizing the Problems of Older Adults

Hoyer (1973) states that "the way in which the aging process is conceptualized will to a large extent indicate the use of a particular intervention approach" (p. 18). It also affects the quality and extent of assessment. Three models used in conceptualizing the problems of the elderly and offering explanations as to why some people cease to perform competently with increasing age are the social, behavioral, and medical models.

The social model attributes changes in behavior, or differences in behavior between older and younger adults, to different roles permitted each of these groups by their culture/society. We tend to expect less responsibility and decreased functional ability on the part of our society's older members. Miller (1979) noted that we accept lesser levels of functioning in these specific areas: self-care behavior, task behavior, and relationship behavior.

The medical model considers deviations from normal functioning as due to illness or disease, most notably, improper physiological functioning that purportedly occurs as a natural (and expected) consequence of aging.

The behavioral model sees behavior as the product of learning, with learning being the result of environmental events occurring immediately before a behavior (antecedent events) and immediately after a behavior (consequence of the behavior, or reinforcers). As one ages, one experiences change in both the antecedent and the consequent events associated with behavior; thus, behaviors change (Baltes & Barton, 1977; Patterson & Jackson, 1980a,b). That is, some appropriate behaviors are gradually lost due to changes in antecedent and reinforcing conditions, and other (perhaps inappropriate) behaviors appear in response to newer environmental antecedents and consequences.

The three models have been viewed as being in conflict, but it is obvious that changes in all three classes of variables occur throughout the life span. All three, therefore, may be considered as causes of change associated with aging (Patterson, 1985). It is necessary to have knowledge of the deficits and excesses within all three classes of variables in order to understand fully the behavior of any older person. Each class of variables contributes to the individual's level of environmental competence. To concentrate solely on any single class of variables results in assessing the individual poorly and not recognizing all contributors to lowered levels of competency. Thus, any type of treatment aimed at the restoration or maintenance of adaptive behavior is not likely to be complete.

Consequences Associated with the Assessment Approach Used

Clinical researchers have long argued that psychological/psychiatric assessment, as traditionally carried out, has not been sufficient for obtaining a valid profile of older adults' functional status (Chacko, 1982; Czirr & Gallagher, 1984; Finney, Moos, & Brennan, 1991; Gallagher, Thompson, & Levy, 1980; Gatz & Hurwicz, 1990; Kane, Ouslander, & Abrass, 1989; Kaszniak, 1990; Knight, 1986; Lawton, 1986; Portnoi, 1982). A common complaint is that even in the face of growing data regarding unique later-life mental health problems, the classification of mental disorders in older adults more often resorts to criteria established for problem areas pertaining to younger populations with different developmental tasks or problems.

The Epidemiological Catchment Area (ECA) Program is a series of five epidemiological research studies performed by independent research teams in collaboration with staff of the Division of Biometry and Epidemiology of the National Institute of Mental Health. Within these sites, research instruments based on the philosophy and signs and symptoms of the *Diagnostic and Statistical Manual of Mental Disorders*, third edition (DSM-III) (American Psychiatric Association,

1980), were used. Although explicated in greater detail, these signs and symptoms have not been changed substantially in later editions of this manual, DSM-III-R (American Psychiatric Association, 1987) and DSM-IV (American Psychiatric Association, 1993). In a study of 1300 older individuals, Blazer, Hughes, and George (1987) found that the traditional DSM-III criteria for defining depression do not seem to capture depression as often expressed by older individuals. Blazer et al. (1987) reported that "though most persons throughout the life cycle who report significant dysphoric symptoms in community surveys do not meet criteria delineated in the *Diagnostic and Statistical Manual . . .* for a specific DSM-III diagnosis of affective disorder . . ., the discrepancy appears greater during the latter part of the life cycle" (p. 281).

Depressed elderly individuals often report physical complaints rather than cognitive or emotional problems. Berkman et al. (1986), reporting on another large-scale epidemiological study of the elderly in New Haven, noted that "while the DSM-III specifically states that depression can be a reaction to a physical illness, research instruments such as the DIS [used in the New Haven ECA study] . . . operationalize the exclusionary criteria of physical illness in such a way that cases of depression may be overlooked in older people who may be prone to attribute their symptoms to physical disorders" (p. 386). The result may be that rates of depression for older people tend to be underestimated by attributing somatic complaints and dysphoric states to the older persons' declining physical status.[1]

Other problems with traditional diagnostic labeling relative to elderly individuals have been reported (Graham, 1986; Gurland, 1973; Kane et al., 1989; Knight, 1986; Lawton, 1986). They include the following: (1) a unidisciplinary, unidimensional labeling process does not attend to the complexity (multiple deficits and supports) of behavior somewhat unique to the aged; (2) in many instances, the primary value of a formal diagnosis is administrative; (3) clinicians are often reluctant to apply certain diagnoses to the elderly; (4) a diagnosis lightly regarded is probably poorly implemented; (5) the labeling process, and its negative connotations, often discourage both assessment and interventions; (6) misdiagnosis is more likely in acute conditions; (7) there are difficulties in the use of labeling criteria in differentiating certain pathologies; (8) personal values and ageism do intrude; and (9) there is poor interrater reliability, particularly across disciplines and across treatment sites.

Importance of Recognizing Person–Situation Interaction

With aged individuals, expressed problems are more likely to be a result of losses or behavioral deficits (i.e., deficits not compensated for by the environment or individual). Environmental factors gain in importance in controlling behavior as the individual's competence (everyday adaptive skills) decreases (Lankford & Herman, 1978). And because environments differ in the degree to which they support altered perceptual and cognitive behavior, the daily behavior of the perceptually and cognitively impaired older person varies highly. Thus, ideally, an

---

[1]This problem remains uncorrected in the DSM-IV draft criteria (APA, 1993).

older person's adaptive behavior should be assessed relative to actual daily living tasks (DeNelsky & Boat, 1986; Goodstein, 1980; Lawton, Whelihan, & Belsky, 1980). The delineation of specific behavioral/environmental deficits should demonstrate the type and degree of support needed for maintaining residence in the "community" in which the person is assessed. Further, it may be necessary to specify a change of residence in order to meet situational requirements congruent with the person's capabilities (Lawton, 1970).

The essential diagnostic product is an indication of the older person's capacity to do things required in his or her own environment. And because major life areas interact, deficits or supports in one area must be examined and interpreted in the context of the whole (Lawton, Moss, Fulcomer, & Kleban, 1982). For example, in a very supportive environment, memory deficit may not result in an incapacity to cope with the demands of one's own milieu. Some environments require more self-management than others. Also, assessment is better conceptualized as being more oriented toward issues of problem solving: how one might either acquire skills necessary to resolve a deficit or compensate for it by acquiring environmental supports. An ecological model of adaptation and aging (Gallagher et al., 1980) is more productive in the sense that context-relevant and necessary care can be determined. Sundberg, Snowden, and Reynolds (1978), in a review of literature dealing with the assessment of personal competence and incompetence in life situations, determined that if assessment of ecological competence is to be useful, it must (1) promote attitudes toward clients that recognize their potentialities based on their current coping skills and ability to learn; (2) develop "age-free" assessment approaches recognizing competence in the elderly; and (3) assess the person along with the nature of present and potential environments.

Lawton (1972, 1978) has developed a useful model that conceptualizes behavior as falling within a number of domains. This model organizes assessment under the construct of competence in such a way that the construct incorporates most behaviors necessary to living successfully in the real world. It appears to be a blending of an ecological approach with behavior analysis. A pathology-oriented approach to the assessment of aging is more consistent with traditional psychiatric and psychological approaches. Even in this latter model, the trend relative to the elderly is toward structured diagnostic interviews. The model, however, emphasizes the need for a comprehensive (and multidimensional) approach that alerts the diagnostician to significant life domains, particularly the influence of situational variables (Fleiss, Gurland, & Des Roche, 1976; Gaitz, 1969; Gaitz & Baer, 1970; Gurland et al., 1970, 1976; Whelihan, 1979). Thus, even though the two models approach assessment from somewhat different perspectives, both emphasize similar needs relative to proper and thorough assessment of the significant and interdependent domains of the older person.

In summary, there are at least four reasons for appraising individual person–situation interactions (with the attendant behavioral/environmental deficits and supports): (1) to match the person's functioning with the requirements of his or her particular environment; (2) to determine the need for particular types of services (support); (3) to prescribe interventions to improve the level of functioning; and (4) to measure change in functioning over time (Patterson & Eberly, 1983).

Value of Age-Free Behavioral Interviewing

In the behavior analysis perspective, human behavior is considered to be alterable (or reversible) until empirically demonstrated not to be. Such an approach is necessary with older adults. It attends to concrete events (deficits/excesses, strengths/weaknesses, antecedents/consequences) as explanations for behavior rather than invoking constructs or labels. It does not place an overreliance on physical entities as the basis for behavior. The smallest units of analysis in relevant diagnostic interviewing of an elderly individual are the mutual and interdependent relations between the individual and his or her environment (Rebok & Hoyer, 1977). Mahoney (1975) asserts that it is more productive to examine the nature of the interdependence than to maintain that one's internal environment has greater priority in terms of behavior than the external environment. Even though physical changes may account for some part of any loss of environmental competence, using a strictly physical model of aging and the diagnostic process based on such an approach is not appropriate. Indeed, the physical model is biased against intervention with older adults by assuming an irreversibility of behavior (purportedly based on aging-related, irreversible physical changes).

Ageism is pervasive and intrudes on diagnostic procedures unless recognized or controlled. This tendency can be countered by using structured diagnostic interviews that guide the clinician over specified life domains (Lawton, 1972), assisting the clinician to identify, understand, and "resolve" problem behavior on an age-free, problem-oriented basis. The fodder of intervention becomes empirically derived knowledge rather than a collection of concepts and biases as to what should be causing nonadaptive behavior among older adults. A comprehensive behavioral interview can generate information (deficits and supports) that more directly explains behavior, needing less specialized interpretation. Diagnostic data needing sophisticated interpretive comments often rely on "experts" and are much more open to professional biases as well as the intrusion of personal biases (ageism). Also, the diagnostic conclusion is based on secondary data, or norms, once again discounting the individuality of the aged. These norms also discount the uniqueness (effect) of the older person's behavior in his or her particular context.

In summary, any reasonable assessment approach relative to an elderly individual must ameliorate cultural and professional ageism, assess diverse areas of the older person's life, and highlight both internal and external antecedents for the expressed problem behaviors. For older adults, appropriate assessment is on a broader scale than for many younger populations, and positive change is predicated on a broad-based assessment of strengths and deficits.

Psychodiagnostic Problems

Because of the increased incidence of dementia in older adults, and also because of the profound impact that this condition has both on the older person and on those associated with him or her, dementia has been a focus of much of the work on diagnostic interviewing of this population. Several standardized mental status examinations have concentrated on diagnosing dementia [e.g., the Mini-mental Status Examination by Folstein, Folstein, and McHugh (1975)]. Although the diagnosis of dementia or cognitive deficit is an important issue in itself, it is a good policy for the interviewer to include some such assessment when interviewing an older adult for the first time regardless of the purpose of the interview. Inclusion of this assessment is to ensure that the interviewee is capable of giving reliable information.

Depression in elderly individuals is also a diagnosis that has generated much recent interest. One reason is that both medical and psychological treatments for this condition have become increasingly effective (Patterson, 1991). A matter of considerable concern has been the distinction among symptoms of depression that may represent only this condition, symptoms that may be secondary to physical illness, depression that may be present with symptoms usually attributable to dementia rather than depression (sometimes referred to as "pseudodementia"), and true dementia, which may be complicated by depression. Bereavement, which may be encountered more frequently in older adults, usually appears much like depression and presents another diagnostic challenge. Obviously, these are complex issues that may require information other than that provided by an interview, including extensive medical and neuropsychological examinations.

Since the subject of this chapter is diagnostic interviewing, these separate but related matters will not be considered here in any detail; rather, some guidelines that have been found to give interviewers information relevant to these diagnostic matters will be discussed. For a thorough review of research relating to these and similar issues, the reader should consult Benedict and Nacoste (1990).

In diagnosing depression in elders, the first question to be considered is whether or not the diagnostic criteria used with younger adults should be used without modification. The reason this question arises is that several kinds of behaviors change normally as we age. For example, older people usually exhibit changes in overall activity level, speed of responding, sleep patterns, sexual activities, and appetite, all of which might be indicative of depression in a young person. Also, older adults are found to have a greater frequency of chronic illnesses that may directly affect the aforementioned symptoms as well as others. As mentioned above, bereavement may also be a matter to be considered.

Czirr and Gallagher (1984) recently considered these diagnostic complications and concluded, on the basis of their research, that the criteria presented in the *Diagnostic and Statistical Manual of Mental Disorders*, 3rd edition (DSM-III) (American Psychiatric Association, 1980), are applicable across the age range of adults. (As previously noted, these criteria have not been changed substantially in later editions of this manual.) However, these authors do suggest several ways in which interviews used to determine the presence or absence of the criteria should differ. Some of these differences will now be presented.

A way in which most of today's elders differ from younger persons is that most of them are not very "psychology-minded," meaning that they may have considerable difficulty in describing and discussing their feelings, especially men. Feelings may be denied, or all problems may be attributed to physical illness. Extensive probing is often required to determine feelings. Also, the nature of existing physical problems may need to be considered in evaluating the nature of many complaints. For example, an elderly depressed man whom the author (Patterson) sees in therapy consistently comes in to complain of back problems. His medical record shows that he is receiving treatment for this illness, but more extensive probing shows that he suffers from general anhedonia and has significant marital and leisure-utilization problems. All discussions with this man must involve his back condition, but the interviewer must be insistent to get this man to consider other aspects of his life. In evaluating loss of interest or pleasure, the proportion of activities that the person engages in and enjoys must be considered, since overall levels of activity may be reduced considerably due to factors other than depression.

Any statements of dysphoria should be followed by inquiries about hopelessness, suicidal ideation, and plans. Older adults are less likely to talk about suicidal ideation or to make gestures, but the suicidal rate for elderly white males is higher than for any other group.

Zarit and Zarit (1983) have published some suggestions useful for distinguishing between depression, delirium (such as may result from a physical illness), and dementia on the basis of a clinical interview. Old people, particularly those who are depressed, frequently complain of memory problems. Many clinicians working with elders consider severe complaints about memory to be highly indicative of depression rather than dementia. However, depressed people do not often make errors on mental status examination items used to determine cognitive functioning. Demented people will usually answer mental status items, but will get them wrong, although they may occasionally give excuses for refusing to answer, such as "I didn't look at a calendar today." Those suffering from delirium will often give rather vague answers referring to conative aspects of a situation (Kahn & Miller, 1978). For example, someone in a hospital, when asked where he is, may say that he is in a hotel or in another hospital located in a different part of town.

As mentioned above, the interviewer should determine early on whether the interviewee is capable of giving a good history because a reliable history is essential in distinguishing between diagnoses. For example, the onset of depression may be related to specific losses in a person's life. If such a condition extends beyond a reasonable mourning time, then depression should be considered. In such cases, the interviewer should look for cognitive distortions regarding the effects of the loss(es) (e.g., "My life is worthless without _____.") Dementia secondary to strokes may also have a sudden onset and not be sufficiently devastating to produce immediate medical attention. With these cases, there are often accompanying weaknesses or dizziness, and there is usually a period of gradual recovery. However, such episodes may be repeatedly accompanied by progressive decline. In contrast, primary senile dementia presents as a long period of more or less steady decline. The latter condition may be accompanied by depression initially, but this depression usually disappears as the disease progresses.

A history of response to treatment, if such was given, is of great diagnostic significance. For example, Patterson (1985) described a case of an elderly woman who had been diagnosed as having dementia on the basis of extensive medical examinations and a failure to respond to inpatient and outpatient medical treatment. Fortunately, this person responded dramatically to a treatment program involving psychosocial rehabilitation using token reinforcement. Depression usually responds very well to medical or psychological treatment, or a combination, as contrasted with dementia, which responds to a very limited extent to behavioral treatment (McEvoy & Patterson, 1986) and not at all to current medical treatments other than palliation.

As the reader has undoubtedly concluded, it is often impossible to derive much of this information from interviewing. It may be necessary to involve collateral sources.

FUNCTIONAL ASSESSMENT

In addition to psychiatrically related diagnosis, interviewing has also been used to obtain information about the functional status of a particular elder and his or her need for and use of resources. The Multidimensional Functional Assessment of Older Adults (Fillenbaum, 1988) developed by a group of researchers at Duke University has been used widely for these purposes. It addresses five areas of functioning: social, economic, mental health, physical health, and self-care. Users of this instrument are trained to administer a standardized interview so as to be able to derive a reliable numerical score in each of the areas. These scores are useful for needs assessments and research purposes, but most of the information that is of practical use for assisting individuals comes from the content of this wide-scale interview. A more practical, shortened form of this interview has been validated by Pfeiffer, Johnson, and Chiofolo (1981).

BEHAVIORAL INTERVIEWING

The authors realize that the types of interviews discussed above have important purposes, notable for prescribing certain types of treatment and for determining needs for resources for individuals. However, we have been primarily concerned with assessing not just the person or his or her environment, but rather the person–environment interaction. Previous approaches seem to have regarded the elderly person as fixed and static, if not inevitably deteriorating. The sole purpose of modifying the environment was to compensate for deficits when it was possible to do so. The diagnostic process to be explained below regards neither the person nor the environment as fixed or inevitably deteriorating. The purpose of the behavioral interview is to determine how the person–environment interaction can be improved to the benefit of the elderly person.

Behavioral Incident Technique

The interviewer of an elderly person is often trying to assess the extent to which the client is involved with a variety of people: medical, government and charitable agencies, social organizations, and commercial establishments. Such involvements are often referred to as *social supports*. The authors find that the term social supports is a bit ambiguous. What is it that is being supported? What we are most often interested in understanding and measuring with regard to older clients is environmental interactions that "support" (i.e., prompt, reinforce, or otherwise help to maintain) maximally independent, organized, and generally adaptive behaviors. The reader should notice here that consistent with our previous discussion, the focus is on person-environment *interactions*. This approach is quite different from more common approaches that treat the elderly person as a mere passive recipient of supports.

Focusing on the person–environment interaction means that both the elderly client's activity and the source of support are crucial. For example, consider the candidate for home-delivered meals. How does this person normally feed himself or herself? Are the deficits causing the eating problem behavioral, financial, medical, or a combination of problems? What can the person currently do to obtain meals? What could he or she do better if given some assistance? What services are really needed?

Obtaining meals is actually a rather simple example compared with the problem of determining the nature and existence of supportive social relationships. Such social relationships are often considered to be of great importance to most people in maintaining a satisfactory personal life. Yet, the *nature* of these relationships is often barely touched on by those working with older adults. It is sometimes determined whether or not the person in question does or does not have some type of contacts and how often such contacts occur. However, this is minimal involvement, indeed. In the case in which there is a relative or friend living nearby who visits or telephones regularly or who lives in the same house, this circumstance is almost always considered a "support." By the definition we are using, such frequent contact with accessible relatives or friends is not necessarily supportive. Frequency of contact tells little or nothing about the *quality* or *effects* of such contact.

Given the preceding considerations, how are social supports to be characterized in the interview situation? Pascal and Jenkins (1961) contemplated similar issues with regard to other populations and developed the Behavioral Incident (BI) technique. This technique was closely modeled after techniques used by Kinsey, Pomeroy, and Martin (1948) and others. Kinsey and his coworkers were startlingly successful in getting ordinary American citizens to reveal many details regarding their sex lives—a difficult task indeed. The basis of the BI technique is to use behavioral shaping to get the subject to describe *actual events* as opposed to opinions and generalities about events. This brief sentence says much that requires explication.

The focus of the interview is on the accurate description of events that reveal the presence or absence of a supportive interaction. Thus, a relevant question might be how a subject obtains weekly medical treatment. The interviewer in this situation would have the task of having the subject explain what he or she did to get the appointment and get transportation, what he or she discussed with the nurse, doctor, and pharmacist, and so on. The interviewer would then be in a position to judge whether or not there were problems or potential problems with necessary support.

Perhaps a more difficult situation might involve the interaction of a depressed female client (who has many physical complaints) and her daughter who visits regularly. The relevant question would be: What is the daughter doing to maintain adaptive, nondepressed, noncomplaining behavior, and what is she doing to maintain the opposite behavior? In this case, the BI would encompass the visit. The interviewer would seek to find out what the two did and what they talked about. Obviously, in this case, reports from both mother and daughter would be useful. From such information (and similar information from other visits), a properly trained interviewer would learn much about which aspects of these interactions were supportive and which were nonsupportive of desirable behavior.

Getting clients to describe actual events in this way sounds much simpler than it is. Most people are not trained to conduct interviews in this way. Indeed, many people are trained to ask for feeling statements and opinion statements rather than behavioral descriptions. Some training and practice in technique is needed before this strategy can be used effectively.

Skillful use of verbal prompts and reinforcers is required to shape appropriate responses in the interview over predetermined content areas (Pascal & Jenkins, 1961; Witherspoon, deValera, Jenkins, & Sanford, 1973). For example, an interviewer may know that an elderly woman has a daughter living in the vicinity. When discussing relationships, the woman may persist in pointing out how wonderful her daughter is and how many interesting things she did as a child. The interviewer should recognize these statements (responding as minimally as necessary to maintain the contact) and as tactfully as possible ask specific questions, such as: "When did your daughter last visit?" "How did she greet you?" "What did you talk about?" Responses to such questions regarding specific behaviors should be responded to with obvious interest by the interviewer in order to socially reinforce the interviewee's responding. In most cases, conscientious prompting and reinforcement will produce a sufficiently detailed portrayal of the interactions between the mother and daughter to enable the interviewer to determine what behaviors were being supported (prompted and reinforced) by the interaction. In many instances, interactions that might be considered "supportive" on the basis of relatively superficial information (such as frequency of contact) or on the basis of opinion statements may turn out to be destructive when BI information is obtained. The opposite is also true. That is, relatively infrequent contacts may serve as important prompts or reinforcers for important behaviors. Also, as is illustrated in the interview presented later in the chapter, opinion statements to the effect that contacts are infrequent or unimportant may not be accurate when compared to more behavioral data.

Although the BI is a very versatile technique and may be used to obtain many types of information, there are several areas of social support that should be of concern when trying to determine the assets and needs of elderly people. Some commonly useful items are discussed next.

Content Areas of the Behavioral Incident

Meals and Food Preparation

It should be determined how, and with what difficulties, the elderly person obtains meals on a regular basis. If the person prepares his or her own meals, then a detailed description of how he or she shops and prepares the food will be needed.

Economic Resources

The person should know where the money comes from, the amount, how the money is protected, and the approximate cost of necessities (e.g., shelter, utilities, food). In addition to the necessities, there is an economic deficit if there is no money for some small personal luxuries.

Social Relationships

Several types of social relationships are desirable that range from the intimate to the superficial. By *intimate* we mean that clients know people with whom they can share their feelings and the important things in life—past, present, and future. Such relationships are supportive if there is an exchange that is mutually enjoyable and serves to reinforce adaptive behaviors. A relationship in which the client only complains or expresses the negative part of his or her life probably serves to promote poor life satisfaction and even depression. Also, the partner in such a relationship will probably find the interaction aversive, and this atmosphere may serve to destroy the relationship.

At another level, it is important for clients to have people with whom they can share leisure activities or just enjoyable light conversation. Also required by older adults are individuals who can be called on when needed for occasional assistance with household tasks, shopping, transportation, and the like.

It is true that one or two people may provide all the previously mentioned interactions, but this is not a very desirable situation. Rather, it is desirable that the different kinds of interactions be maintained with several people so that a more normal social environment with a consequent variety of social behaviors may be maintained.

Health Care

Elderly clients should have solutions to several situations involved in obtaining adequate health care. Obviously, they should have easy access to primary care physicians. Beyond this, they should know how to avail themselves of other public or private agencies providing care. They should know a pharmacist and be knowledgeable as to how to obtain and take needed medications.

Leisure Activities

It is useful for elderly people to enjoy leisure activities of more than one type several times a week. They should be aware of leisure activities that can be carried out *alone* as well as those with another person or a group. Witherspoon et al. (1973) designated hobbies in which one took pride as an important source of support.

Residence

According to Witherspoon et al. (1973), it is important that a person exhibit interest, satisfaction, and even pride in his or her residence. This attitude is evidenced behaviorally by efforts to maintain and decorate it, however simple these efforts may be (e.g., growing plants, displaying personal treasures, crocheting doilies).

Transportation

Support in this area requires that the client have ways of going to shopping sites, medical treatments, leisure activities, and occasional unplanned places and events. Transportation is also needed for various ways of maintaining social contacts. More than one source of transportation is highly desirable, in order to provide for backup, and transportation to an adequate variety of locations.

An interview will now be presented that seeks to accomplish many of the desirable features of assessment as described before.

Case Illustration with Dialogue Comments

The Interview

The person interviewed (Mrs. J) is a 66-year-old divorced woman who was a regular client of the day treatment component of the behavioral treatment program described extensively by Patterson, Dupree, Eberly, Jackson, O'Sullivan, Penner, and Dee-Kelley (1982). This program assesses elderly people, particularly in regard to social skills and daily living skills. The results of these assessments are then used to indicate what types of skills training are needed in order to enhance the life of elderly clients.

This is an *initial* interview in that the interviewer and the patient have never met. Further, the interviewer was not involved clinically in the case. The reader should note that although the interviewer is seeking specific information in the specific categories described previously, the interview was treated as a relatively free-flowing process. To reiterate, the person talking is exhibiting operant behavior. The interviewer has the task of shaping this behavior by proper use of prompts and reinforcers, but the information must and should be free-flowing according to the way the client presents it. It would be a great mistake to try to adhere rigidly to a particular order or style of obtaining the information, such as would be done with most standardized psychological tests and questionnaires. Such adherence to order or style would greatly limit the amount of information obtained. The interviewer in this case prefers to begin by talking about leisure-time activities, because this area is easy to discuss casually. Also, much information about social activities, family, and friends may be given very readily in connection with leisure activities. This occurred in the illustrative interview.

I: Tell me about the last time you did something just for fun.

P: Lately, not much [opinion statement].

I: What are some things you have done recently?

P: Visited the historical district, played cards with the ladies in the laundry room, went window shopping in the mall. I enjoyed going to the airport and people watching. I like to do things when I have the transportation, but I can't do too much because of respiratory problems. I get out of breath very easily. [Comment: The facts seem to contradict the opinion statement that she hasn't done much recently. This became more apparent as the interview continued.]

I: Tell me about the last time you did something just for fun.

P: Well, that was last Friday. My friend and I went to the historical district—spent several hours there in the shops, and we had dinner there.

I: That's a nice outing.

P: It is, there's something there for everyone. There are antiques, there are crafts, and so forth. There are imports—it's a very enjoyable place for a person my age. There are places to get coffee and just sit.

I: Mostly what you did was to visit the shops, have coffee, and go to dinner?

P: Yes, the food was very good and reasonable. That's the last thing I did, other than visit with my daughter and grandchildren.

I: You've done that recently?

P: Yes, last Sunday—and then I went to their house for dinner the next day.

I: When was the last time you saw your daughter before then?

P: They dropped in for an hour a couple days before.

I: How long before then?

P: A week or so. They have two small children, and it's hard for them to come by very often, but I call her. She doesn't call me very often, but I call her. And I had calls from my daughters in Michigan and Pennsylvania.

I: What did you talk about?

P: They were all snowed in and had brutal weather, but the one in Pennsylvania I was concerned about. She had marital problems. I was kind of worried, depressed about her. She told me that they had worked things out and had renewed their marriage vows. Things are going well, and that made me feel much better. Before, she had been calling me complaining about my son-in-law. [She went on to explain the situation of the daughter and the son-in-law. Apparently, the client knew a great deal about what was going on in their lives, although they live more than 1000 miles away.] I had told my daughter that telling friends and family didn't help the problem. She had to discuss it directly with her husband. She did, and they were able to work things out. I feel good about them, and I feel better about myself. I've made several adjustments in the last month here.

I: What have you done?

P: I moved from a trailer in the boondocks back to the apartment where I used to live. I have nice neighbors.

I: Do you see your neighbors regularly?

P: When I go to the laundry or pick up my mail. Sometimes I see them going in or out, and we speak.

I: Tell me about the last visit you had with a neighbor.

P: It's not one of those visiting kind of things where I would go over and have coffee. Sunday, we played cards while doing our laundry in the apartment laundromat.

I: What did you talk about?

P: About how they're repairing the street, and how bad it was that the freeze killed the oranges, things like that.

I: Do you have anyone you see several times a week?

P: No. I have made a reacquaintance with my friend who took me to the historical district. I've seen her twice last week and once this week, and I'll see her again on Friday. She has suggested us going to different places. [Comment: The opinion statement "not much" seems to be contradicted by the events described.]

I: She has a car and you don't?

P: That's right. Transportation is a problem for me.

I: Tell me about your friend. What did you talk about the last time you went out together?

P: She has a very authoritative manner and is very domineering—usually puts me down. I went through a bankruptcy thing and wasn't allowed to work. I used to live in her garage apartment. I felt that she made me feel worse, so I didn't see her for several months. Now we've become friends again.

I: Tell me what you said to each other when you were out together recently.

P: I talked about how the hostages had been released and how good that was. She said that it was all political and racial and that I really don't understand these things. Well, I used to have a very responsible job, and I think I have some understanding of the world. I don't feel like a moron. I feel that I can discuss the news and current events intelligently. Before, when we were friends, I got so many negative comments from her that I began to doubt myself, whether I was really just plain dumb and didn't understand things. I started staying mostly in my room when I lived at her place. I told myself that I had to get out of there because I was damaging myself and getting more and more depressed.

I: That was the only friend you had?

P: Yes, the only close friend. I had had others at work, but when you lose your job you lose contact with them, unless you have a car and can keep up with them. If I were driving I could meet them the way I used to. I gave up driving after I had a stroke—and then I had a heart attack. That led to losing most of my friends.

I: The friend that you had a good time with recently—I guess your conversation was different than it used to be?

P: I explained to her that I had to leave and move for my own benefit. I think maybe it had an impact on her. Maybe she didn't realize what she was doing. We were in one shop the other night where they had things from France—the dresses were very expensive. I was looking through the rack, and she said, "There's no sense in you looking, because you can't afford them." I said, "No, but I can appreciate the workmanship and how beautiful they are." That seemed to stop that.

I: Hm-mmm.

P: It used to be always a put-down.

I: But I suppose you had some pleasant conversation, say, over dinner?

P: We talked about our grandchildren. We talked about Christmas; and of course we both are cat lovers; and we talked about the birds outside of the courtyard. We made plans to get out more often, and I think that was good, because once I asserted myself and let her know that the put-down business was getting to me, and that I didn't feel that I was that kind of person, I think that we got along better. I would never move back in with her. I think that it's her way to do the put-downs. I have to accept her that way.

I: Let me ask you about your daughter who lives close by. You saw her recently. Tell me what you did and what you talked about. Do you remember a conversation you had with her then?

P: Well, we talked about their plans. They were going to a friend's house for a party, and they were going to stay over. They took the children. I told them that was good. We made plans for them to come over the next day so that we could go out for supper. We have a fairly good rapport.

I: You share personal things?

P: Yes. We've shared many personal things. Things that have left deep personal scars on me, but you have to go on.

I: She has told you things that are important in her life?

P: Yes. I try to be fair and listen, but I don't try to interfere between husband and wife. I don't know if this is pertaining to what you are interested in . . . .

I: Yes.

P: [At this point she proceeded to tell how she assisted her daughter financially and otherwise during a period of deep marital conflict. She confided that she has guilt feelings over this matter, because of the way she was involved. However, she revealed that now she is close to the daughter and her family as indicated by the recent visits as previously described.]

I: Now, let's talk about something else. You mentioned that you have transportation difficulties. How did you last get to the food store?

P: I called my daughter, she took me.

I: Is that the only way you can get groceries?

P: Yes. I call her, and she takes me. I don't have any other way. I called Share-a-Van, but they only take people to medical appointments.

I: Any place you can walk to get small items?

P: No. Besides, right now I don't think I'll have even food stamps for this month because of moving. I have to reapply. By the time I pay my rent, $240 a month, $50 a month rental on an oxygen concentrator—then I have my electric, I don't know how much that will be. My son-in-law supplies me with a telephone. It's on his bill. My daughter in Pennsylvania will try to send me $15 a month for my oxygen, which will leave me $10 to $15 each month to spend. It's not much, but it helps. My children have troubles of their own and their own families; I can't expect much help from them. I'm not allowed to work. I'm too ill.

I: Do you have a regular doctor?

P: Yes, Dr. T.

I: Do you have any difficulties seeing him?

P: Well, my daughter used to take me. But she has to take the children to school. I used to make my appointments according to her schedule. She can't do that any more. Now I don't know what I'll do. I guess I'll call Share-a-Van.

I: Your doctor's office is only a block from here. Can you walk that far?

P: No, I can't walk that far. I can't even walk from here [the day treatment program] to the cafeteria. They serve my meals on the unit. I know I'm a pest.

I: We expect that some people will eat on the unit. It's normal procedure. Do you have anything you do just for fun when you're by yourself?

P: I'm an avid reader.

I: You read a great deal?

P: I read a tremendous amount of books, and I knit. I read more than anything, more than I watch TV.

I: Regularly . . . you read every day?

P: Every day I read.

I: Are you reading a book right now?

P: Yes . . . It's a mystery by Mary Stuart. I just finished [goes on to describe several books she's read recently, and mentions authors she prefers and authors she dislikes].

I: That's a good hobby. Do you have any problem getting books?

P: Oh, no. A friend of my daughter goes to one of these half-price exchange places. She knows what I like and just brought me a grocery bag full [goes on to talk enthusiastically about books and authors she likes, then engages in a criticism of television, especially the violence].

I: I need to ask you how you take medicine. I know you take several kinds. Do you have them with you?

P: Oh yes. [Reaches in her purse and pulls out several small plastic bags rubber-banded together.] I put my pills in these little bags and label them according to when I'm supposed to take them. See here? [Shows interviewer a labelled bag.] I'll take this before lunch.

I: How did you get the medicine from the pharmacy the last time?

P: I called ahead, and the pharmacist had them ready when my daughter took me to the doctor. The pharmacy is in the same building. Of course, I'm not sure how I'll get to the doctor now. Maybe Share-a-Van . . . .

I: How do you pay for your medicine?

P: It's paid by the county. There's no problem. I do have a problem with food, though.

I: How's that.

P: I have only $60 per month for food, but I'm a diabetic and have high blood pressure—so I'm supposed to eat mostly fresh vegetables and meats. They're expensive.

I: What did you eat this morning?

P: I had some cereal. Of course, when I come here, I have a good lunch which is prepared according to my diet. That's my main meal of the day.

I: What do you plan to eat this evening?

P: I have some canned soup and rice. I have a bag of fruit which my neighbor brought me. I love fruit, and could eat it all the time.

I: How will you prepare your meal?

P: I have some small pans, but not enough utensils. I don't have any problems opening and heating canned food, or macaroni, or rice, or things like that.

The interview was terminated at this point because the interviewer thought he had obtained sufficient information to complete the assessment.

Summary of the Interview

The interview information will now be summarized and briefly discussed according to each major topic.

Meals and Food Preparation.   Mrs. J has several problems in this area. She does not have the money to buy the kinds of foods she needs, nor does she have money to buy utensils. This problem is currently exacerbated because of the temporary interruption in food stamps. Transportation might be somewhat of a problem because she is dependent on her daughter for shopping. She is unable to buy casual incidentals on her own. Food preparation does not seem to be a problem.

Economic Resources.   Mrs. J has her money carefully budgeted, including a small amount for personal luxuries. There is some contradiction here with problems in buying food. It would be highly desirable for her to have money for taxis, but she does not.

Transportation.   The daughter seems to be the sole source of regularly available transportation, and even this is limited. There is a deficit here.

Social Relationships.   Mrs. J apparently has maintained solid relationships with her daughters. She seems to have maintained her role as someone the daughters trust and can turn to in time of need. It is probable that these relationships are important to Mrs. J in that they may maintain her opinion of herself as an important and useful person. However, these relationships also involve her in the daughter's difficulties. It might be that additional details about interaction with the daughters over an extended period would reveal aspects of the relationships that are not so supportive and might relate to the depression. More than an initial interview would be required for such a determination.

There seems to be a deficiency with regard to friends. Mrs. J has only one close friend, and the relationship with this friend has been at least partially nonsupportive. It seems that this friend has helped to prompt and reinforce Mrs. J's negative self-image. Other than this friend and the daughters, only the most casual relationships were mentioned. These relationships, however, are apparently very supportive of normal, casual, social interactions and are of considerable importance to Mrs. J.

Health Care.   Mrs. J had very high-level skills at taking medicine. Also, other than the problem with transportation as previously mentioned, she has no problems with the doctor or the pharmacy. Her knowledge about her required diet is very good, but she has difficulty affording proper food.

Leisure Activities.   Mrs. J has kept amazingly busy considering her handicaps and economic limitations. She seems to be able to enjoy casual activities with others (the card games and conversation at the apartment and the activities she planned with her friend) as well as when she is alone. Reading is obviously an important pastime, and one in which she takes pride. The limitations here are those of transportation and health.

Residence.   Mrs. J seems to be very pleased with her new apartment and considers it a great improvement over her previous two residences.

In this case illustration, the interviewee freely produced information that is pertinent, specific, and intimate. Thus, the interviewer's style and appropriate use of the chosen interview format appeared to result in cooperation from the client. A useful assessment was obtained that portrays defined domains of the individual's life. These results were not accidental but planned. The interviewer knew both how to use his diagnostic instrument and how to interview an older person. A valid and useful assessment is a product of the chosen assessment approach, the interviewer's knowledge of older adults, and his or her interview style in response to that knowledge.

DO'S AND DON'T'S OF INTERVIEWING OLDER ADULTS

Excellent articles have been written noting techniques for communicating with (and ultimately assessing) older people (Blazer, 1978; Goodstein, 1980; Gurland et al., 1977/1978; Pfeiffer, 1980). Gurland et al. (1977/1978) focused on limiting stress in older adults that is elicited by an assessment interview. Reducing stress leads to a fuller exploration of problems, enhances interviewee cooperation, and more likely leads to a completed interview. Also, limiting stress within the interview setting reduces the likelihood of prompting deficits in behavior suggestive of organic conditions (e.g., apparent memory impairment and disorientation). Potential sources of interview stress for elderly individuals include (1) fatigue as a result of questions that are lengthy or confusing or both, and (2) "the embarrassment of disclosing symptoms which suggest psychiatric disorder or cognitive incapacity (as well as the interviewee's fear that this information might initiate or prolong his hospitalization or stay in an institution)" (Gurland et al., 1977/1978, p. 22).

More recent articles regarding successful assessment and counseling of older adults have emphasized that the skills and techniques needed for aged individuals are much the same as those used with younger populations (Knight, 1986; London & Behncke, 1987; Myers, 1990; Waters, McCarroll, & Penman, 1987). They also noted that while there are many similarities in counseling older and younger persons, there are important differences. It is important that counselors understand these differences as well as their own attitudes toward older adults. Attitudes convey powerful, unspoken messages that color the way a communication is transmitted and received (London & Behncke, 1987).

The major differences that counselors should consider when working with older adults include the older person's reluctance to seek counseling and the need for counselor sensitivity to physical changes. Many of today's older people hesitate to seek counseling assistance, and because of this reluctance to seek formal help, it is important that those who interact with older adults be alert for requests for informal or "by the way" counseling (Waters, 1984). Once this reluctant client is in counseling, Goodstein (1980) recommends certain interpersonal considerations that not only enhance the comprehensive evaluation but also make the client more comfortable: Sit alongside the older client so that he or she can see your face and hear what you say; be respectful, hopeful, and honest; offer friendly nonverbal cues, such as looking in the older client's eyes when talking to him or her; differentiate sympathy and empathy [sympathy makes older people feel like children, whereas understanding (empathy) is favored]; share something of yourself (sharing mutual interests may facilitate the process); do not hesitate to discuss intimate data if presented; permit physical contact (shake hands, pat on the back for support); and know your feelings about aging and how they affect your performance. Blazer (1978) and Pfeiffer (1980) have also delineated effective techniques for communicating with elderly people during the diagnostic interview (some of which overlap those suggested by Goodstein).

Robinson, Smaby, and Donovan (1989), Wilber and Zarit (1987), and Friday (1986) offered additional important suggestions: Address older clients by their honorifics (e.g., Mrs. Smith, Mr. Jones) unless permission is granted to use more familiar terms; show respect for clients and treat them with courtesy; be honest and open; move along at the client's pace; promote initial rapport with clients by using self-disclosure to promote similarity; communicate at the client's level of under-standing (avoid psychological jargon and accommodate to the client's interaction style); familiarize yourself with the older person's culture and values; maintain warmth despite challenges and lack of response; use reflective listening to build trust; and minimize direct confrontations that might be viewed as an attack or lack of sensitivity by older persons.

The aforementioned interpersonal considerations are important and are likely to have a positive impact on assessment, but interviewers working with older adults should also be aware of physical and sensory considerations. Physical changes and sensory loss have an important impact on the ability of the older person to communicate effectively. Individuals with hearing and visual impair-ments need special attention, and a counselor's sensitivity to these limitations may make the difference in effective treatment. These issues have been addressed extensively (Chandler, 1989; Exum, 1980; Ganote, 1990; Hittner & Bornstein, 1990; Salmon, 1987; Waters, 1984), and the recommended do's and don'ts for effective communication with the hearing impaired include these: Select a quiet room (improve acoustics with carpeted floors, covered walls, furniture, and drapes) and minimize background noise (including radio or piped-in music); speak distinctly, slowly, and only slightly louder, but not in a higher range; face the client when speaking; use nonverbal cues; repeat words or phrases when appropriate; and use written communication or visual aids.

The visually impaired require accommodations that include these: adequate lighting and controlled glare; positioning oneself near the patient during inter-action; written materials that are prepared in large type with considerable white space on the page; large clocks and calendars available for orientation; and minimum stairs and areas of extreme light or dark that require quick visual accommodation.

Other physical deficits such as stiffening of the joints and altered urinary functioning may limit the older person's ability to sit for long periods of time, and sessions should therefore be shortened and clients permitted to get up and move about if they feel the need. Also, firm, straight-back chairs are recommended. It is more difficult for older adults to get in and out of soft chairs. Consequently, all professionals who work with older persons should be aware of the physical settings they work in and their own behavior and actions in order to accommodate the physical decrements and sensory problems of the older client population.

Counselees of all ages need both support and challenge from their counselors. They need to know that their helpers respect them and expect them to grow (Waters, 1984). Building trust and respect in a helping relationship is important to the elderly client and to the success of the interaction. Facilitating this type of effective relationship requires acknowledging special needs tactfully to show empathy and providing for the comfort of clients by going beyond common courtesy (Supiano, 1980). For example, Tobin and Gustafson (1987) noted the importance of touching as an extension of the workers' active approach to the elderly's needs. It is something that is readily understood and experienced as a form of caring for those who need help and assurance when in turmoil.

Another method for establishing trust and respect involves a less formal approach. Bernstein (1990) suggests that counselors who are able to laugh and cry with the client, offer the support or a hug or pat on the arm, and share a cup of tea, for example, are often helpful. Additionally, the counselor can contribute to a relationship based on trust and respect by making positive statements such as "Nice to see you"; trying to spend time with the older client, even if this is limited to sitting, holding hands, and so on; making promises and keeping them; not getting angry and criticizing the client for forgetting and not laughing at his or her mistakes; and not changing plans frequently without notifying the client (Pinkston & Linsk, 1984).

These comments refer to general factors in interviewer behavior applicable to any face-to-face communications with an elder. In addition, other clinical researchers in this field have written about specific, practical necessities for productive interviewing.

Due to the widely recognized increased incidence of cognitive losses in elderly populations, the interviewer should obtain early in the process an estimate of the subject's cognitive functioning. The purpose of this estimate is to know better how to relate to the elder as well as to ascertain the utility of the information obtained. This information is often obtained using a brief mental status examination such as that used by Pfeiffer (1975). This examination can be carried out as soon as a reasonably comfortable relationship has been established. For those people with considerable cognitive losses, it may be necessary to use other sources to obtain factual information regarding the older person's situation in life (Fillenbaum, 1988).

Czirr and Gallagher (1984) have also pointed out some practical tactics that are useful for facilitating the interview process and making it more meaningful. First, ensure that the purpose of the interview is made clear to the client. Also, early in the interview process, the interviewer should ask the client for permission to interrupt in order to achieve the stated purpose. These authors have found that most elderly people will readily agree to such interruption and not take offense when it is done with proper courtesy. Such permission is often needed because of the tendency of some older individuals to talk excessively about physical problems, tell stories, or otherwise detract from the purpose of the interview.

There is often need for direct prompting and questioning by the interviewer to obtain certain information (the interview presented above demonstrates this). Such direction is particularly necessary in discussing depression and suicide. As noted above, many older people may suffer significantly from losses, a lack of support, and consequent depression. However, they may be very reluctant to consider these factors and prefer to blame illnesses or some other agent for all their problems. It is necessary for elders to be realistic in order to help solve their difficulties. Suicide is a particularly difficult problem. Elderly white males have the highest suicide rate, but they are less likely to talk about it than other groups. In general, older adults make fewer suicidal gestures or attempts, but are more likely to succeed when they try. It is necessary to ascertain the presence and severity of cognitive distortions in order to determine the existence of an unrealistic reaction to losses and possible depression. One of us (R.L.P.) has met an elderly man who felt his life was absolutely worthless because he had to retire to Florida rather than out west, and another who was guilty of all the sins of the world because of some earlier misdeeds. Still another blamed all his problems on back pain, although he had significant marital and retirement-related problems resulting in depression. Looking for cognitive distortions is a useful tool for us in distinguishing between bereavement and depression. With normal bereavement, there is a severe sense of loss and consequent sadness. Depression occurs when cognitive distortions about the bereaved person's life extend beyond the specific loss (e.g., "my life is worthless," "I can't go on without _____") and persist beyond a reasonable period.

In general, the older adult with cognitive distortions decides that his or her life is completely useless or worthless because he or she no longer can have or do what he or she used to. Such people may or may not show clinically accepted signs of depression, but they need help in becoming more realistic about their situations regardless of these signs.

Summary

In summary, inadequate performance on the part of the interviewer can markedly affect the information produced, which in turn can generate an inaccurate picture of the older client's deficits or supports (and level of performance). Once an appropriate interview approach is formulated, much of the choice of accurate vs. distorted indexes of performance is left to the interviewer's style (whether or not the interviewer is aware of this consequence of his or her interviewing style). It would appear that a clearer picture of the older interviewee is obtained by using a broad-based structured interview in the hands of an interviewer who communicates well with older adults by recognizing and using the previously mentioned interview requisites.

References

American Psychiatric Association (1980). *Diagnostic and statistical manual of mental disorders*, 3rd ed. Washington, DC: Author.

American Psychiatric Association (1987). *Diagnostic and statistical manual of mental disorders*, 3rd ed., revised. Washington, DC: Author.

American Psychiatric Association (1993). *Diagnostic and statistical manual of mental disorders*, 4th ed., draft criteria. Washington, DC: Author.

Baltes, M. M., & Barton, E. M. (1977). New approaches toward aging: A case for the operating model. *Educational Gerontology, 2*, 383–405.

Benedict, K. B., & Nacoste, D. B. (1990). Dementia and depression in the elderly: A framework for addressing difficulties in the differential diagnosis. *Clinical Psychology Review, 10*, 513–537.

Berkman, L. F., Berkman, C. S., Kasl, S., Freeman, D. H., Leo, L., Ostfeld, A. M., Cornoni-Huntley, J., & Brody, J. A. (1986). Depressive symptoms in relation to physical health and functioning in the elderly. *American Journal of Epidemiology, 124,* 372–387.

Bernstein, L. O. (1990). A special service: Counseling the individual elderly client. *Generations, 14,* 35–38.

Blazer, D. (1978). Techniques for communicating with your elderly patient. *Geriatrics, 33,* 79–84.

Blazer, D. G., Hughes, D. C., & George, L. K. (1987). The epidemiology of depression in an elderly community population. *Gerontologist, 27,* 281–287.

Butler, R. N. (1969). Age-ism: Another form of bigotry. *The Gerontologist, 9,* 243–246.

Butler, R. N. (1980). Ageism: A foreword. *Journal of Social Issues, 36,* 8–11.

Butler, R. N., & Lewis, M. I. (1977). *Aging and mental health,* 2d ed. St. Louis: C. V. Mosby.

Chacko, R. C. (1982). Diagnostic dilemmas in geriatric psychiatry. *The Gerontologist, 22(5),* 240.

Chandler, M. H. H. (1989). Teaching interview techniques utilizing an instructional videotape. *Educational Gerontology, 15,* 377–383.

Czirr, R., & Gallagher, D. (1984). Assessing depression in older adults. In P. A. Keller & L. G. Ritt (Eds.), *Innovations in clinical practice: A source book,* Vol. III. Sarasota, FL: Professional Resource Exchange.

DeNelsky, G., & Boat, B. (1986). A coping skills model of psychological diagnosis and treatment. *Professional Psychology: Research and Practice, 17,* 322–330.

Dupree, L. W., O'Sullivan, M. J., & Patterson, R. L. (1982). Problems relating to aging: Rationale for a behavioral approach. In R. L. Patterson, L. W. Dupree, D. A. Eberly, G. M. Jackson, M. J. O'Sullivan, L. A. Penner, & C. D. Kelly (Eds.), *Overcoming deficits of aging* (pp. 7–21). New York: Plenum Press.

Exum, H. A. (1980). Cultural diverse elderly: An overview of the issues. In C. J. Pulvino & N. Colangelo (Eds.), *Counseling for the growing years: 65 and over* (pp. 197–217). Minneapolis: Educational Media Corporation.

Fillenbaum, G. G. (1988). *Multidimensional functional assessment of older adults: The Duke older Americans resources and services procedures.* Hillsdale, NJ: Lawrence Erlbaum Associates.

Finney, J., Moos, R., & Brennan, P. (1991). The drinking problems index: A measure to assess alcohol-related problems among older adults. *Journal of Substance Abuse, 3,* 395–404.

Fleiss, J., Gurland, B., & Des Roche, P. (1976). Distinctions between organic brain syndrome and functional disorders: Based on the Geriatric Mental State Interview. *International Journal of Aging and Human Development, 7,* 323–330.

Folstein, M. F., Folstein, S. E., & McHugh, P. R. (1975). Mini-mental State: A practical method for grading the cognitive state of patients for the clinician. *Journal of Psychiatric Research, 12,* 189–198.

Friday, J. C. (Ed.) (1986). *Geriatric mental health: Assessing and improving the performance of personnel.* Available from Southern Regional Education Board, 592 Tenth Street N.W., Atlanta, GA 30318-5790.

Gaitz, C. M. (1969). Functional assessment of the suspected mentally ill aged. *Journal of the American Geriatrics Society, 17,* 541–548.

Gaitz, C. M., & Baer, P. E. (1970). Diagnostic assessment of the elderly: A multifunctional model. *The Gerontologist, 10,* 47–52.

Gallagher, D., Thompson, L. W., & Levy, S. M. (1980). Clinical psychological assessment of older adults. In L. W. Poon (Ed.), *Aging in the 1980's* (pp. 19–40). Washington, DC: American Psychological Association.

Ganote, S. (1990). A look at counseling in long-term-care settings. *Generations, 14,* 31–34.

Gatz, M., & Hurwicz, M. L. (1990). Are old people more depressed? Cross section data on Center for Epidemiological Studies depression scale factor. *Psychology of Aging, 5,* 284–290.

Gatz, M., & Pearson, C. (1988). Ageism revised and the provision of psychological services. *American Psychologist, 43,* 184–188.

Goodstein, R. K. (1980). The diagnosis and treatment of elderly patients: Some practical guidelines. *Hospital and Community Psychiatry, 31,* 19–24.

Graham, K. (1986). Identifying and measuring alcohol abuse among the elderly: Serious problems with existing instrumentation. *Journal of Studies on Alcohol, 47,* 322–326.

Gurland, B. J. (1973). A broad clinical assessment of psychopathology in the aged. In C. Eisdorfer &

M. P. Lawton (Eds.), *The psychology of adult development and aging* (pp. 343–377). Washington, DC: American Psychological Association.

Gurland, B. J., Fleiss, J. L., Cooper, J. E., Sharpe, L., Kendell, R. E., & Roberts, P. (1970). Cross-national study of diagnosis of mental disorders: Hospital diagnosis and hospital patients in New York and London. *Comprehensive Psychiatry, 11,* 18–25.

Gurland, B. J., Fleiss, J. L., Goldberg, K., Sharpe, L., Copeland, J. R. M., Kelleher, M. J., & Kellett, J. M. (1976). A semi-structured clinical interview for the assessment of diagnosis and mental state in the elderly: The Geriatric Mental State Schedule. II. A factor analysis. *Psychological Medicine, 6,* 451–459.

Gurland, B., Kuriansky, J., Sharpe, L., Simon, R., Stiller, P., & Birkett, P. (1977/1978). The comprehensive assessment and referral evaluation (CARE)—rationale, development and reliability. *International Journal of Aging and Human Development, 8,* 9–42.

Hittner, A., & Bornstein, H. (1990). Group counseling with older adults: Coping with late-onset hearing impairment. *Journal of Mental Health Counseling, 12,* 332–341.

Hoyer, W. J. (1973). Application of operant techniques to the modification of elderly behavior. *The Gerontologist, 22,* 240.

Kahn, R. L., & Miller, N. E. (1978). Assessment of altered brain function in the aged. In M. Storandt, I. Siegler, & M. Elias (Eds.), *Clinical psychology of aging.* New York: Plenum Press.

Kane, R. L., Ouslander, J. G., & Abrass, I. B. (1989). *Essentials of Clinical Geriatrics.* New York: McGraw-Hill.

Kaszniak, A. W. (1990). Psychological assessment of the aging individual. In J. E. Birren & K. W. Schaie (Eds.), *Handbook of the psychology of aging* (pp. 427–445). San Diego: Academic Press.

Kimmel, D. (1988). Ageism, psychology, and public policy. *American Psychologist, 45,* 175–178.

Kinsey, A. C., Pomeroy, W., & Martin, C. (1948). *Sexual behavior in the human male.* Philadelphia: W. B. Saunders.

Knight, B. (1986). *Psychotherapy with older adults.* Newbury Park, CA: Sage Publications.

Lankford, D. A., & Herman, S. H. (1978). *Behavioral geriatrics: A critical review.* Summary of paper presented at the Nova Behavioral Conference on Aging, Port St. Lucie, Florida.

Lawton, M. P. (1970). Assessment, integration, and environments for the older people. *The Gerontologist, 10,* 38–46.

Lawton, M. P. (1972). Assessing the competence of older people. In D. P. Kent, R. Kastenbaum, & S. Sherwood (Eds.), *Research planning and action for the elderly.* New York: Behavioral Publications.

Lawton, M. P. (1978, October). *What is the good life for aging?* Kesten Lecture, University of Southern California, Ethel Percy Andrus Gerontology Center.

Lawton, M. P. (1986). Functional assessment. In L. Teri & P. M. Lewinsohn (Eds.), *Geropsychological Assessment and Treatment* (pp. 39–84). New York: Springer.

Lawton, M. P., Moss, M. S., Fulcomer, M., & Kleban, M. H. (1982). A research and service oriented multi-level assessment instrument. *Journal of Gerontology, 37,* 91–99.

Lawton, M. P., Whelihan, W. M., & Belsky, J. K. (1980). Personality tests and their uses with older adults. In J. Birren & R. B. Sloane (Eds.), *Handbook of mental health and aging* (pp. 537–553). Englewood Cliffs, NJ: Prentice-Hall.

London, J., & Behncke, C. M. (1987). Intergenerational communication skills. In H. S. Briggs (Ed.), *Teaching aging: A series of training modules on aging for educators* (pp. III-1–III-28). Tampa: Human Resource Institute, Center for Applied Gerontology, University of South Florida.

Mahoney, M. J. (1975). The sensitive scientists in empirical humanism. *American Psychologist, 30,* 864–867.

McEvoy, C., & Patterson, R. (1986). Behavioral treatment of deficit skills in dementia patients. *Gerontologist, 26,* 475–478.

Meeks, S. (1990). Age bias in the diagnostic decision-making behavior of clinicians. *Professional Psychology: Research and Practice, 21,* 279–284.

Miller, L. (1979). Toward a classification of aging behaviors. *The Gerontologist, 19(3),* 282–289.

Myers, J. E. (1990). Aging: An overview for mental health counselors. *Journal of Mental Health Counseling, 12,* 245–259.

Palmore, E. (1990). *Ageism: Negative and positive.* New York: Springer.

Pascal, G. R., & Jenkins, W. O. (1961). *Systematic observation of gross human behavior*. New York: Grune & Stratton.

Patterson, R. L. (1985). Senile dementias. In R. J. Daitzmann (Ed.), *Diagnosis and intervention in behavior therapy and behavioral medicine*. New York: Springer.

Patterson, R. L. (1992). Psychogeriatric rehabilitation. In R. P. Liberman (Ed.), *Handbook of psychiatric rehabilitation*. New York: Macmillan.

Patterson, R. L., & Eberly, D. A. (1983). Social and daily living skills. In P. M. Lewinsohn and L. Teri (Eds.), *Clinical geropsychology* (pp. 116–138). New York: Pergamon Press.

Patterson, R. L., & Jackson, G. M. (1980a). Behavior modification with the elderly. In M. M. Hersen, R. M. Eisler, and P. Miller (Eds.), *Progress in behavior modification*, Vol. 9 (pp. 205–239). New York: Academic Press.

Patterson, R. L., & Jackson, G. M. (1980b). Behavioral approaches to gerontology. In M. L. Michelson, M. Hersen, and S. M. Turner (Eds.), *Future perspectives in behavior therapy* (pp. 295–315). New York: Plenum Press.

Patterson, R. L., Dupree, L. W., Eberly, D. A., Jackson, G. M., O'Sullivan, M. J., Penner, L. A., & Dee-Kelly, C. (1982). *Overcoming deficits of aging: A behavioral approach*. New York: Plenum Press.

Pfeiffer, E. (1975). *Functional assessment: The OARS Multidimensional Functional Assessment Questionnaire*. Durham, NC: Duke University Center for the Study of Aging and Human Development.

Pfeiffer, E. (1980). The psychosocial evaluation of the elderly patient. In E. W. Busse and D. G. Blazer (Eds.), *Handbook of geriatric psychiatry* (pp. 275–284). New York: Van Nostrand Reinhold.

Pfeiffer, E., Johnson, T., & Chiofolo, R. (1981). Functional assessment of elderly subjects in four service settings. *Journal of the American Geriatrics Society, 29*, 433.

Pinkston, E. M., & Linsk, N. L. (1984). *Care of the elderly: A family approach*. Elmsford, NY: Pergamon Press.

Portnoi, V. A. (1982). Underrepresentation of geriatric mental health disorders in DSM-III: Need for revision. *The Gerontologist, 22(5)*, 239.

Rebok, G. W., & Hoyer, W. J. (1977). The functional context of elderly behavior. *The Gerontologist, 17*, 27–34.

Robison, F. F., Smaby, M. H., & Donovan, G. L. (1989). Influencing reluctant elderly clients to participate in mental health counseling. *Journal of Mental Health Counseling, 11*, 259–272.

Salmon, H. E. (1987). Counseling older people. In G. Lesnoff-Caravaglia (Ed.), *Handbook of applied gerontology* (pp. 231–248). New York: Human Sciences Press.

Schaie, K. W. (1988). Ageism in psychological research. *American Psychologist, 43*, 179–183.

Sundberg, N. D., Snowden, L. R., & Reynolds, W. M. (1978). Toward assessment of personal competence and incompetence in life situations. *Annual Review of Psychology, 29*, 179–221.

Supiano, K. P. (1980). The counseling needs of elderly nursing home residents. In C. J. Pulvino and N. Colangelo (Eds.), *Counseling for the growing years: 65 and over* (pp. 233–246). Minneapolis: Educational Media Corporation.

Tobin, S. S., & Gustafson, J. D. (1987). What do we do differently with elderly clients? *Journal of Gerontological Social Work, 10*, 107–121.

Waters, E. B. (1984). Building on what you know: Techniques for individual and group counseling with older people. *The Counseling Psychologist, 12*, 63–74.

Waters, E., McCarroll, J., & Penman, N. (1987). *Training mental health workers for the elderly: An instructor's guide*. Rochester, MI: Continuum Center, Oakland University.

Whelihan, W. (1979). *Dynamics of the team interaction in geriatric assessment*. Paper presented at the Conference on Geriatric Assessment, VA Medical Center, St. Louis.

Wilber, K. H., & Zarit, S. H. (1987). Practicum training in gerontological counseling. *Educational Gerontology, 13*, 15–32.

Witherspoon, A., deValera, E., Jenkins, W., & Sanford, W. (1973). *Behavioral interview guide*. Montgomery, AL: Rehabilitation Research Foundation.

Zarit, S. H., & Zarit, J. M. (1983). Cognitive impairment of older persons: Etiology, evaluation, and intervention. In P. M. Lewinsohn & L. Teri (Eds.), *Coping and adaptation in the elderly*. New York: Pergamon Press.

Index